The Brass Tacks of
ANIMAL HEALTH

The Brass Tacks of
ANIMAL HEALTH

James Blakely
Dwight D. King

DOANE AGRICULTURAL SERVICE, INC.
St. Louis, Missouri

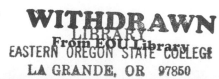

Library of Congress Cataloging in Publication Data

Blakely, James.
The brass tacks of animal health.

Includes index.
1. Veterinary medicine.   I. King, Dwight D., joint
author.   II. Title.
SF745.B64   636.089   78-14371
ISBN 0-932250-00-9

© 1978 by Doane Agricultural Service, Inc.
St. Louis, Missouri

10   9   8   7   6   5   4   3   2   1

Printed in the United States of America

Contents

Preface

This book is written for farmers and ranchers—people who handle livestock routinely, but don't have formal training in animal medicine. It was conceived and written for you, not for veterinarians or college professors. In the pages that follow, you will find that the authors have kept you, the stockman, clearly in mind.

Throughout the book you'll notice the liberal use of examples to help bring key relationships into sharper focus. While a discussion of animal disease and health problems must deal with some fairly technical material, the writing style of this book helps to alleviate the often confusing tangle of drugs, animal anatomy, and technical definitions. Complex subjects have not been oversimplified, but in most cases they are reduced to the key points needed in order to gain a good understanding. You'll find technical terms are also explained in concise, everyday language. The result, we believe, is an easy-to-read book that provides you with what you need to know to care for livestock.

Material is organized so that it is easy to follow and convenient for reference. Concluding sections are designed to ground the reader in the fundamentals of managing a herd health program. For example, the section on drugs should provide a better understanding of the maze of drugs available. The discussion will serve to preface later sections dealing with specific health problems in beef, dairy, swine, and horses.

Cattle producers will find that information common to both dairy and beef cattle has been consolidated under beef cattle, leaving the dairy section to discuss conditions that are unique to dairy herds. This is done to minimize duplication of information and to make the material more easily accessible for reference purposes.

We hope that the information in *Brass Tacks* will find its way directly into your day-to-day management and decisions regarding the well-being of your livestock. This book should also provide a basis for better communication between you and your veterinarian in order to further your common goal —healthy and profitable livestock.

The Doane Editors

Acknowledgment

The authors are indebted to the agricultural extension specialists from all fifty states and Puerto Rico, and to the USDA research publications and the Land-Grant institutions for providing public domain information. Without exception, every request for information, advice, materials, and assistance in compiling data was met with promptness and courtesy.

Although specific charts, photographs, and tables are appropriately credited, much material in this book was summarized and condensed from public documents too numerous to mention. Although permission to use any publication in the public domain is not required, we would like to express a sincere appreciation to the hundreds of extension and USDA specialists throughout the United States and its Possessions for making the system a superb form of communication for the dissemination of information.

This information combined with our own experiences and observations, along with private industry research and publications, constitutes the resource material for this handbook.

Special appreciation goes to the following reviewers for their corrective criticisms and suggestions leading to the finalized material in this book: Dr. Alex Hogg, cattle, University of Nebraska; Dr. James D. McKean, swine, Iowa State University; Dr. Les Waymack, horses, Tarleton State University; Dr. David Hanselka, horses, Texas A&M University.

An Overview of Animal Health

Herd Health

IT STARTS AND ENDS WITH YOU

Every year stockmen lose a staggering number of dollars because of animal health problems. The majority of these losses are preventable. Through close observation plus a few simple techniques and some basic equipment, you can turn many of these losses into profits.

Like most stockmen, you can spot an obviously sick animal, but there is a good chance that the problem goes deeper. For example, how did the animal get sick in the first place? Did it struggle with less severe problems before succumbing to this more serious illness?

An acutely sick animal is usually already quite ill before the signs of the disease are noticed. Therefore, other animals in the herd could be fighting off the same disease agent, causing their productivity to deteriorate. Some disease conditions may go unnoticed except to an experienced eye, or they may require laboratory tests before the problem can be isolated. These subclinical health problems may actually account for a much larger share of the overall losses than those caused by animals that get noticeably sick or even die. Moderate reductions in growth rate, in milk production, or in reproductive efficiency may be difficult to detect, but when spread over a number of animals can amount to a substantial dollar loss.

You are responsible for the health of your animals; and although as an average farmer or rancher you do not have a veterinarian's years of formal training and experience in animal medicine, you as an individual livestock owner or herdsman must recognize that you alone are in charge of the health status of the animals in your care. Your skills, your powers of observation, and your management ability form the first line of defense against disease in your herd. Therefore a considerable amount of time can profitably be spent sharpening these skills and abilities.

Learn to observe the behavior and condition of animals carefully and on a routine basis. Develop the ability to spot problems early, before the condition progresses into one that will require more time and expense to handle. Reduce livestock stresses as much as possible by providing protection against environmental factors, parasites, and injury. By understanding the basics of veterinary care and by developing a keen sense about animals, you will have a sound basis for determining when to call for the assistance of your veterinarian. The material that follows in this book is designed to assist you in making wise decisions, both in handling those situations within your capabilities and in recognizing those that require the help of a professional.

BACK TO BASICS

The ability to identify individual animals in the herd is fundamental to all disease-control efforts. All animals should be marked by brand, ear tag, neck chain, or some other identifying characteristic. Good records must be kept, based on these identities, in order to determine previous health of individual animals as well as to maintain a history of the herd.

A planned program for the health of the herd is important in controlling diseases and in maximizing profits. Vaccination, castration, isolation, sanitation, and herd replacement should be done on a systemized, organized basis. A suggested calendar plan for each of the species covered in this book—beef, dairy, swine, horses—will be presented at the end of each section.

Disease pathogens must be eliminated or controlled before they become a problem; therefore, isolation, quarantine, sanitation, and vaccination are not only tools to be used in the fight for animal health, but tools that must be used at the right time and in the right place in order for them to be effective.

Learn to use the professional advice of your local veterinarians and extension specialists on treatment programs in order to operate at the highest level of efficiency.

Know the capabilities and limitations of animal drugs, administer them via proper routes, and follow the drug restrictions unless your veterinarian advises you otherwise.

Proper equipment and facilities for handling and treating livestock are a great aid and reduce time and labor required to administer an animal health program. Proper housing and restraint make the job much easier.

The number one cause of most diseases is not an attack by some organism, but rather a lack of proper nutrition. Be sure that your animals are fed at the optimum level for maximum performance in order to minimize health problems.

VITAL SIGNS

We can think of a healthy animal as any animal that is free from abnormal structural or functional changes in the tissues of the body. Your veterinarian usually relies on the vital signs to determine if an animal is exhibiting normal health. You should be aware that these vital signs pertain only to three simple things: temperature, respiration rate, and pulse rate of the body. Usually the first signs of disease are slight and may go unnoticed by many people, but by observing a few simple rules you can detect early signs and can initiate proper action either by calling your veterinarian or, if you feel qualified, by taking appropriate action yourself.

Temperature

An animal's abnormal temperature may play a part in your ultimate diagnosis of whether or not a disease is present. When an animal's temperature is above normal limits, it is called a *fever*; when it's below normal, it's called a *chill* or *hypothermia* (meaning below normal temperature). Considerable variations will be found in temperatures of animals depending on their physical activity, stage of pregnancy, time of day, or environmental conditions. However, the normal temperatures for different animals are given as:

HORSE	FOAL
99.5–101.3° F	99.5–102.2° F
CATTLE	SWINE
100.4–103.1° F	100.4–104.0° F

If the body temperature increases by 1° F over the normal upper limit shown above, you can consider this as indicating a mild fever. Elevations higher than that, of course, may show a more severe infection. Usually, even in severe infectious diseases, the temperature never exceeds 106.0° F in horses or 107.0° F in cattle. In horses, high temperatures are seen in cases of influenza, severe tetanus, and heatstroke. High temperatures in shipping fever are often encountered in cattle. However, in many types of animals suffering from heatstroke, the temperature may exceed 110.0° F.

In cattle an increase in body temperature does not always represent the degree of fever, and it may be necessary to consider other signs, such as a chill, pulse rate, respiration rate, appetite, digestion, etc.

Subnormal temperatures may or may not indicate disease. They are seen much less frequently than fevers but do occur in a variety of ailments such as chemical poisoning, indigestion, and paralysis.

Pulse

The important factor in taking a pulse is the frequency. This is determined by counting the number of heartbeats occurring in one minute. Although your veterinarian will be concerned with more than just the frequency of the pulse, you can get a good idea of this important vital sign just by palpating (touching with the fingers) the arteries that can be pressed against a hard or bony structure. Then it is a simple matter of counting the number of beats of the heart felt by the fingers in a timed 60 seconds. The pulse of a cow or horse is usually taken at the external maxillary artery that can be felt just under the jaw. There is a small notch on the jawbone to help you. With a little experimentation you should be able to find the artery by pressing it against the jawbone. If you feel a rhythmic pulse, then you have a place to begin. Don't try to feel a vein because veins do not exhibit this rhythmic pulse. In swine the pulse cannot be felt at all; the heart itself must be palpated directly over the chest cavity.

The frequency of the heartbeat varies among different species and among individuals depending on age, size, sex, breed, time of day, excitement level, etc. The average pulse frequency, or the normal pulse rate, for the species covered in this book is as follows:

SPECIES	HEARTBEATS PER MINUTE
Adult horses	28–40
Newborn foals	100
Foals (6 to 12 months)	45–60
Cattle	40–70
Swine	60–100

Respiration

Respiration is the act of breathing, the taking in of oxygen and the giving off of carbon dioxide. In observing the respiration rate you should begin at the nostrils and work toward the rear. Attention should be given to respiration rate, quality of the breath (foul odors, etc.), nasal discharge, any swelling of the lymph nodes under the jaw, and coughing or unusual sounds coming from the chest. Intelligent observations concerning the process of breathing can give an indication of impending problems.

In examining respiration in an animal, you should look for the number of breaths taken in (inspiration) per minute and the intensity or indication of straining, sneezing, wheezing, rattling, or groaning; and you should pay particular attention to the expansion and relaxation of the ribs and abdominal wall. A sick animal will often be heaving at the belly, flanks, or ribs. A good example of this is "thumps," an iron-deficiency anemia problem in swine in which breathing is so labored that the belly actually slaps the ground, making a thumping sound. Not all respiration problems are this severe, but it gives a good indication of what you should be looking for in respiration, usually on a much milder scale.

It's a good idea, if you have some reservation about your diagnosis of respiration, to check two or three other animals to compare your findings. The normal range in respiratory rates for mature animals at rest is:

SPECIES	BREATHS PER MINUTE
Horse	8–16
Beef cow	10–30
Dairy cow	18–28
Pig	8–18

Learn when you need to call your veterinarian and when you are able to handle a situation without his assistance. There are two sides to every coin. For example, the veterinarian may view his client in the following way. A call is received at 11:00 P.M. The caller describes the symptoms of the sick animal. He says he has already tried remedies of his neighbor, his feed-store manager, and his grandmother—all to no avail. Now he wants the veterinarian to diagnose the problem over the phone and recommend a home remedy that he can prepare from kitchen ingredients and administer himself without being charged for advice. If and when the animal dies, the caller spreads the word about the sorry state of the veterinarian's qualifications. It is a most frustrating experience to deal with.

On the other hand, you, the farmer or rancher, probably view the veterinarian in an equally unfavorable light. You see the veterinarian drive up to the farm or ranch headquarters, and after making a phone call from his air-conditioned automobile, jump out and give a shot in the rump of the animal for an illness that you have already diagnosed for him. Then the good doctor jumps back in his automobile and roars off to treat a race horse for a head cold, before the day ends with a pool-side dinner at his country estate where his accountants are already tallying up the day's receipts.

Neither side of this coin is true, but the exaggeration illustrates the frustration that both the veterinarian and client must experience on some occasions. No one can blame the farmer or rancher for wanting to avoid a veterinary bill. Expenses are always high, and profits in today's agriculture are slim enough without the added expense of unnecessary medical bills. This book is specifically designed to help the farmer or rancher know when professional assistance is required and to give him a better understanding of the complexity of the situations that the veterinarian must face. Even though this book is detailed from a layman's standpoint, it is but a small fraction of the information lodged in the mind and medicine bag of the trained professional.

You must be able to recognize an acute or emergency situation that requires immediate assistance, such as the problems of difficult birth, choking, milk fever, colic in a horse, bloat in a cow, or a prolapsed uterus. There are many other acute situations but hopefully this will give you an idea of the type of serious disorders that there is little time to experiment with.

In other instances there may be time to experiment without fear of causing complications. A few examples of situations that do not require speed are skin problems, runny nose, and mild lameness. If the situation does not improve or actually gets worse, professional help should be called in while there is still time to diagnose the specific cause properly and to treat for the organism or condition causing it. Don't expect miracles from any veterinarian. His greatest ally is time, and you are the only one who can decide how much of it to give him.

You should also know what your veterinarian can do that you cannot possibly do for yourself. Few veterinarians will criticize the abilities of the experienced stockman who has a feel for animals; but remember that your veterinarian has a specialized background and years of training in the field, and furthermore, he devotes 100% of his time to problems that you may encounter only occasionally. He is a walking computer who gathers information on the scene and compares it to research, education, and experience, in order to come up with the most probable diagnosis. He also has available to him tests, tools, culture methods, and diagnostic laboratories to confirm his suspicions.

The best way to use your veterinarian is not to solve a problem once it occurs, but rather to recognize a condition before it becomes serious. With the advice of your veterinarian you should develop a preventive program to eliminate as many disease and disorder situations as possible. This book is divided into sections that cover beef cattle, dairy cattle, swine, and horses. At the end of each section is a herd health program designed to provide a specific program of action. Use the information in this book to help you use the skills of your veterinarian to the maximum potential and at the minimum expense. Knowing when to call for professional assistance will save both animals and money.

Sanitation – Control of Disease Pathogens

Disease organisms can and do live outside the host. Animal quarters are surrounded constantly by numerous organisms such as clostridial bacteria and infective viruses. These organisms must be controlled since we are forced to live with a multitude of them. Controlling the movement of these organisms on our instruments and controlling the level of their population on our premises are important for disease control by sanitation. A disease cycle can be broken by cleaning and disinfecting. In addition, thrifty, clean animals perform their function better.

The cardinal principle for good sanitation is to provide clean, dry quarters with good ventilation and plenty of pure, fresh water. The first step is to remove any buildup of waste material so that proper disinfecting can take place. No disinfectant will cut through a buildup of animal waste or other organic matter. Dirt and manure inactivate some disinfectants and protect most organisms. A cleaning agent such as soap and water may be used for the preliminary cleaning. Use a high-pressure sprayer with pressures adjustable to 1000 psi. Pressure plus the soap and the water will remove manure and filth with great efficiency. Portable steam cleaners may also be used to remove the buildup of organic matter, but you should be aware that steam cleaning does not kill organisms unless the nozzle is held 6 to 8 inches away from the area to be cleaned. Since this is not practical over the entire area, sanitation by chemical means (disinfection and/or fumigation) will have to be carried out after a thorough cleaning has been completed. Disinfection and fumigation will be discussed again later in this chapter.

Idle periods for some facilities provide for a break in the buildup of selected organisms. Idle periods, particularly in the case of swine-farrowing buildings or feed-lot operations, are important because some organisms live only 24 to 48 hours outside the host. By removing the animal hosts, these organisms are without their source of survival and normally decrease rapidly in number. The facility should be kept empty for 3 to 4 weeks or longer, but even a few days is helpful. Thus, by providing for idle periods, certain organisms can be controlled. Other organisms, such as the anthrax bacillus, live for years and are almost impossible to control through this method.

Common sense indicates that new or sick animals should be quarantined. Their movements can be restricted, and observation and treatment with the necessary drugs can be more effectively undertaken.

All dead animals should be disposed of quickly and properly. For large animals, rendering-plant operators offer the best solution for sanitary removal. Alternate methods include deep burial (6 feet at least) with a proper covering of quicklime, or cremation. In the case of small pigs, large drainage tile can be sunk in a high, sandy area supplying good bottom drainage. The dead pigs may be dropped in and covered with quicklime for good sanitary disposal. A tightly fitting lid should be made to keep out children, dogs, insects, and other predators.

Controlled access to some farms, such as SPF (specific pathogen free) hog operations, is necessary to restrict the movement of humans, birds, small animals, rodents, and vehicles that might inadvertently carry in an infectious organism, thus contaminating an otherwise clean area.

In order to obtain proper sanitation and control of disease pathogens, it is necessary to (1) clean up before applying a disinfectant; (2) use an effective disinfectant; (3) clean floors regularly, say twice a week; (4) properly dispose of manure, bedding, and dead animals; and (5) allow buildings to remain free of animals for at least 3 weeks if possible to break the disease cycle. These methods are especially needed in cases where continuous use and high concentrations of animals indicate potential problems. Dairy calf-raising facilities and swine buildings are especially vulnerable.

MATERIALS AND METHODS USED IN SANITATION

Cleaning eliminates most of the problems in livestock sanitation. However, in the case of a disease outbreak or for precautionary measures, a disinfectant may be necessary to create an environment unfavorable for the survival of certain organisms.

Characteristics of an ideal disinfectant are:

Stability—should not lose its effect upon contact with organic substances, soaps, detergents, or common materials found in nature.

Solubility—should dissolve readily in water.

Deadly to microbes—should be able to kill a variety of organisms.

Right amount of toxicity—should be toxic to lower life forms such as bacteria and protozoa, but harmless to higher forms of life such as man and animals.

Noncorrosiveness—should not react with tin or metal substances such as barns and instruments.

Penetrating power—should be able to go to depths as far as necessary to destroy organisms.

Economical cost—should be comparable to other forms of disinfecting such as steam cleaning.

For use in dairy barns, a disinfectant must have the additional quality of being free from strong odors to minimize the possibility of milk contamination. Another consideration is that a disinfectant that will decontaminate a building may be too toxic or irritating to the skin of man and animal.

Specific examples of chemical disinfectants and other techniques for pest control follow.

Alkalies

Alkalies work on the principle of a pH greater than 9, which inhibits most bacteria and is destructive to many viruses. The most common active ingredient of alkalies is sodium hydroxide (lye).

Dry lime (calcium oxide, unslaked lime) is a very popular, inexpensive disinfectant widely used around livestock. Scattered over yards or concrete floors, it is a good disinfectant. Since it does have the disadvantage of drying out skin and hoofs of animals, excessive amounts should be avoided because cracks in the skin sometimes invite foot rot in livestock exposed to large amounts of lime.

Sodium phosphate detergents are also included in this category and are the most commonly used sanitation compounds for sterilizing bottles and milking equipment in dairies.

Slaked lime (quicklime added to water) is effective because of the active ingredient calcium hydroxide. This material (calcium oxide) added to water and made into the form of a whitewash (calcium hydroxide) in a 0.5% solution is one of the better known and most common bactericidal compounds available. It will kill bacteria and also viruses, especially in stronger solutions. It has properties that will control such contagious diseases as foot-and-mouth disease and hog cholera. It is used in weaker solutions to sterilize milking equipment and to disinfect milking parlor stanchions and farrowing houses.

Lye (soda lye) contains about 94% sodium hydroxide and is normally used as a 2% solution in hot or boiling water (one pound of lye to 5.5 gallons of water). A 5% solution is recommended for use on the anthrax organism because its spores are highly resistant to destruction. Concentrated lye is a caustic poison and should be handled with extreme care. Solutions of lye may damage paint or varnished areas. Textiles may also be damaged if the solution is in contact with them for any length of time. Lye does not injure bare wood, enamelwear, earthenwear, or metals except aluminum.

Phenols or Phenol-Related Compounds

The active ingredient in most phenols (also referred to as coal and wood-tar derivatives) is carbolic acid. Mixed with water or glycerine, it is very effective even in a 0.5% solution. It is one of the most potent of the sanitation liquids available.

Phenol is effective against most types of bacteria but is generally considered too expensive and toxic for general use. Concentrations of more than 2% phenol are dangerous to man and animals because of absorption through the skin.

Cresol (Lysol) in a 1 to 5% solution is a phenol-related compound that is used around barns, pens, and trucks and is very effective in sanitizing numerous items and equipment even in the presence of large quantities of organic matter. It has great killing and penetrating power. It is inexpensive and efficient as a disinfectant. Mixtures of cresol with soap are used to form more soluble solutions for easy applications. Cresols are not suitable for use in dairy barns because of the possibility of contamination of milk. However, for disinfecting animal quarters, carriers, and facilities, a dilution of 4 ounces per gallon of water is recommended. A pressure sprayer with adjustable pressures up to 1000 psi provides the most efficient application.

Sodium orthophenylphenate is widely recognized as an official disinfectant for use in dairy barns. It is particularly effective against the tuberculosis organism, is readily soluble in water, and has good germicidal properties. It is active in the presence of detergents and is usually mixed with them. Care should be used in application because the material is irritating to the eyes, but it has no objectionable odor.

Quaternary Ammonia Compounds (Surfactants, Soaps)

Quaternary ammonia compounds are alkaline in nature, providing a double action because of the fact that they are bactericidal as well as alkaline, both of which characteristics control the spread of bacteria. This type of compound is primarily used as a sanitizer on dairy utensils after mechanical cleaning. It is also used to disinfect instruments for castration. This compound is antibacterial, but it is readily neutralized by soaps. Therefore, any surfaces to be disinfected should first be rinsed thoroughly.

Several forms of quaternary compounds are available. Two common ones are Zepharin and Roccal.

Anionic soaps also fall into this category and are most effective against Gram-positive bacteria. Phisohex (hexachlorophene) is the most common soap. You have probably seen your veterinarian using it as a disinfectant on his hands during routine procedures. Phisohex is acid in nature and should not be used in combination with the previously discussed alkaline compounds because when used together, they neutralize each other, allowing a film to develop under which bacteria can survive.

Heavy Metal Compounds

Compounds made of many of the heavy metals are used to sanitize equipment as well as areas on the animal itself.

Mercurial compounds can be used as bacteriostatic solutions, although they are not effective against spore-forming organisms. Copper sulfate is a heavy metal solution used to control foot rot and algae. Zinc oxide is used to treat skin infections caused by bacteria. Silver nitrate is a heavy metal compound used in weak solutions to treat against bacterial invasion, especially in the eye.

Halogens

Halogens are very strong oxidizing agents. A few of the more common ones are discussed below.

Chlorine.   Chlorine is a common product used in swimming pools and various other areas where a good safe sanitizer is needed. It is also a good spore killer and is used most commonly on dairy utensils. Its effectiveness is substantially reduced by the presence of dirt or manure, so preliminary cleaning is essential before chlorine will be of any benefit. Used on clean material, it takes action rapidly against bacteria, spores, fungi, and viruses.

Powdered chlorinated lime is a chlorine-type product used in contaminated livestock quarters as a powerful disinfectant and deodorant. It should be stored in an airtight container because it deteriorates upon prolonged contact with the air.

Iodine.   Iodine is a bactericidal, viricidal, fungicidal skin disinfectant of unmatched quality. A 2 to 7% tincture of iodine solution is probably the most effective skin disinfectant available in animal medicine. Iodine offers the added benefit of changing color upon losing its disinfecting properties.

The activity of iodine solutions is directly related to the amount of free iodine present. Tincture of iodine refers to a 2% solution of iodine in alcohol. It is a very effective antiseptic. A 7% solution is a strong tincture of iodine preparation that has more killing power but is somewhat irritating to animal tissues.

Idophores (tamed iodine).   Idophores are not as good as iodine but may be used as a substitute for a good sanitizer and topical dressing. Idophores are commonly used in the disinfection of dairy utensils and equipment and for teat dipping after milking. They are combinations of iodine and solubilizing compounds. They are nonstaining and nonirritating in general; however, idophores containing phosphoric acid, prepared for use on equipment, should not be used on skin because of the irritating properties of the acid.

Chlorhexidine (Nolvasan)

Chlorhexidine is a nontoxic product, soluble in water and broad-spectrum in action. It can be used on both wounds and equipment; it is very effective and highly recommended. It is widely used to sanitize udder cloths and milking equipment, as a wound-treatment germicide, and for teat dipping.

Fumigants

Fumigation is the most effective of all the methods for killing fungi, spores, bacteria, and viruses. Formaldehyde solutions can be purchased in liquid form containing about 40% formaldehyde under the common name of Formalin. The principle involved in fumigation is the release of a toxic gas, so it is necessary to have an airtight building or to make it airtight for the period of time that fumigation takes place.

A concentration of 4% formaldehyde gas is extremely potent; it is lethal to highly resistant anthrax spores within 15 minutes. Fumigation in this manner has been popular for use in large swine units for many years. It may be used on other buildings as well, provided animals are removed and kept from the premises for at least 48 hours. Proper disinfection depends on a lengthy exposure in the proper concentration and humidity. Because the gas condenses at low temperatures, the fumigation procedure is unreliable below 18° C (65° F). Buildings should be thoroughly cleaned first and allowed to air out for 48 hours before reuse.

Two methods of fumigating with formaldehyde gas are commonly in use in the United States. The first method employs wide-bottomed buckets placed every 10 feet throughout the length of the building. In each bucket, 10 level tablespoons of potassium permanganate are placed; then $1\frac{1}{2}$ cups of a 40% solution of formalin are poured over the permanganate. Care should be taken not to breathe this mixture, but no undue concern is needed provided the treatment is carried out by starting at one end of the building and progressing with reasonable haste, in order, to the other end. Under proper conditions, each bucket of this mixture will generate enough gas to disinfect 1000 cubic feet of space.

The second method involves a white powder called *paraformaldehyde*; gas is released from the powder by heating with electrical units.

With either method, all surfaces to be disinfected should be moistened about 15 minutes before fumigation and the building made airtight for at least 8 hours.

Foot Baths

Many synthetic foot baths are on the market under different trade names. Most of them are the phenol compounds previously discussed. Foot baths are used commonly in SPF hog operations and other places where a control of organisms is necessary. Most foot baths are used in a concentration of 500 parts per million (ppm) as a sanitizing agent and 1000 ppm as a disinfectant. They are effective against Gram-positive and Gram-negative bacteria, most types of fungi, and some forms of viruses, although they are not effective against bacterial spores. They have rapid killing properties, good activity in the presence of organic debris such as dirt on footwear or feet, and good residual activity. Some formulations are affected by hard water, so this should be checked out beforehand; or make sure you have soft water to mix your foot bath. Foot baths are not compatible with most soaps; so your best bet is simply to mix the product with soft water.

Miscellaneous Disinfectants

Hydrogen peroxide solution is an effective disinfectant that releases free oxygen rapidly upon contact with wounds containing exudates (pus). It is most often used in cleaning an old wound by a boiling action (no heat involved), releasing oxygen in the wound and chemically cleansing the wound, without much germicidal activity. In spite of its nongermicidal activity it is a very effective cleansing agent.

Other miscellaneous compounds as well as a summary of disinfectants and suggested applications are covered in Table 2-1.

Rodenticides

Numerous bait-type materials are on the market that provide an anti-coagulant mixed with grain to lure rats and mice to consume enough of this product to cause them to bleed to death internally. One beneficial effect of these products is that they work slowly, so the animal has time to crawl off somewhere to die. The material also has a drying effect on the carcass, thus creating little or no offensive odor in the event rats or mice should die while inside a building.

Bird Control Techniques

Control of birds is a difficult situation out-of-doors. Most feed-lot operations use a repelling system of a "feed-lot gun," a device fueled by acetylene gas that causes a minor explosion and a very loud report about like a shotgun blast. The guns may be timed to go off every minute or so to repel birds. Interestingly enough, feed-lot cattle get used to the noise and pay little attention to it.

Indoors, birds may be attracted to fine seeds such as grain sorghum, which can be treated with poisons. See your local county agent for specific recommendations in your area. Bird control is important, particularly in cases where heavy concentrations exist because birds are common carriers of lice, mites, and other disease organisms that could contaminate domestic livestock. Birds are especially known to serve as a host for the virus that causes sleeping sickness in horses.

Table 2.1 Disinfectants—Suggested Application

DISINFECTANT	STRENGTH	APPLICATION	REMARKS
ALKALIES Lye	2 percent (one 13½ ounce can to five gallons water)	Farrowing pens to control infectious organisms and parasites. Pens and stalls following outbreaks of hog cholera, vesicular exanthema and erysipelas.	Very caustic—rubber garments and goggles should be worn to protect the face, eyes and hands. Be sure pen floors and walls are thoroughly dry before allowing animals to enter, or leave lye solution in contact with pens and walls for at least 8 hours and then rinse thoroughly. Not effective against the organism of Johne's disease or tuberculosis. Effective virucide.
	5 percent (one 13½ ounce can to two gallons water)	Pens and stalls following outbreaks of anthrax, malignant edema and blackleg. Also used as a cold soak for milking machine inflations.	
Lime (white-wash)	Slaked quicklime (38 pounds) with 15 pounds salt. Enough water for spraying or brushing.	Annual disinfection of barns, poultry houses and pens—controls spread of warts, ringworm and miscellaneous diseases that may be harbored in cracks of walls, floors and wood fences.	Addition of 4 percent saponated cresol or 1 pound lye to approximately 5 pounds lime is often helpful. Commercial white-wash preparations containing insecticides are also available. Should be used when fresh.
Lime (unslaked)	Liberal applications uniformly applied over entire area	Spread liberally on soil of poultry and livestock yards. Cover dead animals or poultry before burying to prevent spread of disease by rodents. Useful in the control of footrot. May be spread with 5 percent copper sulfate where cattle or sheep will walk through daily, or by water and feed trough.	May cultivate into soil. Exposure to air will destroy disinfection value.
Sal soda	10.5 percent (13½ ounces to 1 gallon water)	Effective for organisms of foot-and-mouth disease and vesicular exanthema	May be used in place of lye.
Soda ash	5 percent (1 pound to 3 gallons water)	Same as sal soda.	Most effective in hot solution. May be used in place of lye.
HALOGENS Iodine (tincture)	2 to 7 percent	Navel or skin disinfectant. Treatment of ringworm or warts.	Very good skin disinfectant. If used too frequently or in too strong a solution, it will become irritating. Corrosive to metal. Never use on sharp instruments.
Iodophore (tamed iodine)	75 to 150 parts per million of available iodine	Dairy utensils.	Use as iodine plus detergent. Release of iodine is controlled. Germacidal action is destroyed by organic material.
Chlorines (sodium hypochlorate) (Chlorine-T)	200 parts per million	Dairy utensils. Udder wash. Wounds.	Action decreased by organic materials. Disagreeable odor. Irritating to skin under prolonged use or too high concentrations.
Chlorinated lime	20 percent solution	Destroy disease organisms in dead animals, droppings and mixed in organic material. Sanitize washing, drinking and feed containers.	Action destroyed by organic materials. Good disinfectant and deodorant. Loses chlorine when exposed to air. Very irritating to nose and throat.
DETERGENTS Anionic detergents (Soaps)	Liberal amounts	Skin disinfectant. Disinfectant for feed and water utensils and hands.	Removes dirt and infectious agents. Low toxicity. Low antiseptic action.
Cationic detergents Benzolkonum Choride-zephiran (Roccal) Cetyl pyridimum (Ceepryn)	1:1,000 to 1:2,000	Udder wash, skin disinfectant and instrument disinfectant. Ringworm treatment. Dairy utensil sanitation. Feed and water utensils. Hands.	Active in the presence of organic matter. Non-irritating. Detergent action plus antiseptic action. Low toxicity. Action neutralized by common soaps.

MERCURIALS	Mercury bichloride (Corrosive sublimate) (Mercuric chloride)	1:1,000 solution	Instruments. Water and feed utensils Soil—1 gallon per 10 square feet.	Unreliable as a germ killer. Toxic when taken internally. Never use on metals. Value decreased by organic materials.
	Merbromium (mercurochrome)	2 percent	Skin wounds.	Has good penetration.
	Nitromersol (Metaphen)	.5 percent	Mucous membranes.	
COAL and WOOD TAR DERIVATIVES	Phenol	5 percent	Cauterize infected tissue.	Very toxic and costly as a disinfectant. Not practical to use as a disinfectant.
	Cresol (Cresylic acid) Saponated cresol solutions (Lysol)	2 to 4 percent (one cup to 2 gallons water makes 4 percent solution)	Foot bath, pens and housing unit or vehicles. For general annual disinfection or following outbreaks of brucellosis, hog cholera, shipping fever, erysipelas or tuberculosis. Disinfection of surgical instruments such as for castration, dehorning, tattooing and docking.	To determine quantity needed for building, multiply length of building times width and divide by 500. This sum equals the number of gallons needed for floors, walls, ceiling and equipment. More bactericidal and less toxic than phenol. Readily absorbed in milk, meat and eggs. Mixes best in soft water. Saponated creosols are readily soluble; soap dissolves grease. Both have good penetration. Possibly best universal farm disinfectants.
	Creosote	Undiluted	Some bacterial action.	Mixture of phenols from wood tar. Two to three times as effective as phenol. Poorly soluble in water.
	Pine tar	Undiluted	Antiseptic action. Used in bandaging. Repells insects on wounds.	Very poor solubility in water. Effects are due to phenols.
MISCELLANEOUS	Formaldehyde	½ to 1 percent solution	Foot disinfectant to treat foot rot or use as walk-through bath for foot rot prevention.	Must be used cautiously as it will harden tissues and may cause injury.
		Gas produced by adding 1½ pounds potassium permanganate to 3 pints formaldehyde. Sufficient for 100 cubic feet.	Fumigation of incubators and poultry houses.	Requires high humidity, temperatures of at least 65 degrees and a well sealed building to prevent gas escape.
		4 to 5 percent	Effective against bacteria and viruses. Applied to contaminated buildings or incubators.	Toxic upon oral intake. Requires at least 8 hours contact to be effective. Bad disinfectant.
	Alcohols	70 percent	Skin and instrument disinfectant.	Most effective at 70 percent.
	Boric acid	6 percent solution	Wash for eyes and other sensitive body tissues.	Weak antiseptic. Prevents organisms from growing.

Reprinted with permission from Dr. I. A. Schipper, *Preventive Veterinary Medicine*, Minneapolis, Minn.: Burgess Publishing Co., 1975, p. 18.

17

EQUIPMENT AND FACILITIES

Steam Cleaning

With the exception of some organisms that are thermophilic (those that live in hot-water springs or tropical soils), the majority of organisms may be killed with moist, high temperatures. However, as mentioned earlier, the steam blasts must be held 6 to 8 inches from any surface to kill organisms, and steam is considered a cleansing agent, not a disinfectant. In steam cleaning, the three major requirements are: (1) high pressure for deep penetration, (2) soap or some type of detergent to act as a cleaning agent, and (3) the proper temperature to kill as many organisms and spores as possible. Dry steam heat at a temperature of 100° C (212° F) will kill most organisms in the vegetative stage but will not assure the destruction of spores. It is therefore recommended that moist heat be used as opposed to dry steam cleaning. Use a high-pressure application with a minimum temperature of 121° C (256° F) to assure control of both the organisms and the spores.

The volume of pressure on a steam cleaning rig should always be at the upper level of the pressure gauge (some go to 1000 psi) in order to get maximum penetration from pressure and steam.

Soaps and disinfectants may be added to the steam cleaning operation through the use of disinfectant metering devices that attach directly to the outlet hose, thus affording the operator the capability of adding soaps or disinfectants as an additional aid to the cleaning action of steam and heat.

Some small items may not be suited to steam cleaning and may be sterilized with dry heat in an oven for 2 or 3 hours at 106° C to 170° C (224° F to 360° F).

High-Pressure Sprayers

Through the use of plain high-pressure water hoses it is possible to do a great deal of cleaning in the absence of steam heat. If hot water is available, it is even more effective as a cleansing agent. The key point to remember is to have plenty of water, preferably warm or hot, at pressures up to 1000 psi. In the event soaps or disinfectants can be attached to the outlet hose, they should also be used as an added cleansing agent.

Sick Pens

The location of the sick pens should be far enough away from other animals to prevent contamination through contact. The pens also should be in an area that does not drain into streams or onto pastures that might be contaminated by organisms from the sick animal, thus allowing grazing animals to pick up the disease. A separate water and feed supply should be assured so that there is no cross-contamination by water, feed, drainage, or other forms of pollution. A dry, isolated, well-drained location is essential for the confinement of diseased animals while treatment is going on.

3

Animal Drugs and Proper Administration

The purpose of this chapter is to acquaint you, the stockman, with various drugs—their differences, uses, and methods of handling. The intent is not to educate you so that you may be able to prescribe your own drugs, but to enable you to better understand and use the multitude of drugs and drug-type materials on the market.

Most drugs used by veterinarians and stockmen to combat disease may be classed as either biologicals or pharmaceuticals. These drugs differ in their use: biologicals are primarily used to prevent disease, and pharmaceuticals are most often used to treat disease or help problems that already exist. Other classes of drugs include vitamins, minerals, hormones, etc.

BIOLOGICALS

The biological drug is designed to stimulate the animal's own immunizing mechanism so that he can protect himself against a certain disease. The action involved with the drug is basically defensive.

In order to establish and maintain an immunity to a virus or bacterium, a small amount of the virus or bacterium is carefully injected so that natural body immunities will be stimulated to produce antibodies strong enough to repel a future attack by the disease organism.

Vaccines

Vaccines are normally used to stimulate an animal's immunizing mechanism for protection against a particular bacterium or virus. Bacteria are actually small living organisms that have many different functions in nature. Certain of these bacteria have the ability to produce disease in animals. These are what we call *pathogenic* or *disease-producing* organisms. Vaccines prepared against these organisms are usually very effective and have been used for many years. Bacterial organisms and bacterial diseases also usually respond well to antibiotics and other products such as sulfa drugs that are used to treat disease.

Many vaccines are also produced to protect against viral-induced diseases. A virus is much smaller than a bacterial organism. Bacteria can be seen with the aid of a regular light microscope, whereas to see viral organisms you have to use an electron microscope that magnifies many times more than an ordinary microscope. A normal bacterium or animal cell is approximately 30 times larger than a virus particle.

There are several different types of vaccines and each is used for a particular disease. As a general rule, vaccines should not be mixed in the same syringe because the preservative in one vaccine might inactivate another vaccine. Each of the vaccines to be described below has different margins of safety because of the type of material being utilized to create immunity. For instance, a modified live virus vaccine (attenuated) has a much greater potential for producing a disease than does a killed virus. On occasions a modified live virus vaccine may actually produce clinical signs of disease in an animal, but the manufacturers are careful to gauge the dosage so that it is only a light case in most instances, and recovery occurs in a short period of time with immunity resulting for the specified period of time.

There is always some risk associated with any live vaccine, and certain hazards should be recognized. There is the possibility that the vaccination could cause the disease, or a mild form of the disease, should a mistake be made in measuring the dosage or should there be a change in the virulence of the disease-producing portions of the vaccine. In severe reactions, disease outbreaks could occur; there also could be abortions, fetal defects, or stress created through the injections. For these reasons it is extremely important for the stockman to read very carefully the instructions given with each vaccine. Drug companies are very good about warning people of the hazards and proper use of their products. Familiarize yourself completely with the vaccine, its limitations, and specific instructions, and the products will work extremely well to produce the desired results.

Modified Live Virus (attenuated). The disease-producing properties of a modified live virus have been reduced so that the strength of the virus is reduced, and the immunity of the body is stimulated with little danger of producing even a light case of the disease.

An example of attenuation is *serial passage*—a process of growing an organism on a particular medium or cell culture several times so that the organism loses its disease-producing character but not its immunity-producing properties. An actual live virus is seldom used unless it has been modified in some manner to make it safe. (Otherwise, it would be just as well to expose the animal to the real disease.)

The technique of a live virus is sometimes used in the manner of a cross-immune reaction. For instance, dogs are immune to the live human measles virus, but an injection of live human measles virus into a dog will create an immunity to distemper in the dog. Thus, in certain cases, a live virus taken from one host and injected in another host can produce the desired immunity without producing the disease.

Killed Virus. In the case of a killed virus, the virus is destroyed as far as its live properties are concerned, and there is no danger of a disease outbreak. This is a very safe type of vaccine; it creates an immunity through the immune body reaction to the killed virus particles that are not capable of doing further damage through growth and development.

Live Bacterial Vaccine of Reduced Virulence. In live bacterial vaccine of reduced virulence, the bacterium has been processed so that it lacks the disease-producing capabilities but retains the ability to stimulate an immune reaction. The brucellosis vaccine is an example of this type; it produces a more lasting immunity than bacterins (vaccines made from dead bacteria; see section on Bacterins below).

Live Bacterial Spore Vaccine. In live bacterial spore vaccine, a culture is grown on a medium and is allowed to sporulate, but the virulence is lowered by cultivation under higher than normal temperatures. After spores form, the cells are washed away, and the suspension is heated to destroy vegetative forms. The living spores stimulate the desired immunity better than bacterins.

Bacterin. Bacterin is a vaccine that works only against bacteria, not viruses. It is usually a killed bacterial preparation that is used without fear of creating an outbreak, but is still capable of developing an immunizing response due to the presence of the organism in the injection. Mixed bacterins consist of several different organisms in one dose to protect the animal against a multitude of bacterial invasions. Example: Shipping Fever bacterin.

Autogenous bacterins are vaccines made from specific organisms isolated from the herd itself, which are then injected back into the herd to help create immunity.

Forms of Vaccines

Vaccines may come already mixed with liquid. In this case there is little to be done except to fill a syringe with the liquid and inject it into the animal. Previously mixed vaccines are usually made from killed products that have good storage life in the liquid mixture in which they are suspended. Precaution should be taken to keep the material refrigerated and out of sunlight or as directed by the instructions. Most vaccines against bacterial diseases such as Blackleg and Redwater come in this form.

Vaccines made from most live and modified live viruses come in a dried cake preparation, which is a precautionary measure to retain the virulence of the product. Usually another bottle will accompany the dried preparation to be used as a dissolving agent for the dried cake. This liquid is most often sterile water, and the preparation should be used within a relatively short period of time after reconstitution. It is recommended that no more be mixed than will be used up in 30 minutes. Modified live virus vaccines should be protected from the ultraviolet rays of direct sunlight.

Multiple-dose vials are made by the pharmaceutical companies for ease of injection in small-to-large operations. Vials can be purchased that range from 5-dose capacity to 100-dose capacity for maximum number of inoculations with the minimum time involved.

It is possible and sometimes necessary to increase the immunity-producing potential of a vaccine by the addition of an adjuvant (a substance added to a drug to aid its action). Examples of materials used as adjuvants are alum, aluminum hydroxide, lanolin, oil and water emulsions, and killed mycobacteria or extracts of these mycobacteria in bacterial toxins. Such materials are mildly irritating to the tissues, causing the immunity-producing particles to be held in the injection area longer. This brings about a longer period of release and a longer period of stimulation of the immunizing mechanisms of the animal's body. The result is the production of a greater quantity of antibodies.

Antiserums

Antiserums provide only very temporary protection. Basically, an antiserum means taking one animal's blood serum that contains antibodies and injecting it into another animal to help immunize against a specific disease after exposure is confirmed. An antiserum usually provides protection for approximately 1 to 2 weeks after injection.

To produce antiserums, the animal's immunizing mechanism is stimulated to the fullest, blood withdrawals are made, and the serum portion of the blood is removed to be made into a preparation suitable for injecting into the patient. Antiserums can be produced to protect against a variety of diseases such as Shipping Fever and Blackleg.

Toxoids

Toxoids are prepared from a potent toxin (poison produced by live organisms), which is detoxified by chemical treatment to remove its poisonous properties. The immunizing response factor is retained. In this way an injection can be given to protect the animal before a problem arises. It is a precautionary measure to guard against such common problems as lockjaw (tetanus). Example: Tetanus toxoid.

Antitoxins

Antitoxins are designed to counteract the toxic effects of particular organisms. In most cases they are only effective against a specific toxin such as tetanus. An antitoxin would be used in the event an animal had not been protected by a precautionary toxoid injection. Example: Tetanus antitoxin.

It is very important to have fresh products. If a vaccine is shipped packed in ice and the shipping is delayed, it should be checked very carefully and refused if there are indications that the vaccine was without refrigeration or has been exposed to extreme heat. It is better to reject any "suspect vaccines" than to take a chance on using a product that has lost its effectiveness. Cooling packs are often sent through the mail and are subjected to unnecessary delays or heat. Feel the cooling pack upon receiving the package to be sure that it is indeed still cool. If a vaccine package has been in transit an unnecessarily long time such as a week, do not accept it. Send it back and ask for a faster form of transportation.

Vaccines once received should always be refrigerated according to instructions. They should not be frozen since freezing could destroy the potency of the material. Most vaccines come in brown bottles in order to protect them from the light. The bottles should be kept out of sunlight and should be stored in a dark place in addition to being refrigerated.

There will often be some material left in the vaccine bottle when vaccination is finished. Discard any unused vaccine because the contents may have become contaminated by the needle used to withdraw the vaccine.

If needles are reused (after disinfection with alcohol or some other chemical), be sure that all of the disinfectant is out of the needle before introducing it into a vaccine bottle because the disinfectant may inactivate the vaccine. It is best not to use chemical disinfection of needles and syringes. Boiling in distilled water is the preferred method.

The expiration date on any vaccine is plainly listed on the label. This should be observed and followed with common sense. It should be recognized that these expiration dates are determined by the pharmaceutical companies by simply putting the material in storage for a specified length of time, trying it, and if immunity still results, guaranteeing it for that period of time. This does not mean that the immunity will be void on the exact expiration date. Usually a wide margin of safety is allowed by the company. Therefore, if the date is only 1 or 2 days over the expiration date on the bottle, the material could still be used. For obvious reasons, the expiration date should not be tested much past the guaranteed period. The available biologicals of practical use to you in combating the various disorders are listed in Table 3-1. The dosage, available form, route of administration, and what disease it is used to combat are covered in Table 3-2. This list does not include every drug available, but it is a good, practical reference.

PHARMACEUTICAL PRODUCTS

Pharmaceuticals are used for treatment of a disease once the illness occurs. These would include such materials as antibiotics, steroids, etc.

Pharmaceuticals are available in a variety of forms, including drenches, boluses, powders, food additives, and liquids.

Table 3-1. Available Biologicals
(Vaccines, Bacterins, Bacterin-Toxoids, Antitoxins, Toxoids, and Antiserums)

CATTLE PRODUCTS

Clostridium perfringens (overeating or enterotoxemia types B, C, D,
CD toxoids, antitoxins, or bacterin-toxoids)
Corynebacterium pasteurella bacterin
Staph-Strep (staphlococcus-streptococcus)

Cattle Products with Clostridium

Blackleg and Malignant Edema (CCS or *Clostridium chauvoei-septicum*)
Triple Bacterin or Blackleg, Malignant Edema, and False Blackleg
   (CCSP or *Clostridium chauvoei septicum, Pasteurella*)
Clostridium novyi (CN)
Clostridium novyi-sordelli (CNS)
Clostridium chauvoei-septicum-novyi (CCSN)
Clostridium chauvoei-septicum-novyi-sordelli (CCSNS) (Four-way Blackleg)
Five-way Blackleg
Seven-way Blackleg
Clostridium chauvoei-septicum-leptospira-pomona
Clostridium haemolyticum (CH)—Redwater Disease
Clostridium chauvoei-septicum-novyi-septospira-pomona

Cattle Respiratory Products

Pasteurella multocida and/or *haemolytica*
Shipping Fever (*Parainfluenza*-3 or SF-4)
Red Nose, or IBR (infectious bovine rhinotrachetis)
   or IPV (infectious pustular vulvovaginitis)
BVD (bovine virus diarrhea)
PI$_3$ and Pasteurella
PI$_3$ and Lepto
IBR and Lepto
IBR and BVD
BVD and Lepto
Pasteurella and Lepto
PI$_3$, IBR, and BVD
PI$_3$, IBR, and Lepto
BVD, IBR, and Lepto
PI$_3$, IBR, BVD, and Pasteurella
PI$_3$, IBR, BVD, and Lepto

Other Cattle Products

Reo-Viral Calf Diarrhea (*Scour Vax-Reo*)
Reo-Corona Viral Calf Diarrhea (*Scour Vax II*)
Antibacterial Serum—Bovine Formula 3
   (*E. coli-Pasteurella-Salmonella Typhimurium* antiserum)
Vibriosis (*Vibrio fetus*)
Vibriosis and *Leptospira pomona*
Anaplasmosis (Anaplaz)
Anthrax Spore Vaccine

Table 3-1. (*Continued*)

25

PHARMA-
CEUTICAL
PRODUCTS

Wart Vaccine
Staphylococcus aureus
Mixed Bacterin Bovine Formula 1, 2, or 3
Corynebacterium pasteurella Antiserum
Pasteurella multocida Antiserum
Autogenous Bacterins (Lab-prepared vaccine from cultures submitted
    by veterinarians or farmers)
Leptospirosis or Lepto (*Leptospira pomona*)
Leptospira canicola-icterohaemorrhagiae
Three-Way *Lepto—Leptospira pomona-grippo-hardjo*
    (*Leptovac-GHP, Leptomune-GHP*)
Leptospira hardjo (Hardjomune)
Leptospira grippotyphosa (Grippomune)
Brucellosis or Bang's disease (*Brucella abortus*)
Tetanus (toxoid or antitoxin)

SWINE PRODUCTS

Erysipelas bacterin or vaccine
TGE vaccine (TGE-Vac)
Atrophic rhinitis (B-B Vac for *Bordetella bronchiseptica*)
Erysipelas Serum
Jowl Abscesses (Streptococcus, Group E Vaccine)
Mixed Bacterins—Porcine (Formula 1 and 2)
Leptospirosis or Lepto (*Leptospira Pomona*)
Leptospira canicola-icterohaemorrhagiae
Three-Way Lepto—*Leptospira pomona-grippo-hardjo* (*Leptovac-GHP,
    Leptomune-GHP*)
Leptospira hardjo (Hardjomune)
Leptospira grippotyphosa (Grippomune)
Brucellosis or Bang's disease (*Brucella abortus*)
Tetanus (Toxoid or Antitoxin)
    Clostridium perfringens (overeating or enterotoxemia types B, C, D,
CD toxoids, antitoxins, or bacterin-toxoids)
Corynebacterium pasteurella Bacterin
Staph-Strep (Staphlococcus Streptococcus)
Coli-Staph-Strep Bacterin
Autogenous Bacterins (Lab-prepared vaccine from cultures submitted
    by veterinarians or farmers)

EQUINE PRODUCTS

Encephalomyelitis Vaccines, eastern, western, and Venezuelan strains
    (killed or modified live virus)
Tetanus Antitoxin
Tetanus Toxoid
Equine Influenza Vaccine (killed virus)
Equine Rhinopneumonitis (modified live virus or live virus)
Normal Serum of Equine origin

Table 3-2. A Practical Guide to Selected Drug Use

Drug	Usage or Activity	Route of Administration	Form	Dosage
Chloramphenicol*	Antibiotic	IV	Sol., pv.	All species: approx. 5 mg/lb/da
		IM	Susp.	All species: approx. 5 mg/lb/da
	Growth promoter	In feed	Premix	S: 10 gm/ton
Chlortetracycline hydrochloride	Antibiotic for susceptible pathogens	IV	Sol., pv.	All species: 2–5 mg/lb/da
		Oral	Pv., tab.	
		Local	Oint.	All species: to effect
Dextrose	Hydration	IV	5% sol.	All species: up to 4–8% of body wt, depending on other fluid
	Dehydration	IV	50% sol.	All species: approx. 1 gm/lb
	Antiketosis, antitoxemia	IV infusion	20–50% sol.	H, C: 100–200 ml/hr Sh, S: 15–60 ml/hr
Diethylstilbestrol	Abortifacient	IM	In oil	
	Promote fattening	In feed	Premix	Fattening cattle: 5–10 mg/da
		Sub Q	Pellet	Fattening cattle: 60 mg
Epinephrine injection	Anaphylaxis	Sub Q, IM	1:1000 sol.	H, C: 4–8 ml
			1:10,000 sol.	Sh, S: 1–3 ml
Hexachloroethane	Fasciolicidal (Liver flukes)	Oral	Susp.	C: 10 gm/100 lb
			Bolus	Sh: 15 gm
Lidocaine hydrochloride	Anesthetic, infiltration	Sub Q	pv.	H, C: 1–2% sol., to effect
	conduction	IM, Sub Q	pv.	H, C: 5–10 ml of 3% sol.
	epidural	Epidural	pv.	H, C: 5–10 ml of 2% sol.
Methylene blue	Nitrite poisoning	IV	4% sol.	C, Sh: 4 mg/lb

Milk of Magnesia	Cathartic	Oral	Susp.	Foal, calf: 30–60 ml Lamb, pig: 10–20 ml
Oxytetracycline hydrochloride	Antibiotic for susceptible pathogens	IV	Sol., pv.	All species: 2–5 mg/lb/da
		IM	Special sol., pv.	All species: 2–5 mg/lb/da
		Local	Oint.	All species: to effect
	Growth promoter	In feed	Premix	Swine: 10 gm/ton Calf: in milk, 15–20 mg/100 lb body wt; up to 4 mo of age 5–15 mg/lb feed
Oxytocin	Obstetrics	IM, IV	Sol.	H, C: 75–150 u Sh, S: 30–50 u
	Milk letdown	IM, IV	Sol.	H, C: 75–150 u Sh, S: 5–20 u
Penicillin G, sodium or potassium	Susceptible pathogens	IM	Pv.	All Species: approx. 5000 u/lb every 4 hr
Penicillin G, procaine	Susceptible pathogens	IM	Aqueous susp.	All species: approx. 5000 u/lb/da
	Growth promotion	In feed	Premix	Poultry: 2–4 gm/ton
Penicillin G, repository salts	Susceptible pathogens	IM	Aqueous susp.	All species: approx. 5000–10,000 u/lb
Piperazine adipate	Antinematodal (dewormer)	Oral	Pv.	H: 10 gm/100 lb to max. of 80 gm Calf: 0.1 gm/lb

Table 3-2. A Practical Guide to Selected Drug Use

Drug	Usage or Activity	Route of Administration	Form	Dosage
Phenothiazine	Antinematodal	Oral dose	Susp.	H: 30–300 mg/da C: 10 gm/100 lb to max. of 80 gm Sh, goat: 25 gm Lamb, kid: 10–15 gm
		Continuous feeding	Salt, feed	H: 2 gm/da Colt: 1 gm/da Dairy cow: 1.5–2 gm/da Sh: 1 part to 10 in minerals or salt
Prednisolone	Antiketosis	IM	Sol.	C: 200–400 mg
Prednisone	Antiketosis	IM	Sol.	C: 100–300 mg
	Antiinflammatory	Within bursa, tendon sheath, or joint capsule	Sol.	H,C: 50–250 mg
		IM	Sol.	H,C: 100–300 mg
Procaine hydrochloride	Anesthetic, infiltration	Sub Q	Pv.	H,C,Sh,S: 2% sol., to effect
	conduction	IM, Sub Q	Pv.	H,C,Sh,S: 5–10 ml of 4% sol.
	epidural	Epidural	Pv.	C: 10–15 ml of 2% sol.
Sulfonamides	Susceptible pathogens	Oral	Pv., sol., susp.	All species: approx. 1 gr/lb or 1 gm/15 lb/da
		IV	Sol., sodium, salt	All species: not to exceed 0.5 gr/lb/da
		IP	Sol., sodium, salt	Baby pigs: 0.5–1 gr/lb/da

Drug	Indication	Route	Form	Dosage
Sulfamethazine sodium	Urinary tract pathogens	Oral	Pv., tab.	All species: 0.5 gm/lb/da
	Coccidiostat	Oral	Pv.	C: therapy, 1 gr/lb followed by 0.5 gr/lb on 2nd, 3rd, & 4th da; repeat on 3rd & 5th wk
Tetracaine hydrochloride	Anesthetic, mucosa	Topical	Sol.	H,C: 2–4% sol., to effect
	eye	Topical	Sol.	H,C: 1% in sol., to effect
Tetracycline hydrochloride	Susceptible pathogens	IV	Sol, pv.	All species: 2–5 mg/lb/da
		Topical	Pv., oint.	All species: to effect

*Not cleared for use in animals used for food.

The following symbols or abbreviations have been employed:

H—horse
C—cow
Sh—sheep
S—swine
D—dog
alc.—alcohol
da—day
gm—gram
gr—grain
gal—gallon
hr—hour
IM—intramuscular
IP—intraperitoneal
IV—intravenous
lb—pound or pounds of body weight unless otherwise specified.
ml—milliliter
Oint.—ointment
Premix—a concentrated commercial mixture of drug and diluent for further dilution in the ration.
Pv.—powder
Sub Q—subcutaneous
Sol.—solution
Susp.—suspension
to effect—the drug is administered until the desired effect is produced.
Tab.—tablet
u—unit

Antibiotics

The name antibiotic implies a material that is "against life." This medical tool is against a specific form of life—pathogenic bacteria. Antibiotics are ineffective against viral organisms; they are used chiefly to treat diseases that are caused by bacteria. Therefore they would not be used in the treatment of viral diseases except when an animal is weakened by a viral disease and becomes susceptible to secondary bacterial infection.

The reason there are so many different antibiotics on the market is that there are so many types of bacteria in the environment. One antibiotic may be effective against a certain bacterium or group of bacteria, but may be completely ineffective against another. Since there are so many types or groups of bacteria, there is the necessity of many types of antibiotics used to combat their effects.

There are also broad-spectrum antibiotics on the market that are designed to control a variety of different bacterial organisms all at the same time. The more commonly available antibiotics on the market are:

Chlortetracycline (Aureomycin)

Oxytetracycline (Terramycin)

Neomycin

Erythromycin

Tylosin (Tylan)

Lincomycin

Penicillin (synthetic and natural)

Streptomycin

Spectinomycin

Gentamycin

Novobiocin

Bacitracin

Penicillin-streptomycin

There are several ways to classify antibiotics according to their effect on certain organisms in animal husbandry. One type of classification of an antibiotic depends on its ability to control Gram-positive or Gram-negative organisms or both. Most bacteria belong to one of these two groups—Gram-positive or Gram-negative. Some antibiotics are specific in their effects on Gram-positive organisms, while others are specific in their control of Gram-negative organisms. A broad-spectrum antibiotic such as tetracycline or chloramphenicol may be effective against *both* Gram-positive and Gram-negative organisms in a shotgun approach. Although a broad-spectrum antibiotic may not be the most potent or the best control for a specific bacterium, it usually is the best place to start. If the organism cannot be controlled with a broad-spectrum agent, then a culture may have to be made, the organism identified, and experiments conducted with various antibiotics to find the specific one to control the bacterium.

The second type of classification for antibiotics is according to how the antibiotic affects the growth and destruction of the organism. The two divisions here are referred to as *bacteriostatic* and *bactericidal*. The difference is that the bacteriostatic group inhibits growth of an organism but does not destroy it immediately. This group usually interferes with the metabolism or the reproductive ability of the bacterium, forcing it to eventually die out. The bactericidal group is much more potent; it exerts a direct killing action on the organism.

Penicillin. The first antibiotic to be used was penicillin; it was discovered by the British bacteriologist Fleming about 1928. He noticed that a mold had contaminated a bacterial culture in his laboratory and was inhibiting the growth of the bacteria. This was quite an accidental observation. The mold was one that he had been watching and, strangely enough, had been originally found growing on a cantalope rind in a garbage can. It wasn't until about 1940 that this mold, after 10 or 12 years of experimentation, was purified and perfected to the state that we know it today. Although some organisms have developed a resistance to penicillin, it is still effective as a selective bactericidal medication with some bacteriostatic properties. Penicillin is much more effective against Gram-positive than Gram-negative organisms. Examples of Gram-positive organisms are the clostridia, staphylococci, streptococci, and corynebacteria. Although penicillin will also inhibit most Gram-negative organisms, some organisms that are not affected by it are members of the *E. coli*, *Salmonella*, *Klebsiella*, *Proteus*, and *Pseudomonas* genera.

Ampicillin, a more recently developed form of penicillin, has a broad-spectrum action and is effective against both Gram-positive and Gram-negative organisms.

Penicillin is given most commonly as an injection, but it may also be given orally. However, the oral form should be recognized as an inhibitor of organisms in the digestive system of ruminating animals, and any use made of it in this form must be considered as inhibiting beneficial bacteria as well. In other words, an oral dosage to cattle could be harmful by destroying the rumen bacteria that help digest cellulose and fiber. Penicillin is also used in many of the mastitis preparations for treatment by intramammary infusion.

The withdrawal period for most antibiotics before an animal may be slaughtered varies, depending on the product used and the method of administration. It is very important to read the label before an animal is slaughtered for meat or before milk is made available for human consumption.

The range of dosage for penicillin is much safer than for other antibiotics, which is what has endeared it to the average stockman. It is usually recommended to use the highest level suggested on the bottle label. In fact, you can even double the dosage recommended in severe cases and need not be concerned about the toxic effect. Such dosages would not be recommended for other antibiotics, but it is all right in the case of penicillin.

The difference in price of various injectable forms of penicillin may cause you to select a form simply because it is cheap. This is not always the best buy because of differences in potency levels and because the cheaper injection forms usually have a shorter injection interval. For example, there are forms that must be injected every 12 hours and others, naturally more expensive, that need only be given at 48-hour intervals. Read the label carefully so that you know what you are buying. The more expensive forms usually are longer acting. It is important to use a high initial dosage of penicillin, but also to continue its use for at least 5 to 7 days to be sure that all susceptible bacteria are controlled.

You should not use penicillin indiscriminately even though it is a very safe, effective drug. If you use it for every little cough and sneeze, the organisms could develop resistant strains and then the drug would lose its effectiveness.

Streptomycin. Streptomycin is another antibiotic; it is more effective against Gram-negative than Gram-positive organisms. For this reason, streptomycin is often mixed with penicillin because they complement each other to form a good antibiotic combination.

There has been some criticism of this combination because streptomycin is only effective for about 4 hours, whereas penicillin is good for about 12 hours. Thus, by the time the penicillin wears off, the streptomycin has long since been depleted. But it is a good product to have on hand and is generally recommended. Several companies make it. It is all similar, so check the expiration date and get the best price.

Streptomycin alone is particularly effective against Pasteurella, Brucella, Hemophylus, Salmonella, Klebsiella, Shigella, and Leptospirosis. The recommended dosage of streptomycin is 5 mg per pound of body weight, repeated every 8 to 12 hours. Caution: Don't use for more than 5 consecutive days because of inner-ear problems that often develop with long-term use.

Tetracyclines. There are several forms of tetracyclines that have basically the same action. These are chlortetracycline or the trade name Aureomycin, and oxytetracycline or the trade name Terramycin.

The tetracyclines are wider in their spectrum of activity than penicillin. They are most effective against rickettsiae and a few of the viruses belonging to the psittacosis group. The tetracyclines are bacteriostatic.

The normal use for this antibiotic is as an intravenous injection. It is available in injectable, oral, and topical products, but is normally used as an intravenous injection because of the burning sensation it causes when given intramuscularly. If injected into the muscle, the injection should be deep because of the discoloration to the skin and meat, in the event of slaughter, and because of the discomfort to the animal. The dose generally recommended is 2 to 5 mg per pound of body weight once per day, or twice per day in certain cases.

Neomycin. Neomycin is most often used for intestinal problems because very little of it is absorbed from the intestinal tract. For this reason, it is not effective against systemic diseases when given orally. It is used mostly in intestinal disorders and is administered orally either as a bolus or liquid.

Tylocin. The trade name for tylocin is Tylan®. It is used for respiratory diseases in cattle and is especially recommended for foot rot, pneumonia, and uterine infections. It is equally effective in calves and adult animals. The recommended dosage is 1 to 2 mg per pound of body weight.

For swine, tylocin is recommended as a treatment for erysipelas, pneumonia, vibrionic dysentery, and arthritis due to mycoplasma organisms.

There are many antibiotics on the market today that are not discussed in detail in this chapter. They are usually used for more specific purposes and don't have as wide a spectrum as the antibiotics described above.

Sulfonamides

The common name used in reference to the sulfonamides is *sulfa*. Discovered early in the 1900s, sulfas were the first drugs to be used to treat bacterial infections directly. Sulfas are not classified as antibiotics, but they do have antibacterial properties and are still considered very effective drugs against certain organisms. Sulfas have generally been replaced by antibiotics, but they still have their place in animal medicine, and many sulfas remain on the market today.

The characteristics of sulfas are that they are bacteriostatic, meaning they are able to prevent the reproduction of certain bacterial organisms, thus giving the body a chance to heal. They are broad-spectrum in nature, inhibiting both Gram-positive and Gram-negative bacteria.

Sulfas are most effective against intestinal problems in animals, such as diarrhea. This drug is normally given orally, as a bolus or drench. Sulfas are also used in the treatment of bladder infections and are particularly effective against coccidiosis. When given intravenously, sulfas can be effective against some respiratory infections, and they are used for this purpose.

Care must be taken when injecting sulfas intravenously because toxic problems can be encountered. If the product is given too rapidly or in too large a dose, the typical response for cattle is an inability to focus the eyes, muscular weakness and incoordination, collapse, and sometimes death.

Some of the common sulfonamides are sulfamethazine, sulfathiazole, sulfamerazine, sulfapyridine, and sulfacetamide. These sulfa drugs are often used in combinations of two, three, or more types given in one preparation in order to get as broad coverage as possible in the control of the organisms in question.

The dosages may vary, depending on the type of sulfa drug to be used, the combination of drugs it contains, and the condition that is being treated, as well as whether it is being given intravenously or orally. For these reasons, a specific recommendation is not very practical. Read the manufacturer's instructions carefully and follow them faithfully. Do not exceed the recommended dosage.

Corticosteroids

Commonly called *steroids*, the corticosteroids are anti-inflammatory drugs used in combination with antibiotics to reduce inflammation. The effects are many, some of which are not completely understood. There is an inhibition of the body's ability to fight infection and to develop immunity when steroids are administered. For this reason extreme caution is recommended. For example, steroids should not be used in combination with a vaccine because the drug will inhibit the body's ability to produce immune bodies and therefore will cancel out the positive effect of the vaccine. Steroids may also inhibit the body's ability to fight off chronic infections over the long run and may do more harm than good. A great deal of experience is needed in order to use steroids properly, and for this reason they are not easy drugs to obtain on the open market. And once obtained, it is not easy to determine when these drugs may be properly employed.

Steroids are usually used by veterinarians in conjunction with an antibiotic for some infectious disease. They are also used as an antishock drug.

The more common steroids on the market are generally referred to by their trade names. Although there are many others on the market, the following are the best known: dexamethazone (Azium®), flumethazone (Flucort®), prednisone, and prednisolone.

Steroids are used to reduce inflammation and alleviate lameness in animals, but recently other drugs, nonsteroidal in nature, have appeared on the market that do about the same thing although they are not classified as steroids. The trade names of some of these newer products are Butazoladone® (phenylbutazone), Arquel® (product of Parke-Davis), and Equiproxin® (product of Diamond).

Antihistamines

Histamines are products that are released by the body tissues in arthritic conditions around the joints; but they are more commonly released in the skin when the body exhibits an allergic reaction. A rash, sneezing, respiratory problems, or similar conditions caused by allergins are brought on by the release of histamines. Therefore, an antihistamine agent is a drug that works against the histamines that bring on the clinical signs of allergic reactions.

Antihistamines are used by some veterinarians, but steroids are used more commonly because of their anti-inflammatory properties and because they show more effective control of allergies in animals.

Coagulants and Anticoagulants

Coagulants are used to stop the flow of blood in such operations as dehorning and castration in the event that excessive bleeding occurs. Coagulants are merely an aid in helping the body's natural mechanism and do not completely inhibit the flow of blood. There are many topical products available for use, especially in dehorning operations. These powders normally go under a trade name such as "hemostatic powder," etc. They act by clotting and by chemically cauterizing the blood vessel, thereby slowing the flow of blood so that normal clotting can occur. These products do have a place in the average operation, but their limitations should be understood.

Anticoagulants have the opposite effect in that they prevent clotting. They are rarely used in veterinary medicine and find even less use on the average farm and ranch.

Anesthetics

An anesthetic is a drug used to induce sleep or insensitivity to pain for surgical purposes.

A local anesthetic is used to deaden the sensitivity of an area for a skin incision, for minor operations such as dehorning, and for minor eye surgery, etc. It is very important to use a sterile technique and follow the exact recommended dosage. The layman may safely use local anesthetics for certain limited procedures, if he takes the time to learn the locations of major nerves to a given area of the body.

On the other hand, general anesthetics, mainly barbiturates, are not recommended for use by the average farmer or rancher because of a vast number of complications that can arise without the assistance of a knowledgeable veterinarian. General anesthetics can be extremely dangerous if used without the proper background and training.

Proper Handling of Antibiotics and Other Pharmaceuticals

The manufacturer wants the product you are using to work. He wants to sell it to you again. Therefore, we cannot stress enough the need to read the instructions carefully and follow them faithfully with the few exceptions that we have noted in the previous discussion. Always follow a sterile technique in the use of these products, and you will not be disappointed in the results obtained. It is important to refrigerate those products that need refrigerating, but do not refrigerate those products that do not require it. Those drugs and vaccines that should be kept out of the sunlight should be protected as recommended. The date indicating the last day of the guarantee should be noted, and any product that is out of date should be used with knowledge of its limitations. Again, it should be stressed that a day or two out of date probably makes little or no difference, and common sense is needed to determine whether a product is still effective.

Most liquid products come in containers that have a rubberized cap and also a cover for the cap. The cover should be used in storing products, and care should be used to maintain sanitary conditions when withdrawing material from bottles. Use of a cotton swab soaked in alcohol is always recommended to wipe off the rubberized cap before insertion of a needle for withdrawal of material. A new needle and syringe, or a sterilized one, is recommended when withdrawing from multiple-dosage bottles that are to be kept for later use. Do not keep material that has been used several times without the use of a sterile syringe and needle, and especially if the material is kept for a period of time.

Do not expose drugs to extremes of temperature, either freezing or very hot weather, such as when a product is exposed for a long period of time in the cab of a pickup truck. Follow the manufacturer's recommendations for maintaining the proper range of temperature, and if this is exceeded at either extreme, the product should be considered for disposal.

OTHER ANIMAL DRUGS

Vitamins and Minerals

Vitamins and minerals are discussed here not from a nutritional standpoint, but rather from a medical determination of their function and proper application. (Chapter 5 will cover the subject of vitamins and nutrition.)

A vitamin is an organic substance required in small amounts to regulate the body processes for natural growth, health, and reproduction. There are also occasions when vitamins are recommended for clinical purposes in which nutrition may or may not be a part. In the case of starvation, of course, vitamins along with other nutrients will be deficient, and should be replaced as part of the therapeutic return to health. However, there are certain conditions such as heavy parasitism and diseases in which blood deficiencies result (anaplasmosis), where nutrition was sufficient but the stress caused by the disease produced a vitamin deficiency.

Cattle with stress-induced vitamin deficiencies will have the same appearance as those with vitamin deficiencies that occur naturally. They will normally be thin, rough-haired, and perhaps evidence a bottle-jaw appearance. In these cases the animals are often given very large quantities of vitamins in order to help their systems overcome the disorder and return to normal health.

As a preventive measure to help cattle and calves through rough winters, vitamins A, D, and E are often recommended because of the liver's inability to store these vitamins for more than a few months time. If adequate nutrition is available, no vitamin supplementation is recommended. However, there are extremely rough ranges in many parts of the country, especially in the mountainous western states, where adequate nutrition is not available, due to bad weather and poor foraging conditions. In these cases, vitamin therapy of A, D, and E is often recommended for bringing cattle through the winter in good health. Normally, injectable A, D, and E vitamins are given along with iron to counteract anemia, which usually accompanies poor nutrition.

Most vitamin therapy recommendations are in the form of injectable vitamins. The concentrations of commercially available vitamin supplements are normally 500,000 I.U. of vitamin A, 75,000 I.U. of vitamin D, and 5 I.U. of vitamin E per cc of material. The product is injected intramuscularly according to the manufacturer's recommendations, for example, 2 to 3 cc per adult cow every 2 to 3 months. Recommendations for other species may vary somewhat from this, and the manufacturer's instructions should be followed.

Oral vitamins are also available and are considered quite effective. "Downer" cows should be given oral vitamins to supplement the stressful condition placed on the body and boost the system to return to normal health. However, 50% or more of the downer cows will not regain their feet regardless of what you do. Therefore it is extremely important to watch cattle and other animals and to use the vitamin booster before this stage is reached —if at all possible. Vitamins in combination with glucose are available for this purpose. The glucose gives an extra energy boost, and the vitamins regulate the functions described in later nutrition chapters, for each of the species covered in this book.

Weak baby calves are good subjects for vitamin therapy. Calves may be given products containing vitamins A, D, and E, and also vitamin B_{12}, which stimulates appetite in most animals. Once calves begin to nurse, the vitamins may be stopped.

Minerals are also needed in very small amounts but generally are not recommended to be injected into the animal. Rather, they are fed in an oral form, usually free choice (always available), mixed with salt to control intake. Minerals are discussed in more detail and recommendations are made in Chapter 5 and in other nutrition chapters for specific species.

Hormones

Hormones are products produced by the endocrine glands (thyroid, ovary, adrenal gland, etc.) for specific effects on the activity of virtually every organ in the body. Nature has seen to it that these hormones work extremely well, except for special situations that require manipulation by man. For instance, the regulation of heat so that all females come into estrus at the same time is desirable for artificial insemination and calf-grouping. Therapeutic hormones are also given in some instances to correct malfunctions.

The action of hormones is very complicated because of the many interactions that occur between the organs and the specific hormones produced. It is very easy for an untrained person to do more harm than good through the indiscriminate use of hormone therapy.

An example of some hormones that are used by veterinarians are testosterone, estrogen, oxytocin, epinephrine, and progesterone. Testosterone can be prescribed to improve male sexual desire. Estrogen is a female hormone used to stimulate heat. Oxytocin has a dual effect on the body: First, it stimulates milk letdown* when the calf begins to nurse or when the milkers are applied to a milk cow or the udder is massaged. Second, it stimulates uterine contractions during the birth process. Synthetic oxytocin can be used in an injectable form during difficult deliveries to give the uterus an extra push to expel the fetus.

Epinephrine is the fright hormone. It momentarily increases muscular strength. It is used in veterinary medicine to treat anaphylactic shock and also to stimulate the heart.

Progesterone is used to synchronize heat periods of all females in a herd so that artificial insemination can be concentrated within a few days. There are numerous hormones on the market that are available for a great variety of purposes; but no hormone is recommended for use by the farmer or rancher unless he knows what he is doing or unless he is under the supervision of somebody who does. It is extremely easy to create an undesirable condition with these potent products.

Energy Sources—Glucose

Glucose is a form of sugar that is used to provide a quick source of energy for the animal. It may be given in an oral form or intravenously. Glucose is normally recommended for animals that are weakened—for those who are already down or about to go down. It is preferable that the glucose be given *before* an animal goes down because it is doubtful whether any treatment can be effective enough to return an animal to its feet.

Several combinations of glucose, electrolytes (a source of minerals), and amino acids (a source of soluble protein) are available on the market. These combinations are usually oral or injectable products that give the animal the necessary protein, energy, and minerals to stimulate a good appetite and a resumption of normal functions.

A common mistake in the use of glucose and electrolytes is to under-dose the animal, especially in the case of injectable products. The animal will require several liters in most instances to do any good at all. Since this intravenous form is very expensive, the common mistake is to hold back on the dosage.

A more usable form is the prepackaged oral combinations of glucose, electrolytes, and amino acids. These are also expensive but not so much as the injectable forms, and they are generally easier to handle and safer to regulate.

In the case of a forced austerity program, a good home remedy—to be used as an oral drench—is one quart of Karo syrup or honey dissolved in one gallon of water. To this add 1 tablespoon of baking soda and 3 tablespoons of salt. This will provide energy and a close substitute for minerals. It may be

---

*The release of secreted milk for ease of extraction.

given with a dose syringe or stomach tube to provide the necessary boost when an animal is not eating. If a downer cow is the patient, be sure not to dose the animal on its side with a dose syringe because it is very easy to put this material into the lungs and produce "foreign body" pneumonia. It is always best to prop the animal up on the breastbone before dosing with a dose syringe or drench bottle. A stomach tube may be a safer method because usually it is fairly easily inserted down the esophagus. If the stomach tube is forced into the lungs by mistake, the animal will usually cough, and this should be taken as a sign to try again. Also, the feel of the tube will be different if it is inserted down the windpipe as compared to the esophagus. In some instances there may not be a cough, but the feel of the tube will be smooth with no restriction if it goes down the windpipe. If it is going down the esophagus, where it should be, there will be some resistance felt on the tube because it has to open the esophagus as it goes along to the stomach.

ADMINISTERING DRUGS

Some products may be given intramuscularly; others may be given intravenously; still others may have a different form of application. There may also be some drugs that can be injected in a variety of ways. It is important to determine from the label how the drug is to be used. For example, an intravenous drug given intramuscularly can cause a sloughing of the skin, damage to muscle tissue, and pain. An intramuscular drug given intravenously may cause severe reactions including shock or death. Therefore, you must read the label and follow instructions.

Some people may recommend an alcohol wipe prior to giving an injection, but it is not recommended for either intramuscular or subcutaneous injections because it is neither practical nor necessary under most farm conditions. It may, in fact, do more harm than good because it takes alcohol about 15 minutes to destroy any skin contaminants. By wetting the area and immediately puncturing the skin you may mobilize these contaminants in a liquid form, providing them an easier entry into the body. An abscess could result.

When considering the administration of injectable products, several decisions must be made.

Needles

The needle size and length will vary depending on the type of medication to be given and the volume of injection. The diameter or size of the hole in the needle is very important because thick material will not go through a very small-bored needle; and the larger the diameter of the needle, the more pain inflicted on the animal. Try to use the smallest diameter needle that is suitable to the product that is being injected. The way to tell what diameter you have is by reading the gauge printed on the outside case of any needle. The gauges will range from 27 down to 10 gauge. The larger the number, the smaller the bore; so a 22-gauge needle would have a very small bore or diameter. Another thing to consider when selecting needles is the length. If an injection is to be given subcutaneously, a short, approximately $\frac{1}{2}$ in. to 1 in. needle will work very nicely. If an injection is to be given intramuscularly, you will want to use a longer needle (about $1\frac{1}{2}$ in.) to make sure that you get through the skin, the subcutaneous tissue, and into the middle of the muscle tissue. If an intravenous injection is being given, it is recommended that a $1\frac{1}{2}$ in. to $3\frac{1}{2}$ in. needle be used so that the needle can be threaded down into the vein. Shorter needles tend to pop out of the vein if an animal moves.

Syringe Type and Size

Stockmen often use one of the old metal, glass-barrel syringes that hasn't been cleaned since the day it was purchased. These syringes do work; but if they're going to be used, they should be cleaned and sterilized between each use. A more practical method is to use disposable plastic syringes. They are very economical and can be discarded after use. The size of the syringe is important and should match the dosage of the medication to be given. Disposable syringes are available in all sizes—from 1 cc up to 65 to 70 cc. So here again is a good reason to use disposable syringes, that is, they provide a wider selection of sizes, as well as being much more economical in the long run.

Methods of Injection

Intramuscular (IM) (Figure 3-1). The proper technique for an intramuscular injection is to use sterile, disposable needles and syringes or ones that have been chemically sterilized or boiled in water for 30 minutes to

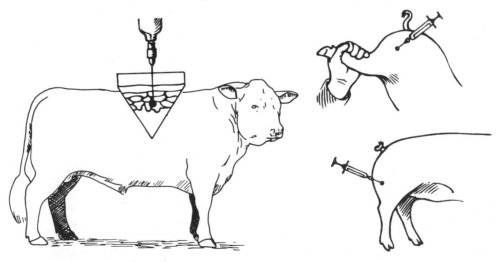

Figure 3-1. Procedure for making an intramuscular injection (IM). Using a needle at least 3/4 in. long, insert needle deeply into large muscle (thigh).

create sterile conditions. Since needles and syringes are cheap, we recommend disposable syringes and needles, using them only once to assure sterility.

The site of an intramuscular injection should be on the heavily muscled part of a back leg for several reasons. First, the animal is less likely to develop a chronic abscess in this area. Second, this area is less likely to experience lengthy soreness. A site is selected halfway from the hipbone to the stifle (knee). The needle is removed from the syringe and held in the hand much as one would hold a dart. A spot is selected on the backside of the leg, and the heel of the hand is used to slap a couple of times to get the animal adjusted to being hit in that spot. On the third slap, the needle is forced through the skin up to the hilt. Animals injected in this way seldom flinch or even feel the needle. The syringe is then applied to the needle and the injection made slowly. The needle is removed quickly, and the finger is used to stroke the point of injection two or three times to prevent any leakage and to seal the hole made by the needle.

A common, preferred injection site for horses is the neck (Figure 3-5). Draw an imaginary triangle with three points represented by the poll, withers, and point of the shoulder. The center of this triangle is the point of entry for the unattached needle. The same slapping technique previously described works equally well with horses. Then attach the syringe. The neck is a preferred site for horses because few nerves or vessels are located in this outer area, making it a safer spot than most.

The more common injectable products that are given intramuscularly are antibiotics, vitamins, and hormones.

Subcutaneous (Sub Q) (Figure 3-2). A subcutaneous injection is an easy, fast, efficient way to give an injection. It will hit no specific nerves or blood vessels, and is relatively safe and easy for anyone following a few simple rules.

A subcutaneous injection means depositing the point of a needle in the fatty tissue between the skin and the muscle area. This is done by picking up a handful of skin between the thumb and middle fingers to assure a large enough area with which to work. Then press in an area with the index finger to make a small pocket between the index finger and the thumb. Slide the needle with the syringe attached into this pocket at a 45° angle, just in front of the index finger. If you get the wrong angle with the needle, it may make an intradermal injection (within the skin) instead of a subcutaneous one (just under the skin). The product works much better if it is placed beneath the skin layers so you should point the needle in the right direction, as well as working with a large enough pocket to assure by looks and feel that you are in the fatty tissue between the skin and muscle. Subcutaneous injections are common with some antibiotics and many vaccines.

Intraperitoneal (IP) (Figure 3-3). In cattle, if for some reason you cannot hit the vein or if you lack the technical training to do so, most materials designed for intravenous injections can be given intraperitoneally. An intraperitoneal injection does not work quite as fast as one given in the vein, but it is a good alternate site for injection.

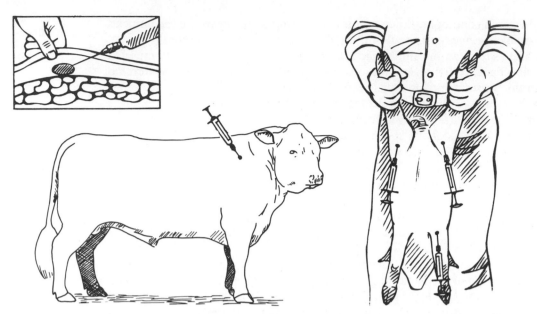

Figure 3-2. Procedure for making a subcutaneous injection (Sub Q). Injection is made in any area where skin fits loosely (neck, chest wall, "armpit," or flank). Pick up skin to facilitate needle entry, insert through skin, and discharge dosage. Massage area to facilitate distribution.

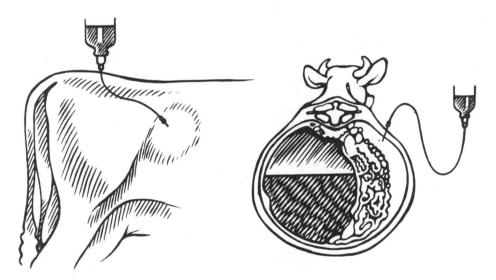

Figure 3-3. Procedure for making an intraperitoneal injection (IP). Use a 16 gauge × 2 in. or 14 gauge × 3 in. needle. Warm solution to body temperature prior to administration, using sterile precautions. For cattle, insert needle into right flank at a point in the center of the triangle formed by the loin, last rib, and a line from the top of the last rib to the hip bone. For swine, insert needle into abdominal cavity at a point in the upper one-third midline area of the abdomen while the pig is hanging head down.

In order to inject into the peritoneal cavity of a cow, you must inject on the right side just below the point of the hook (hip) bone in the hollow indentation. Use a 3 to 4 in. needle and pop it through the skin first, as described at the beginning of this section. After the needle is through the skin, up to the hilt, attach the intravenous tube or syringe to give the injection.

Vitamins, minerals, electrolytes, and glucose may be given in this manner when you want to load up an animal without the risk of overloading, as is possible with large doses by the intravenous route. Normally, an intraperitoneal injection is used only when for one reason or another a vein cannot be hit—which would be the preferred method.

Intravenous (IV) (Figure 3-4).   In the cow or horse, there is an indentation between the muscle layers that outlines the jugular vein. This is called the *jugular furrow* and is readily seen by the trained observer. The untrained observer may pick it up by following a line from the base of the jaw to just above the chest area on either side of the neck. The jugular will run along this furrow.

Pull the animal's head slightly to the opposite side from the site where the intravenous puncture will be made. Press with the fingers at the base of the jugular furrow where it enters the chest to block off the blood that is returning to the heart. This causes an accumulation much like a dam in a river, making the vein stand out and be more visible. Maintain this pressure with the hand for 15 to 30 seconds. In this case an alcohol wipe is recommended, not necessarily for sanitary purposes but to slick the hair down so

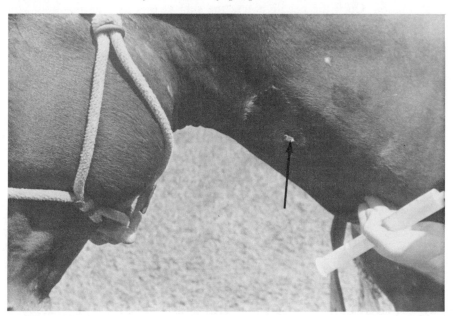

Figure 3-4. Procedure for making an intravenous injection (IV). Press with the fingers at the base of the jugular furrow for 15 to 30 seconds. This allows the vein to stand out. Note needle already in place. Syringe is attached for injection.

the vein is more easily seen. Use the free hand to stroke along the furrow area of the neck. You can feel and see the ripple where the vein is located using this method, and you get a much better idea of the exact location of the jugular. Take the needle off the syringe, and, still maintaining the pressure, make a quick stab completely through the skin and into the vein at a 45° angle so as not to go completely through both sides of the vein. Some people may suggest going through the skin first and then trying to locate the vein with the needle. This is not recommended because of the damage that could be done in probing with a sharp instrument. It is considered much better to make a quick stab at the angle described, going through the skin and the vein in one motion. You can tell if you have hit the vein because blood will begin to flow from the needle. If a flow of blood is not apparent, then you may have gone completely through the vein, in which case pulling back slowly may position the point properly. Once proper needle placement is assured, the IV tube or syringe is attached, and the solution is given as directed.

Intradermal (ID) (Figure 3-5). Some vaccines, especially those associated with the horse, must be given intradermally. In the case of some tests such as tuberculosis and Johne's tests, an intradermal injection is the method utilized.

Using a very short needle, approximately 22 to 25 gauge, pick up the skin, spread it with your fingers, and slide the needle along almost parallel with the skin until it penetrates. The slope of the needle point should be aimed to the outside so that the sharp point makes an easy entrance with this sliding motion. Once the needle enters the skin at this parallel position, you can usually tell if you are in the skin rather than underneath it by a small blister that will be visible at the point of the needle, after a small amount of the material has been injected. If this happens, then you know the needle is properly positioned, and the injection may be completed.

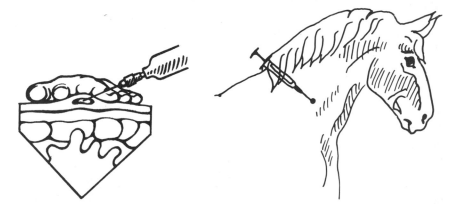

Figure 3-5. Procedure for making an intradermal injection (ID). Inject a 20 to 26 gauge needle into skin after shaving hair. An intradermal injection should raise a blister.

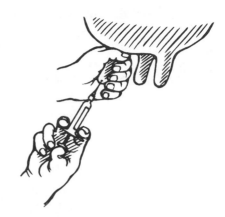

Figure 3-6. Procedure for making an intramammary infusion (IMM). Disinfect teat, depress teat to open sphincter muscle, insert sterile cannula, and force medication into teat canal. Disinfect teat after infusion.

Intramammary or Udder Infusions (Figure 3-6). Intramammary infusions are discussed in detail in the cattle section on mastitis, Chapter 12. Udder infusions are not very common in other species.

Boluses or Tablets. The key to giving either boluses or tablets is "restraint." The animal should either be in a squeeze chute or be held securely by halter or mugging (by hand). A squeeze chute for cattle is much preferred; however, other species may be held by rope and halter. In either case, the animal is restrained. Nose tongs are preferred in cattle for ease of entry of the balling gun through the side of the mouth and over the top of the tongue to the back of the throat, where the trigger mechanism of the balling gun releases the bolus or tablet. The animal will usually swallow at this point, assuring consumption. Watch the throat area to determine if the material was swallowed. Caution should be used because rough handling with a balling gun can produce tender areas in the mouth, making the animal go off feed or causing problems of a more serious nature.

Topical Applications. A variety of products are available to treat wounds, cuts, abrasions, etc. There are many antibiotic powders, sprays, and ointments available to promote healing. Other products are found in similar preparations to protect the wound or repel insects, etc. The key to using any of these products is to get a good even layer of coverage, whether it is with a powder, spray, or ointment applied with a swab. Use the material as indicated, don't abuse the application, and there should be no problems. These materials are generally not recognized as having much value other than protection from minor problems while natural healing is going on.

Drenches. The dose syringe is a very handy instrument for administering liquids. The proper technique includes good restraint of the animal so that it doesn't jump. The tip of the dose syringe should be inserted into the side of the mouth between the teeth and over the tongue and directed into the back part of the throat. The liquid should then be dispensed at a moderate rate so that the animal has time to swallow the material, rather than causing an overload, which could cause fluids to be aspirated into the lungs through the trachea. Another problem with dose syringes is that in careless hands severe damage can be inflicted to the roof of the mouth when the tip of the syringe is gouged rather than gently placed in the back part of the throat.

Implants. It has become a common practice to implant stilbestrol or stilbestrol-like products in animals to produce faster rates of gain. The proper technique for implanting is to insert the needle approximately $1\frac{1}{2}$ to 2 in. from the base of the ear, above or below the midline of the ear. After the needle is inserted, the point should be directed to within $\frac{1}{2}$ to 1 in. of the base of the ear. It should be possible to feel the point of the needle under the skin. As the trigger is squeezed, the operator should be able to feel the pellets as they are discharged from the gun. Improper implantation can lead to poor absorption, usually caused by (1) gouging of the cartilage of the ear; (2) intradermal rather than subcutaneous implantation; or (3) severing one of the veins of the ear, causing a hemorrhage.

BASICS IN DRUG THERAPY

Basically, drug therapy in this discussion refers to the use of various antibiotics, any one of which may have a different level and period of time for its effective action to take place. Adequate dosage and proper intervals, according to the recommendations of the manufacturers or the attending veterinarian, are basic points to consider in adequate drug therapy. Treatment should be continued long enough to completely control the infection. If treatment is given for 1 to 2 days and then withdrawn, even though response has been seen there is the chance that a relapse will occur, and the condition will be worse than it was in the beginning. If the antibiotic is given over too long a period, alteration of the bacterial flora of the intestinal tract can occur, plus drug toxicity and other related problems. So it is very important to administer drugs at the proper dose, at the proper interval for additional dosage, and for a sufficient period of time to be effective. You are cautioned to select the probable antibiotic based on recommendations from your veterinarian and stick with that until such time as it is obvious no response is being produced. Some antibiotics may be combined; but in general when you are using one you should not be using another.

ADVERSE REACTIONS TO DRUGS

Injectable products may create adverse reactions, and you should be aware of what could happen and what it takes to correct the condition once it is observed. Quick reaction is normally required, or death may be the end result.

Allergic reactions can range from a minor rash to difficulty in breathing, to a more severe reaction such as anaphylactic shock. If the allergic reaction is as simple as a rash or difficult breathing, a quick acting steroid such as Dexamethazone or Flumethazone, injected intravenously, will stop the reaction within 10 to 15 minutes.

47
DRUG
RESTRIC-
TIONS
AND LABELING
REQUIRE-
MENTS

If this injection does not stop it, the condition may progress to anaphylactic shock in a matter of minutes. The antidote for this severe allergic reaction is epinephrine, given intravenously, at the rate of 1 to 2 cc of 1 : 1000 strength for an adult animal. This should be given as quickly as possible. If it is given quickly, response can be positive, rapid, and dramatic. The animal could be back to normal within 10 to 15 minutes. If the injection is not given, the animal is likely to die. Anaphylactic shock can happen with vaccines, serums, antibiotics, etc. Any injectable has this potential. It is very uncommon and should not be a source of extreme concern, but you should be aware of what could happen and be prepared to deal with it in the event an unusual case develops.

It is advisable to have antidotes such as steroids and epinephrine on hand for allergic reactions. These products are highly recommended. Epinephrine, especially, should be on hand for emergency use by the average stockman in the event a serious condition such as anaphylactic shock occurs and there is no time to seek professional help.

Damage to the tissue caused from an injection should be minor except when an injectable is given differently from the way in which it was designed to be given. For instance, if an IV product is given intramuscularly, it could cause abscessing, draining sores, and sloughing of the skin.

Sterilized needles and syringes should always be used, or you will risk transmitting disease and starting an infection. Infections, especially in a horse, are quite easy to induce with a dirty needle. Even though a small lump may not appear to be of serious concern, this lump often is the outer sign of a deeper abscess that affects the muscles, making the horse very sore and unwilling to run or work. Similar possibilities exist in cattle and swine for an infection's developing into a serious abscess that would need proper lancing, drainage, and prolonged antibiotic therapy to clear up.

DRUG RESTRICTIONS AND LABELING REQUIREMENTS

The manufacturers of drugs provide adequate information on the label accompanying the product. If you will take the time to read and study this material, it will answer most of the questions that will ever arise concerning a product's use. The leaflets accompanying drugs usually tell what is in the drug, the active ingredient, the recommended dosage, the side effects and potential hazards, the theory of its action, and the antidote should a difficulty arise. This gives the veterinarian as well as the stockman a working knowledge of the product and its limitations.

Drug residues should be monitored carefully according to the instructions of the manufacturer. Condemnation of milk or beef is possible if the restrictions for drug withdrawal are not noted. If the withdrawal recommendations are not followed in horses, a racing purse may be lost and an innocent owner labeled a scoundrel when blood or saliva tests indicate the presence of a drug.

Concern over drug residues in meat has increased markedly in recent years. This presents a challenge to stockmen to see that all drugs are used in accordance with prescribed procedures. Residue violations leave the producer open to punitive actions and also increase the risk that a valuable drug will be removed from his arsenal of medications by the government if these violations cannot be controlled.

If residues are discovered, the owner could lose the value of the condemned animal at the very least. Often these incidents are much more costly. The producer may be prohibited from marketing any animal for slaughter until all are found clear of residues. This can involve quite a lengthy interval because of the laboratory testing involved and may result in a substantial financial loss. Where residues result from intentional misuse of drugs, the owner may also be subject to legal proceedings. The cardinal rule should always be: Follow the label!

4

Restraint of
Domestic Animals

In order to restrain and handle any type of livestock, it is essential that safe, calm handling be a major consideration. Death or injury, either to the handler or the animal, is prevented through proper handling and restraint. Injuries to the animal also result in carcass damage and can rob the owner of profits because of bruises and condemnation. If you want to "rodeo," it is a good idea to use someone else's stock because these habits become ingrained in the animals and they become trained to react in a wild manner. However, in the stockman's situation, you will come to appreciate animals that are trained to behave in a positive manner. Therefore, any "rodeoing" should be left to the professional arena where people pay to see the action.

One of the pet peeves of veterinarians and professional stockmen who work constantly with livestock is a lack of handling pens or poorly designed facilities. Good health care is greatly improved when adequate materials and equipment are available. However, even under the most primitive conditions, livestock can be handled safely, calmly, and efficiently by using a little knowledge and the right type of equipment.

Safe handling and restraint of any type of livestock can be accomplished by the following three methods: (1) use of physical strength; (2) use of ropes, chains, or belts; and (3) use of mechanical restraints.

The following illustrations give examples of normally safe, proper handling and restraining methods for the different species of livestock.

BEEF CATTLE–RESTRAINT EQUIPMENT, PSYCHOLOGY AND TECHNIQUES

Designing an effective corral system is essentially a problem of organizing different parts into a working unit that fits your needs. The component parts of an effective livestock-handling system are: holding pens, crowding pen, working chute, squeeze chute or head gate, and loading chute. If needed, the system can also include a scale, spray pen, cutting gates, and dipping vat.

Start by preparing a scale drawing. Your agricultural engineering department at the state university can assist you with drawings and ideas. Keep in mind the habits and preferences of the cattle while you are planning, and prepare several designs before making your final decision.

It is important to select a location for your handling facilities near an all-weather road. Good drainage at the site and a knowledge of the prevailing winds should be utilized in order to prevent any undesirable odors or environmental pollution problems in the area. If possible, position the facilities so that cattle moving through the chutes will be heading back toward the direction from which they came. This aids movement by taking advantage of the animals' desire to return to a familiar area.

The first rule to remember in handling cattle is to make the first attempt at restraint successful whenever possible. Cattle soon learn from negative input—that is, if they have managed to escape from a head gate, squeeze chute, or other situation, they become much more difficult to get in position to repeat the attempt at restraint. If using a head gate, try to catch the animal's head on the very first attempt. If cattle are in a squeeze chute that does not "feel solid," they have a tendency to fight the restraint and may eventually tear up equipment or injure themselves.

When working with cattle, it is necessary to understand a few basics about their psychology in order to outsmart them. First of all, cattle follow a curved path much easier than a straight line because they are unable to see the squeeze chute at the end of it until they are practically in it. Also, animals are always looking for a way to escape and tend to follow the leader. Thus, a curved alley leading to a squeeze chute is generally considered to be superior to other types.

Cows have panoramic vision. They can see behind themselves as well as in any other direction without turning their heads, giving them a distorted view—similar to a view through a fisheye lens. This makes fences and other straight lines appear curved to them; therefore a curved chute has no disadvantage whatsoever.

Because of their wide-angle vision (360°), they are easily spooked by moving objects. For this reason many cattle owners use a solid fence in their chutes leading to the head gate or other desired location. A solid fence prevents animals from seeing men, dogs, equipment, other animals, etc., and provides less distraction and calmer handling. The principle of a solid fence is to keep the cattle looking straight ahead and free from distractions, so that while they are searching for an escape route, they cannot see very much until they progress to the furthermost point. This is good psychology because you don't want them to see very much, just enough to keep their curiosity aroused in order to keep them moving.

In some facilities, it is difficult to drive animals through a gate because the gate also is solid like the fence. The reverse psychology should be used here; the gates should be made of expanded metal or bars spaced far enough

51
BEEF CATTLE—
RESTRAINT
EQUIPMENT
PSYCHOLOGY,
AND TECH-
NIQUES

apart so that the cattle can see through the gate, giving them a false impression of a way out. Gates should be free swinging and located in the corners of pens. Gates should close in the direction cattle are moving unless they are cutting gates, in which case they must swing in either direction.

Fences in the holding pen can be 5 ft high but should be 6 ft in areas where cattle are worked or crowded.

Although cattle have panoramic vision, they have extremely poor depth perception and therefore often spook themselves at simple things like a shadow on the ground. To cattle a shadow may appear to be a deep hole. Therefore, diffuse light should be available inside barns where cattle are to be worked. The reason cattle will not cross a cattle guard is usually because of the inability of the animals to see depth brought about by a contrast in light and dark areas. In many feed lots where snow fencing is used for shade areas, cattle have a tendency to shy away from the contrast in light and shadowed areas until they have become accustomed to the situation. If they are driven into a new place where these shadows fall in the working area, it could lead to problems in movement of the cattle to the restraining equipment.

Anything that creates a grid pattern on the floor or ground can prevent cattle from moving across it. Therefore, drains and other similar outlets should be placed well out of the path of cattle-handling facilities. The cow's fear of stepping on a grid pattern is so great that some of the western states have capitalized on this fear by doing away with cattle guards and simply painting a grid on the highway.

The same effect occurs inside a barn when material is suddenly changed from wood to metal or from solid to wire, creating a contrast. It is a good idea to paint all the facilities inside the same color to help alleviate this problem.

Cattle often refuse to enter a building because it is darker inside than the daylight outside. A simple solution to this problem is to move the cattle in late in the evening and turn the lights on in the barn, making it the lightest area. Generally no problems will be found when this method of handling is utilized. Moving in late in the evening also has a tendency to reduce fighting that occurs when new animals have to find their place in the social order. Darkness of night tends to have a calming effect so that all cattle may be more easily worked the following morning.

In areas of large concentrations such as feed lots or packing plants, it has been found that cattle are much easier to get into a building if they are lined up single file for a distance of 10 to 15 ft before entering the opening to the building. A single file chute has thus been found to be very effective when it extends from the wall of the building for 10 to 15 ft before entering the desired area.

Some handlers make the mistake of overusing electric prods. These devices are to be used as sparingly as possible; however, they are very effective when used as a last resort. The key to handling livestock with an electric prod is to leave the cattle alone as long as they are moving. When you get an animal that cannot be persuaded to move by any other method, a prod may be just the thing to motivate it to proceed.

People standing in the wrong place at the wrong time also are a deterrent to effective livestock movement. A simple way to handle this is to build shields so that operators of head gates and squeeze chutes may hide behind them for the few strategic moments needed to restrain the animal.

Wrangling Techniques

A few well-chosen illustrations perhaps explain livestock handling and restraint much better than a wordy discussion. Therefore the following illustrations should give the operator a good idea of how livestock may be handled, whether through the use of extensive, expensive handling facilities or through very simple devices such as ropes.

Casting methods vary from a tilt-table or squeeze chute to several forms of rope casting. Range cowboys in the old days used the head and heel method, which is still practiced on larger western ranches today. One cowboy ropes the horns of a cow or steer to prevent choking the animal and pulls it along while a partner throws a loop in front of the hind legs. Through a combination of pulling from the front and rope artistry from behind, cattle can be stretched out by horns and back feet (head and heel) for any purpose.

Another method using the rope is to throw the animal as shown in Figure 4-1 (a). The principle is to make a loop over the neck, a half-hitch around the heart girth, and a half-hitch around the flank-loin area. Another rope or halter holds the animal to a post or fence. By pulling straight back on the rope, the half-hitches are tightened, resulting in paralysis in the hind legs due to pressure on the nerves. An alternate method [Figure 4-1 (a)] of crossing the rope over the back and between the legs is also illustrated. A very large animal can be thrown to the ground in this way with surprising efficiency and can be worked on with ease. This method is commonly used in Mexico, in Central and South America, and in other areas where less sophisticated equipment is available or desired because of remote ranches.

For more gentle cows even a simple loop over the flank area [see squeeze restraint, Figure 4-1 (f)] is effective in reducing mobility.

Flanking can be used on calves up to 300 lb in weight by the average size man. A rope is usually used to catch the calf. Reach across the back and grasp the opposite front leg of the calf with one hand, placing your other hand on the opposite flank; by using your knees for leverage, lift the calf off its feet and throw it to the ground with enough pressure to slightly knock the wind from it. Then, with one knee placed on the calf's neck, curl the calf's front leg back in a position allowing you to hold the calf down by placing most of your weight on the calf's neck and applying most of the pressure to one front leg.

Hand restraint on relatively large calves is very efficient with two people. One person holds down the head and neck while applying pressure to

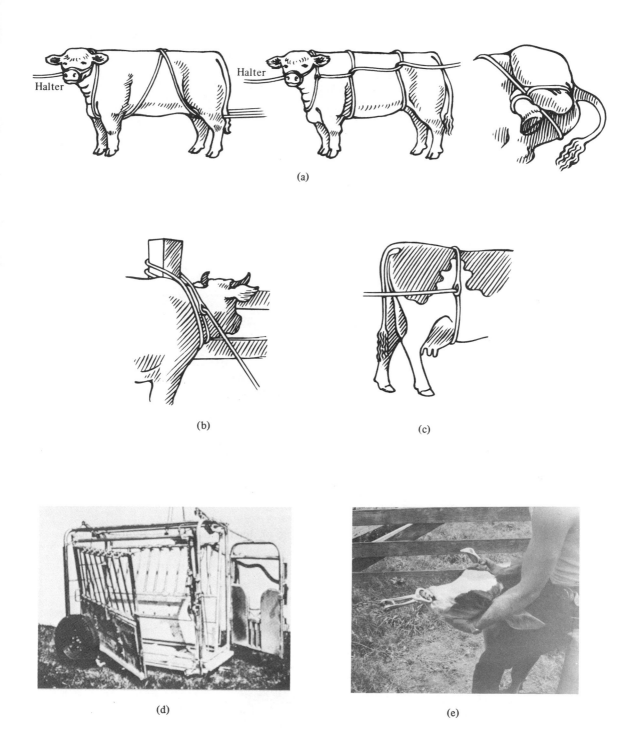

Figure 4-1. Cattle restraints: (a) rope restraints, (b) dehorning restraint, (c) squeeze restraint, (d) mechanical restraint, (e) nose leads, (f) grasping the nostrils, (g) tail restraint, (h) castrating restraint.

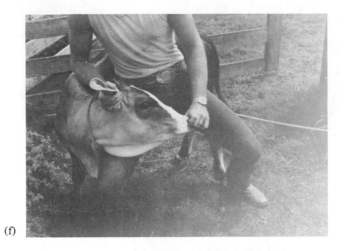

(f)

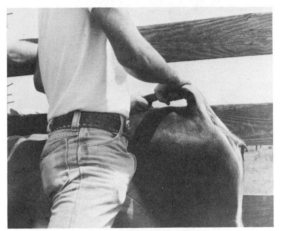

(g)

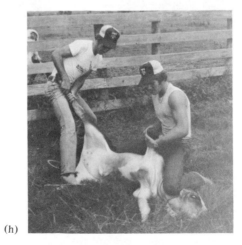

(h)

Figure 4-1 (*Continued*)

the curled front leg from the back of the calf, and a second person places his feet on the hock of the bottom leg and pulls back on an extended top leg while sitting on the ground behind the calf.

Nose tongs are very efficient in handling even large animals because of the tenderness of the nose area. This is also a very humane form of restraint and has a calming effect on the animal. Very large animals can be controlled provided the tongs close in the proper fashion. If the tongs are slightly too large, one side could tear out part of the nostril, causing pain to the animal and danger to the operator.

Use of the tail for restraint is effective even with large animals. By grasping close to the base of the tail, cattle can have forward pressure applied without harm to the animal. Always stand to one side to prevent getting kicked. This hold is especially good for moving a balky animal forward or preventing an animal from backing up in the chute.

Pens and Equipment

Pens and lots should be built to contain the required number of cattle and provide for efficient movement through the working area. A minimum of two holding pens is needed: one for holding cattle before working, and one for cattle after they have been worked. Table 4-1 shows size specifications of holding pens for the number of cattle to be processed in one group.

Table 4-1. Suggested Dimensions for Beef Handling Equipment

Space Requirements	Below 600 lb	600–1200 lb	Over 1200 lb
Holding area (per animal)	14 sq ft	17 sq ft	20 sq ft
Crowding pen	150 sq ft or space for 1 truckload		
Working chute (vertical sides)			
Width	18 in.	22 in.	26 in.
Desirable length (min.)	20 ft	20 ft	20 ft
Working chute (sloping sides)			
Width at bottom	15 in.	15 in.	16 in.
Width at top	20 in.	24 in.	26 in.
Desirable length (min.)	20 ft	20 ft	20 ft

Loading Chute (all weights of cattle)	
Width	26 to 30 in.
Length	8 ft (min.)
Rise	$3\frac{1}{2}$ in./ft
Height	
Gooseneck trailer	15 in.
Pickup truck	28 in.
Van-type truck	40 in.
Tractor-trailer	48 in.
Double-decker	100 in.

Beef cow operations should use dimensions for over 1200 lb. Large exotic breeds may require another 2 in. in chute width—bulls an extra 4 in.

55
BEEF CATTLE–
RESTRAINT
EQUIPMENT
PSYCHOLOGY,
AND TECH-
NIQUES

Position the crowding pen for direct access from holding pens into the working chute. Most layouts utilize a funnel-shaped or circular crowding area to make use of a free-swinging gate for pushing the cattle forward into the working chute. Figures 4-2 and 4-3 give a few examples to illustrate the point.

The size of the crowding area will determine the number of cattle that can be worked in one group. Pen size should be 150 sq ft or larger if you want to be able to work a full truckload at a time. If desired, the crowding pen can also do double-duty as a spray pen or sorting area.

The working chute should be a minimum of 20 ft in length to handle four or more animals at once.

Head gates of an endless variety are available and widely used across the United States. Although there is a great variation, most head gates have either a V-type arrangement with a straight-out exit or a drop-plate arrangement (a side exit requiring backing up). The V-type is used by those cattlemen who have larger cattle with horns, while other cattlemen may prefer the type that drops a plate from overhead to a fixed plate under the neck. This latter type should be watched closely because of the possibility of an animal being held too tightly, causing strangulation.

Stanchions are used as a restraining device but normally only with tamer animals, such as dairy cows, that have been accustomed to being restrained. An untrained or wild animal will normally destroy a stanchion.

The squeeze chute has received wide acceptance in the U.S. cattle industry and may vary in price from $800 to $1500 or more. The selection of a type of squeeze chute will vary depending on your own situation and the adaptability to your program. The type selected depends on the structure of other pens; the length of the chute to be assured the cattle are not too big for it; the type of exits (side or front exits); whether the chute is portable or stationary; the type of head gate or drop head gates; whether your cattle have horns; and whether palpation is to be done (if so, a rear gate will need to be considered). Many chutes have a rear gate that slides from side to side; others have an overhead gate. The overhead is definitely not recommended for palpation because of the possibility of its dropping on the operator. Palpation gates are also available and should be considered so that the palpator does not have to climb over a fence each time he wishes to check a cow. Chutes should also be studied for removable bottom panels if footwork is necessary, and a chute should be studied for a quick release if a downed animal is choking or in other serious difficulty.

Two common mistakes that farmers and ranchers make in selecting or using a squeeze chute have been noted during the author's general practice. First of all, the posts used to secure the squeeze chute as well as structural posts in the crowding chute should always be on the outside. Many cattlemen place them inside, creating a prime situation for scrapes and injuries. Second, the selection of a chute too small for the breed or type of cattle is a common mistake. Some chutes may be too high or too short for your type of operation. The average chute should be about $4\frac{1}{2}$ to 6 ft tall, at

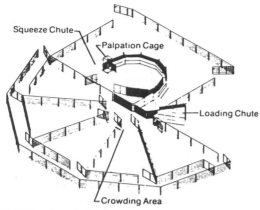

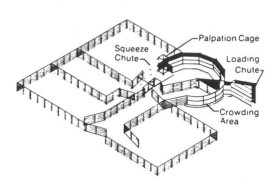

70-400 head or more.

Circular crowding pen and curved working chute. Expand from 1 to 4 pie-shaped holding pens, which require more fence than rectangular ones. Careful construction is needed.

USDA 6229. Expansible corral.

70-400 head or more.

Circular crowding pen and working chute. Good sorting and loading arrangement. This layout can be a hospital area, receiving lot, or combination. Consider roofing over the working area.

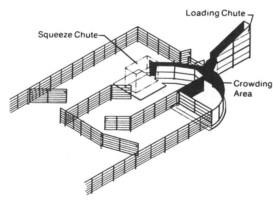

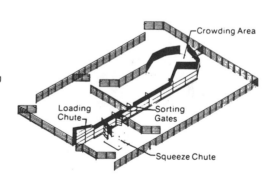

25-75 head.

Circular crowding pen and working chute. Good layout for loading and sorting. The plan is adapted to only limited expansion and has no ideal scale location.

USDA 6230. Corrals with working facilities.

Up to 200 head.

Circular crowding pen. Straight working chute to loading chute or squeeze. Holding pens next to the crowding area. There is poor crowding for loading and restricted expansion.

Figure 4-2. USDA corral plans 6229 and 6230. Many existing corrals can be improved by using the handling areas shown in these two plans. They can be ordered from the addresses listed at the end of this chapter.

57

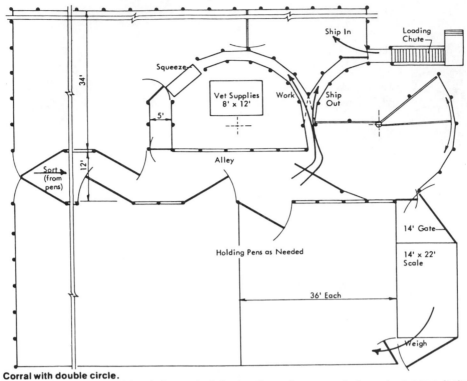

Corral with double circle.
Adapt length of chutes around the circles, and relative locations of squeeze, chute, and gates to suit site. Consider roofing over the work and treatment areas.

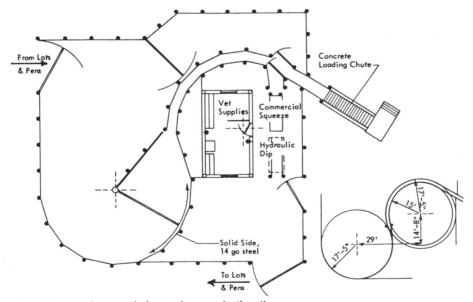

Crowding pen in one circle, work areas in the other.

Figure 4-3. Corral with double circle (top); crowding pen in one circle, work areas in the other (bottom).

58

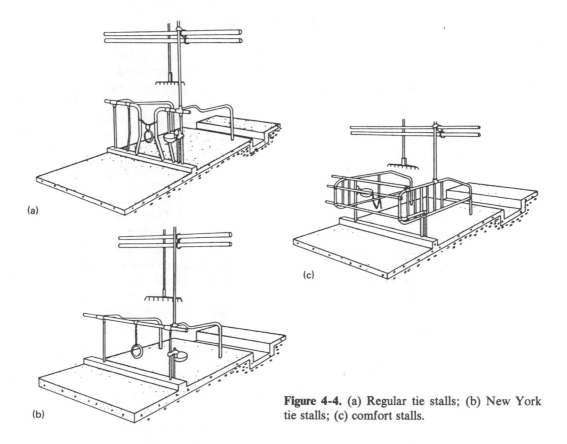

Figure 4-4. (a) Regular tie stalls; (b) New York tie stalls; (c) comfort stalls.

least 6 ft long, and may range from 24 to 30 in. in width. Be sure to select one that will allow the greatest ease for your type of operation.

Hydraulic tilt-tables are used mostly in purebred operations and are generally too expensive to be considered by all except registered breeders who of necessity must have them. When hoofs are to be trimmed or there is need to perform other operations, the tilt-table is without equal. The use of this device allows as gentle handling as could be expected. Care should be taken not to leave an animal on its side for a prolonged time on a tilt-table because of the possibility of bloat being induced due to this abnormal position.

Work with cattle requires facilities for vaccinating, pregnancy checking, dehorning, and treating specific illnesses, and for artificial insemination. A complete system should include facilities to load, weigh, sort, confine, spray, and treat cattle. Figure 4-3 offers ideas for arrangements to gather, direct the flow, and restrain cattle for most needs, large or small. Further information is available from the Midwest Plan Service.*

---

*Midwest Plan Service, Agricultural Engineering Department, Iowa State University, Ames, Iowa 50011.

RESTRAINT OF DAIRY CATTLE

A basic knowledge of a cow's social life and her senses of smell, sight, and hearing can be utilized to move or restrain dairy cattle as needed.

Cattle have a well-defined social order, especially under total confinement situations such as dairy operations. Boss cows are evident in any herd and dominate other cows by continually pushing and crowding others away from feed bunks and water and mineral boxes. One way to reduce the disruption caused by these boss cows is to provide plenty of space for feed and water. See Table 4-1 for recommendations concerning spacious conditions that will allow both dominant and subservient cows to get their full share. The desire by dominant cows to assert their authority is most evident right after cattle have been moved or regrouped. Therefore, it is important to reduce movement to once a month, in most cases, after DHIA (Dairy Herd Improvement Association) production records are returned to the farm.

Docile, calm cows are generally the best producers, as opposed to the dominant cows; so it is doubly important to handle them easily in order to keep milk production at a peak.

Cattle are very sensitive to the odors that surround them. In the past this sensitivity enabled them to find a mate and to select plants suitable to their diet. This condition is still evident in the spring when new grasses erupt and the grazing gets greener on the other side of the fence. For this reason fences should be kept in good repair. When moving cows, the calves should be kept downwind or a substantial distance away, because cows may otherwise feel that they are being permanently separated from their calves.

As previously discussed in the beef cattle section, cattle are very sensitive to visual contrasts and light patterns. Sharp changes should be avoided in colors of buildings by utilizing a similar color scheme with as few shadows or bright spots as possible. One dairyman reported a vastly improved control situation with his cattle guard simply by painting the bars bright yellow in contrast with the darkness below. Although cattle are colorblind, the difference in the contrast of the colors used on the cattle guard made it an effective guard because of the cows' inability to perceive depth.

Chutes and fences should be made of similar material, since when board changes to wire, the cattle sense a difference in contrast and often will balk at that area. Good lighting inside dairy barns is especially recommended to prevent any balkiness on the part of sensitive cows who must be calm in order to produce the maximum amount of milk. Fluorescent lights are well-suited for dairy barns to give an even, diffused light.

The restraint of dairy cattle is not nearly as difficult as that of beef cows. Since dairy cattle are handled so frequently, they rarely require restraint other than common stanchion facilities, halters, and pen systems, with some of the beef cattle facilities such as squeeze chutes for treating situations requiring immobility of the animal. The stanchion designs and equipment shown in Figure 4-4 offer commonly utilized in dairy operations. Further information is available from the Midwest Plan Service.

RESTRAINT OF SWINE

Poor handling and loading facilities can result in many lost hours, bruised carcasses, and financial loss to the swine industry. The largest loss is due to shrinkage of hogs brought about almost entirely by rough handling, fear, and excitement. It is essential to handle swine quietly and calmly.

A few simple suggestions in handling hogs will result in more efficient movement and less loss due to shrinkage and/or injury. If pigs cannot be loaded directly from the pen, they should be driven into a truck or trailer from a narrow passage such as a loading chute, which is easy to make on the farm. The loading chute is most effective when it has solid sides or has sacks hung in such a way as to prevent the pigs from seeing out.

A rough-surfaced floor or plenty of straw added to the loading ramp prevents slippage and excitement. A gradual slope is easier to climb, and hogs will show less reluctance than when on a steep slope. Pigs can be driven easily if a solid board or sack is moved along close behind them. An electric prod is sometimes used in stubborn cases, as well as a canvas slapper that makes lots of noise but produces no injuries. In some cases the scattering of manure from the pigpen onto the loading ramp and edge of the truck is effective in overcoming strange odors that may make the pigs balk at the entrance.

An old trick in handling a stubborn hog is to place a bucket over its head and back it into a trailer, because a hog invariably will try to back out of a place into which it cannot see.

In restraining pigs for such procedures as clipping needle teeth, ear notching, and castrating, it is important to know how to catch pigs and properly restrain them.

Small pigs are best seized by grabbing one or both back legs, placing one hand between the back legs and supporting the abdomen, while using the other hand in the middle of the back to hold them in place. Figure 4-5 gives illustrations of this and other methods commonly used in restraining relatively young hogs.

Weanling pigs can be grasped by the hind or front legs and held in the position shown in Figure 4-5 (a, e, g, h). Larger boars and sows are often quite dangerous to handle and should be held by rope trusses or by the use of a "pig paralyzer," shown in the illustration as a commercial hog-holder or noose-holder [Figure 4-5 (b) and (c)]. The commercial hog-holder is especially effective because of the nylon-covered steel cable that is slipped well back over the upper jaw and pulled tight. Pigs of all sizes can be kept completely under control in this manner.

Pigs can transmit brucellosis and erysipelas to humans; therefore it is important to wash hands carefully when handling pigs, or preferably to wear gloves.

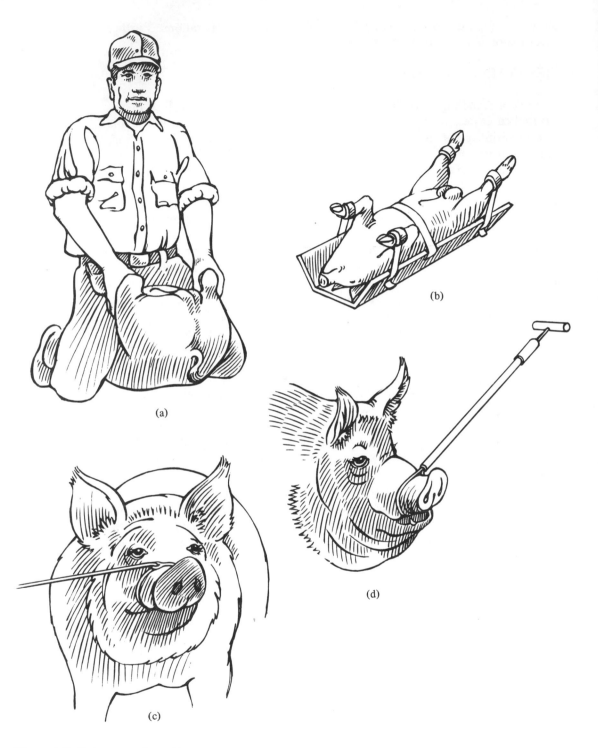

Figure 4-5. Swine restraints: (a) castrating restraint; (b) commercial hog-holder; (c) noose-holder; (d) mechanical restraint. Procedure: (e) Seize the pig by one or both hind legs and swing it clear of the floor.

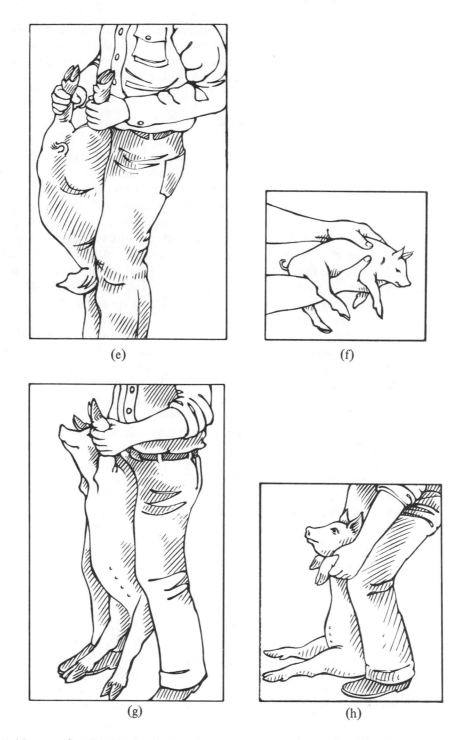

(e)

(f)

(g)

(h)

Figure 4-5. (*Continued*) (f) Hold small pigs this way. (g) Squeeze the pig's sides firmly between your knees. (h) With the pig on its haunches or rump, clamp your knees against its ribs.

In restraining hogs you must take into consideration the various needs for sorting, working, confinement during gestation, confinement during farrowing, and growing-finishing on solid or slatted floors. Detailed plans for swine handling equipment and systems are available from the Midwest Plan Service.

RESTRAINT OF HORSES

Every time a human being catches and uses a horse, he uses psychology because his strength cannot hope to match that of the horse. However, if he doesn't use superior psychology, he may find the situation reversed. It is the role of the handler to anticipate the probable behavior of horses and to establish conditions that encourage responses consistent with his goals.

Survival of the early horse depended on its hiding, running away, and adapting to constantly changing conditions. Hard to catch domestic horses have become that way either from being handled insufficiently to overcome their fear of man, or from bad treatment they have experienced after being caught. Therefore, in restraint and handling of horses, as with other species, it is important to be as calm and reassuring as possible.

Survival of the horse among its natural predatory enemies depended on its sight, reflexes, speed, memory, herd instincts, feeling of vibrations from the ground, hearing, and sense of smell. All these factors come into play when handling horses. A few simple observations and a little knowledge of the evolution of the horse will help the handler understand the situation in which the horse can most effectively be controlled.

Horses see rather poorly, and they adjust their range of vision by lowering and raising their heads much as a human does in the use of bifocal glasses. Although horses see well enough for grazing and other necessary functions, their vision is relatively inefficient when it comes to judging height and distance. For this reason horses are quite often cast as excitable when they balk at entering a dark barn or dark trailer. Horses taken to a trailer for loading may first lower their noses to the floor and then raise their heads rather high. This is done to give themselves the best possible vision. A trailer is regarded by a horse much as its ancestor regarded a dark cave that might be full of predators. Only the calmness, patience, and reassurance of the horse's owner will overcome its natural instinct of fear. Allow plenty of time for loading young horses until they are well-trained. A good system is to park a trailer in a horse lot and feed young horses in it.

Horses are colorblind. In looking at a landscape they see only different amounts of light reflecting from it. Objects that remain still convey little information to them, but they see movement instantly and react accordingly. This has given rise to the term *spooky* horses, but in reality this trait is a reaction to temperament, experience, and/or confidence in the rider. Instill confidence in horses by gently urging them to come near objects they fear. If they are concentrating on the feared object and are punished, they assume the object caused the pain and their suspicions are reinforced. Handling under this kind of situation will always be difficult.

The horse has blind spots both in front and back. This is why you should not approach a horse directly from the rear, and you should speak to the horse using sound as a guide to your position when passing behind it. Most horses do not see objects directly in front of their faces without moving their heads. They do not see the feed they eat or the ground they step on when their heads are in a normal position. For this reason, when handling a horse, allow free movement of its head in negotiating obstacles so the horse will have good vision. After horses have been handled in a difficult spot several times, they develop a very good memory for it and will calmly pass by the obstacle because of previous, uneventful occasions.

"Flighty" horses should be handled with strong equipment and not hurried into a new or strange situation. Even though they are under control at home, they may not be when under different surroundings such as a fair or horse show. The object in handling these horses is to impose the handler's will without provoking a difficult confrontation with the horse.

A few signs will warn the handler when a situation is serious from the horse's viewpoint. Ears pinned backward indicate anger or, in some cases, faked anger. They warn the handler that he will be bitten or kicked. Old horses sometimes fake anger. Experience will eventually provide the owner with enough information to distinguish faked anger from a real situation. However, mares with newborn foals are probably not bluffing when they have their ears pinned back and should be left alone.

A well-trained young horse never forgets his training. Neither does a poorly trained one. For this reason bad habits should be recognized and corrected before they become fixed.

Idle horses tend to seek activity, some of which may involve gate latches. Once they succeed, their good memory keeps them trying to open doors. For example, when they get the grain bin open, they remember only the joy of eating. They can't associate overeating with the following bellyache from colic or damage to hooves from founder (see Chapter 6).

Horses are gregarious by nature; that is, they band together. This tendency has practical applications. For instance, it is much easier to move a group of horses than to move one by itself. Wise old ranch horses learned they were more likely to be roped from the remuda for the day's work if they were near the edge. Therefore they sought the center of the circle. This gregarious nature is still evident today and can be utilized by the handler in moving large numbers of horses to the proper place.

Fear of ground vibrations is a hangover from the prehistoric horse. Being alerted to an approaching animal by vibrations was one of the tools of survival. Today it is mostly a headache to horse owners, as some horses tend to shy away from areas because of vibrations from motors, machines, or even from other horses.

Most animals in the wild state have a good sense of smell. Research has shown that a horse under domestic conditions can find his way directly homeward from a downwind distance of 5 miles, even when confused by being driven in a trailer over a circuitous route. Young colts being saddled for the first few times should be allowed to smell the saddle and blanket before

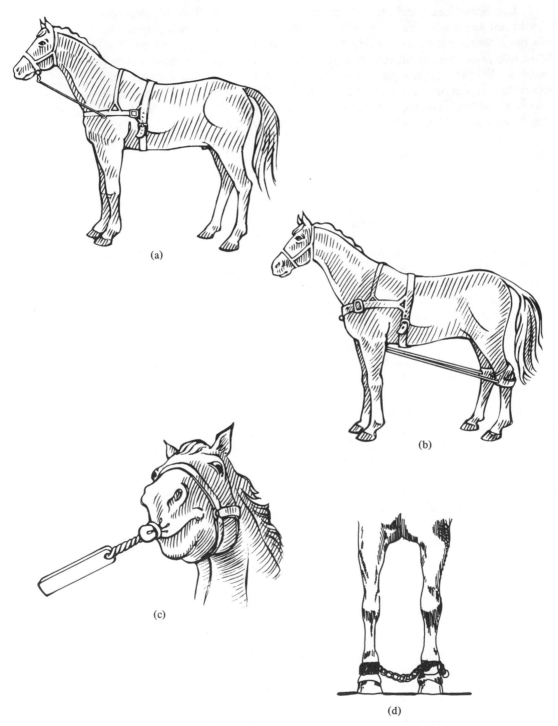

Figure 4-6. Horse restraints: (a) side stick; (b) breeding hobbles; (c) twitch; (d) hobble.

saddling. This reassures them that these items are not dangerous and that they have been used by other horses.

The most sensitive spots on horses seem to be the mouth, feet, flanks, neck, and shoulders. Knowing where these areas are allows the handler to utilize the proper restraining method while creating the least amount of pain.

Figure 4-6 gives illustrations of some of the more simple methods for restraining horses. The side stick is used to prevent the horse from nibbling at its legs and other areas that may be under treatment. The breeding hobbles and the traditional hobble are used either to prevent a mare from kicking a stallion or to enable the owner to catch a horse loose in a pasture.

In addition to halters, ropes, and mechanical devices, one of the oldest and most effective means of restraint is the twitch, shown in the Figure 4-6 (c), capitalizing on one of the sensitive areas previously mentioned. This simple method allows almost total restraint of a horse and is highly recommended.

A common method used for restraining anesthetized stallions for castration is illustrated in Figures 4-7 and 4-8. A horse is a very powerful animal and may inadvertently injure the handler even though under the influence of anesthesia. A precautionary rope restrains all four feet together or only the one most likely to do damage. Note that in both cases the handler stands on the back side of the horse out of respect for the strength of the equine.

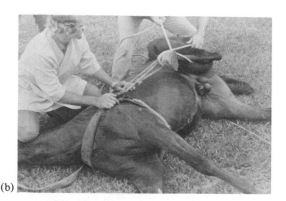

(b)

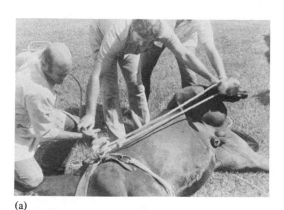

(a)

Figure 4-7. A method of restraining an anesthetized stallion. Note that only a breast collar and a rope with a ring are needed.

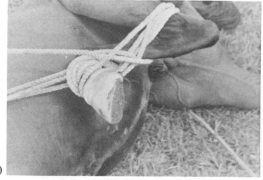

(c)

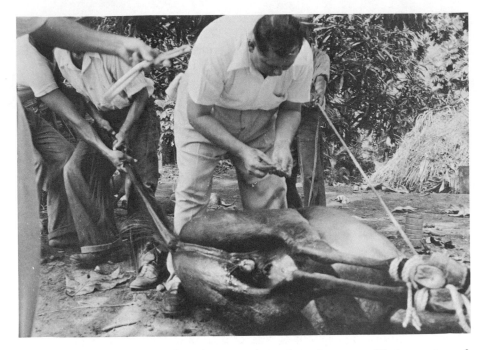

Figure 4-8. Restraint of a stallion for castration using only a rope. (Photo courtesy of Dr. Carlos Gaztambide Arillaga, University of Puerto Rico)

Designs for many forms of pens and numerous ideas for restraint and handling of animals, including beef cattle, dairy cattle, swine, and horses, are available through the Midwest Plan Service at any of the following land-grant universities: University of Illinois, Purdue University, Iowa State University, Kansas State University, Michigan State University, University of Minnesota, University of Missouri, University of Nebraska, North Dakota State University, Ohio State University, South Dakota State University, and University of Wisconsin. Consult your local county extension agent, who may also have access to individual issues of the housing and equipment handbooks offered through this service. These handbooks cost about $3 each for beef, dairy, swine, and horses. The publications are available at all the universities listed above. However, outside these states the best advice would be to contact the Midwest Plan Service staff at the following address: Midwest Plan Service, Agricultural Engineering Department, Iowa State University, Ames, Iowa 50011.

SPACE REQUIREMENTS FOR LIVESTOCK

The following table, Table 4-2, lists space requirements for livestock. Providing the proper amount of space for livestock is essential for optimum production. Overcrowding reduces performance, jeopardizes health, and increases management problems. Too much space increases housing and fencing cost and can also magnify management problems.

Table 4-2. Space Requirements for Livestock

BEEF CATTLE

Situation	Space Required
FEED LOT	
Lot surfaced, cattle have free access to shelter	20 sq ft in barn and 30 sq ft in lot per head
Lot surfaced, no shelter	50 sq ft per head
Lot unsurfaced except around waterers, along bunks and open-front buildings, with a connecting strip	150 to 800 sq ft per head
Sunshade (amount needed)	20 to 25 sq ft per head
BUILDINGS WITH FEED LOTS	
600 lb to market	20 to 25 sq ft per head
Calves to 600 lb	15 to 20 sq ft per head
Bedding (amount needed)	$\frac{1}{2}$ ton per head annually
COLD CONFINEMENT BUILDINGS	
Solid floor, bedded	30 sq ft per head
Solid floor, flushing flume	17 to 18 sq ft per head
Totally or partly slotted	17 to 18 sq ft per head
Calving pen	100 sq ft
Calving space	1 pen per 12 cows
FEED BUNKS	
All animals eat at once:	
Calves to 600 lb	18 to 22 in. per head
600 lb to market wt.	22 to 26 in. per head
Mature cows	26 to 30 in. per head
Calves	14 to 18 in. per head
Feed always available:	
Hay or silage	4 to 6 in. per head
Grain or supplement	3 to 4 in. per head
Grain or silage	6 in. per head
Creep or supplement	1 space per 5 calves
Bunk throat height:	
Calves	Up to 18 in.
Feeders and mature cows	Up to 22 in.; 30 in. only if hogs will run with cattle
Bunk width:	
If fed from both sides of bunk	48 in.
If bunk is divided by mechanical feeder	54 to 60 in.
Bottom width if fed from one side of bunk	18 in.
WATERERS	
In dry lot	40 head per available water space
CORRALS	
Animals to 600 lb	14 sq ft per head holding corral; 6 sq ft crowding corral
600 to 1200 lb	17 sq ft per head holding corral; 10 sq ft crowding corral
1200 lb and heavier	20 sq ft per head holding corral; 12 sq ft crowding corral
ISOLATION & SICK PENS	40 to 50 sq ft per head. Allow space for 2% to 5% of herd
MOUNDS	25 sq ft minimum per head

Table 4-2. (*Continued*)

HOGS

Situation	Space Required
FEEDER AND WATERER SPACE	
Self-feeders	One space per 5 pigs
Supplement feeders	One space per 15 pigs
Sow feeders	1 ft per sow self-feed; 2 ft per sow all fed at once
Waterers	One space per 20 to 25 pigs
BUILDING FLOOR SPACE	
Sows and boars	15 to 20 sq ft per head
Pigs starting through finishing:	
12 to 60 lb	4 sq ft per head
60 to 125 lb	6 sq ft per head
125 lb to market	8 sq ft per head
100 lb to market	5 sq ft per head under roof plus 13 sq ft on outside paved lot
Sow and litter	
Slotted floor, full confinement	26 sq ft per sow
Indoor-outdoor system	32 sq ft per sow inside plus 42 sq ft outside
PASTURE SPACE	
Gestating sows	10 sows per acre
Sows with litters	7 sows per acre
Growing-finishing pigs	50 to 100 pigs per acre
SHADE SPACE	
Sow	15 to 20 sq ft per sow
Sow and litter	20 to 30 sq ft per sow
Pig under 100 lb	4 sq ft per head
Pig over 100 lb	6 sq ft per head
FLOOR AND LOT SLOPES	
Slotted floors	usually flat
Farrowing, solid floors: without bedding	$\frac{1}{2}$ in. to $\frac{3}{4}$ in. per ft
with bedding	$\frac{1}{4}$ in. to $\frac{1}{2}$ in. per ft
Finishing—Paved lots	$\frac{1}{4}$ in. to 1 in. per ft
Paved feeding floors:	
Indoors	$\frac{1}{4}$ in. per ft minimum
Outdoors	1 in. per ft
Building alleys:	
Cross slope for crown	$\frac{1}{2}$ in. per ft
Slope to drain	$\frac{1}{10}$ in. to $\frac{1}{4}$ in. per ft
Gutters and pits:	
Slope to drains	1 in. per 25 ft to 1 in. per 100 ft
Slope for flush gutters	18 in. per 100 ft
SLOT WIDTHS IN SLOTTED FLOORS	
Newborn pigs	$\frac{3}{8}$ in. and 1 in. (cover slots during farrowing)
12- to 60-lb pig	$\frac{3}{4}$ in. to 1 in. (3-in. slats preferred over wider widths)
60 lb to market wt.	1 in.
Sows and boars	1 in. to $1\frac{1}{4}$ in.

Table 4-2. (*Continued*)

DAIRY COWS	
Situation	*Space Required*

STALL BARN DIMENSIONS

  Alley width:

Flat manger feed alley	5 ft 8 in. to 6 ft 6 in.
Feed alley with step manger	4 ft to 4 ft 6 in.
Service alley with barn cleaner	6 ft
Cross alley	4 ft 6 in. (taper end stalls inward for 6 in. at front for added turning room for feed cart)

  Manger width:

Cows under 1200 lb	20 in.
Cows 1200 lb and heavier	24 in. to 27 in.

  Gutters:

Width	16 to 18 in. or as required for barn cleaner
Depth, stall side	11 to 16 in.
Depth, alley side	11 to 14 in.

FREE STALL DIMENSIONS

  Calves:

6 weeks to 4 months old	2 ft wide by 4 ft 6 in. long
5 to 7 months old	2 ft 6 in. wide by 5 ft long

  Heifers:

8 months to freshening	3 ft wide by 5 ft 6 in. long

  Cows (average herd weight)

1000 lb	3 ft 6 in. wide by 6 ft 10 in. long
1200 lb	3 ft 9 in. wide by 7 ft long
1400 lb	4 ft wide by 7 ft long
1600 lb	4 ft wide by 7 ft 6 in. long

TYPICAL FREESTALL ALLEY WIDTHS

Feeding alley between a bunk and front of a stall row	9 to 10 ft
Feeding alley between a bunk and back of stall row	10 to 12 ft

  Resting alley between backs of 2 stall rows:

Solid floors	8 to 10 ft
Slotted floors	6 to 9 ft

COW STALL PLATFORM SIZES

  Stanchion stalls:

Cows under 1200 lb	4 ft wide by 5 ft 6 in. long
1400-lb cows	4 ft 6 in. wide by 5 ft 9 in. long
Cows over 1600 lb	Stanchion stalls not recommended

  Tie stalls:

Cows under 1200 lb	4 ft wide by 5 ft 9 in. long
1400-lb cows	4 ft 6 in. wide by 6 ft long
Cows over 1600 lb	5 ft wide by 6 ft 6 in. long

SLAT SPACING

Elevated calf stalls	$\frac{3}{4}$ in. slot between 1 × 2s on edge
Calves, wide slats	$1\frac{1}{4}$ in. slot
Cows, wide slats	$1\frac{1}{2}$ in. to $1\frac{3}{4}$ in. slot

Table 4-2. (*Continued*)

DAIRY COWS	
Situation	*Space Required*

FEED BUNKS

All animals eat at once:

Situation	Space Required
Calves to 600 lb	18 to 22 in. per head
Heifers	22 to 26 in. per head
Mature cows	26 tc 30 in. per head

Feed always available:

Situation	Space Required
Hay or silage	4 to 6 in. per head

Bunk capacity

Situation	Space Required
Animals fed twice daily	1 cu ft to $1\frac{1}{2}$ cu ft per ft of bunk length, minimum

Bunk throat height:

Situation	Space Required
Calves	Up to 16 in.
Heifers	20 in.
Mature cows	24 in.
Mature cows on unscraped, flat apron	30 in.

WATERERS

Situation	Space Required
In confinement	40 head per available water space (pave at least a 10 ft apron around waterers)

HORSES	
Situation	*Space Required*

DIMENSIONS OF STALLS
INCLUDING MANGER

Box stall

Mature mare or gelding:

Situation	Space Required
Small animal	10 ft × 10 ft
Average animal	10 ft × 12 ft
Large animal	12 ft × 12 ft
Brood mare	12 ft × 12 ft or larger
Foal to 2-year-old (avg. size)	10 ft × 10 ft
Foal to 2-year-old (large)	12 ft × 12 ft
Stallion	14 ft × 14 ft (work stallion daily or provide 2- to 4-acre exercise paddock)
Pony	9 ft × 9 ft

Tie stall

Mature mare or gelding:

Situation	Space Required
Average animal	5 ft × 9 ft
Large animal	5 ft × 12 ft
Foal to 2-year-old (avg. size)	4 ft 6 in. × 9 ft
Foal to 2-year-old (large)	5 ft × 9 ft
Pony	3 ft × 6 ft

The space requirements and design recommendations in this chapter were furnished by the Midwest Plan Service, Iowa State University, Ames, Iowa, and are based on popular types of buildings and equipment.

2

Beef Cattle

5

Nutrition

Although you may not normally consider a lack of certain feed ingredients as being the cause of disease, nutrition is the number one problem in animal production today, and a lack of nutrition in proper form and variety precipitates more diseases and disorders than any other factor. In the United States we have less than an 85% calf crop; at least 5% of calf losses occur at birth, and estimates have run as high as 250,000 head of cattle that starve each year due to inadequate feeding. Estimates of 1.5 million calves dying with the so-called weak calf syndrome are considered close estimates. The weak calf syndrome is nothing more than inadequate levels of energy supplied by the mother cow due to inadequate levels of her energy intake. If losses could be curtailed, it has been estimated that our productivity could easily be increased by 25% without increasing our breeding stock.

Nutritional deficiencies influence the course of infectious diseases by weakening the host, facilitating invasion by secondary organisms, and delaying recovery of the host once a disease has been arrested. It is a documented fact that well-nourished animals not only resist disease but also recover faster when stricken. The level of protein and vitamins in the feed is known to affect the immunizing response.

Viruses develop and reproduce only within the cells of animals. Those hosts deficient in protein and vitamin B complex are particularly susceptible to disease. The effect of nutrition in combating bacterial invasion is commonly known among researchers and veterinarians. Nevertheless, energy deficiencies are the most common cause in adult cattle of the various metabolic disorders that occur, such as grass tetany, ketosis, and "downer cow syndrome." Nutritional deficiencies are also considered a contributing factor in the severity of common scours outbreaks in calves.

Internal parasites influence the ability of an animal to absorb nutrients; they also damage internal tissues, reduce absorptive capabilities, absorb food destined for the animal's use, mechanically obstruct blood vessels and parts of the digestive tract, produce wounds through which bacteria can invade, secrete harmful substances, and predispose the animal to attack by other parasites. Many nutritional deficiencies may come about because of internal parasite infestation; therefore, nutrition and health are closely related. Nutritionists working with management must attempt to compensate for reduced disease resistance and lowered appetites by providing feed intakes of rations containing higher levels of key nutrients. It is much more sensible to feed animals adequately in the first place so that their disease resistance will be at a maximum.

The stress of disease also depletes the reserve of nutrients; so high-performance diets are doubly important to an animal's recovery from a disease or illness once it strikes.

In order to understand nutrition and related problems, you have to understand the digestive system and the peculiar requirements of different animals brought about by different digestive arrangements.

DIGESTIVE SYSTEMS OF VARIOUS ANIMALS

Farm animals are classified as *ruminants* (complex-stomached) and *nonruminants* (simple-stomached). The nonruminants are swine and horses, which will be covered in later chapters. The ruminating animals are those that are able to consume relatively coarse-type roughage and regurgitate it in order to chew it again. A bolus or "cud" is formed by this regurgitation. Mixed with bacterial preparations from the rumen (paunch or fermentation vat), the cud is reswallowed for more complete digestion and absorption. Chewing of the cud is the chief visual factor in watching the marvelous system of a ruminating animal in action. Beef and dairy cattle are the ruminants that will be discussed in this book. They are alike in action, and most of the theories that are set forth in this chapter on cattle can also be applied to sheep.

Most cattlemen think of cattle as having four stomachs. This is not exactly accurate, as there is only one true stomach. It is more like four divisions of a digestive system; but from the layman's standpoint, it will not hurt to think of this system as four stomachlike divisions. However, it is important to distinguish between the activities that take place in these four compartments.

It is very hard to visualize the ruminant system unless you look at an artist's conception and then the real thing. Imagine as you look at Figure 5-1 that the cow's head is to your right. If we trace the flow of feed through this system, it may shed some light on the function of each compartment. Feed such as grass or grain is chewed very little by cattle. It is mixed with saliva to provide lubrication for passage down the esophagus. The feed comes first to the *rumen*, also known as the *fermentation vat*. This is a very large compartment where most of the digestive procedure begins due to the action of bacteria and protozoa. The rumen may be as large as 20 to 50 gallons in capacity. It is filled with water and other fluids, creating a vat that may be

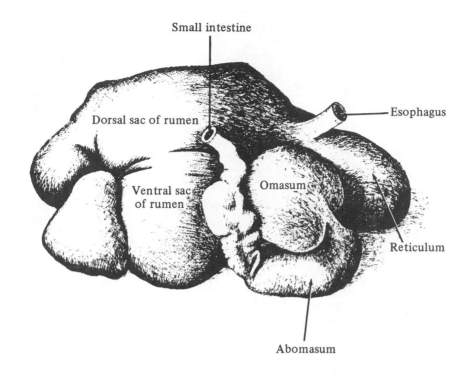

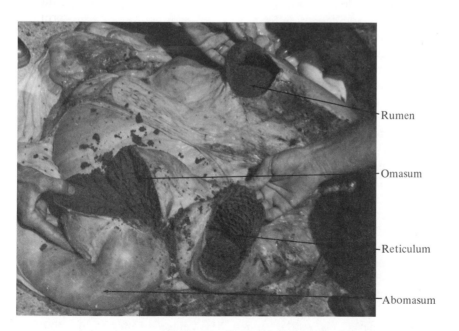

Figure 5-1. The ruminant's digestive system. (From Blakely and Bade, *The Science of Animal Husbandry*. Reston, Va.: Reston Publishing Company, Inc., 1976)

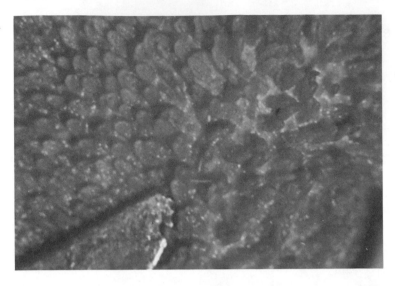

Figure 5-2. Villi line the wall of the rumen. (From Blakely and Bade, *The Science of Animal Husbandry*. Reston, Va.: Reston Publishing Company, Inc., 1976)

thought of as an average-size gas tank. There is a flow, or "tide," in counterclockwise direction that allows the feed to sink slowly, settle toward the bottom, and then move forward to compartment number two, the reticulum. Little absorption takes place in the rumen, most of this occurring in later stages of digestion. However, there are fingerlike projections called *villi* (see Figure 5-2). Some energy in the form of *volatile fatty acids* (VFA) is absorbed directly from the rumen through these villi. The villi are mentioned here because high-concentrate feeds can cause a corroding of these tiny projections, which produces all sorts of gastrointestinal disorders including bloat. Roughage, such as hay, provides the coarse materials that serve to scrape clean these avenues of absorption. It is also speculated that roughage stimulates nerve endings in the villi to cause *eructation* (belching of gas).

The feed next comes to the *reticulum*, also called the *honeycomb* because of the beehive appearance of the inside (see Figure 5-3). The reticulum also has the less well-known name of *pacesetter*. It has a rhythmic contraction similar to but much slower than the heart. This contraction causes small portions of the feed that has been delivered to it by the "tide" to be regurgitated (the reverse of swallowing). A bolus or "cud" is formed, chewed thoroughly, and reswallowed. Upon reswallowing, the material is so heavy that it does not float in the rumen "tide" but sinks directly to the third compartment, the *omasum*.

The omasum is also called the *manyplies* because it has numerous folds similar to the plies on a tire (see Figure 5-1). The function of this section is to absorb most of the water from the feed.

The fourth compartment is the *abomasum*, or true stomach, where all of the important digestion takes place. The microorganisms that attacked the forages and other feeds in the rumen have died. At this point they are themselves digested and absorbed as nutrients.

If you should cut out surgically the first three parts of this digestive system, you would have the same inefficient monogastric system (simple

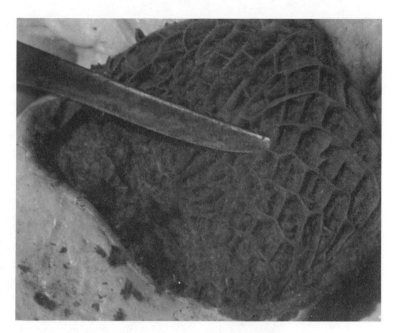

Figure 5-3. The wall of the reticulum (honeycomb). (From Blakely and Bade, *The Science of Animal Husbandry*. Reston, Va.: Reston Publishing Company, Inc., 1976)

stomach) possessed by the pig, dog, or human. Researchers have actually surgically removed everything from the esophagus down to the true stomach in cattle and have found that the animals lose their ability to digest roughage, creating severe diarrhea and necessitating the use of concentrates only for mere survival. A similar cause–effect relationship may exist in natural digestive disturbances that can be applied as a diagnostic tool to make a few educated guesses as to cause and treatment. For instance, compaction of the rumen with mesquite bean hulls has been observed to destroy the animal's ability to digest roughage, and cattle could literally starve on lush pasture. It is very important to understand the workings of the ruminant digestive system if you are going to evaluate disorders that arise.

Any ruminant must receive a sufficient *quantity* of feed, and that feed must be of a certain *quality* or it will not meet the animal's requirement. Sometimes, quality may be supplemented by the peculiar nature of the ruminant's digestive system. At other times, man's management has to take care of the needed supplementation. In either case, *feeds* are divided into *concentrates* and *roughages*. Either of these two types of *feeds* may produce an inefficient ration from the standpoint of *nutrient requirements*. In the following pages, the nutrient requirements are broken down for ease of explanation into the six major categories known to make up these requirements.

WATER

Although water is a very cheap nutrient, it is a very necessary part of adequate growth, reproduction, fattening, and lactation. The average cow consumes about 12 gallons of water per day and can exist on a surprisingly poor quality of water.

A number of observations have been made concerning saline (salty) livestock waters. At high-salt concentrations, increasing levels of salinity may cause an increased water consumption, even though at first animals refuse to drink for a short period of time. On the other hand, at very high salinities cattle may refuse to drink for several days, followed by a period when they drink large amounts and suddenly sicken and die. Older animals are more resistant to saline waters than are the young. Cattle do seem to have the ability to adapt to saline waters quite well. Whenever an alternate source is available to them, even every 2 or 3 days, cattle will avoid excessively salty waters. If cattle should suffer from the effects of saline waters, the recovery can be complete and rapid when allowed water from a source low in salt.

Salt is sometimes used in feeds to control intake, especially in the western states, with the use of protein supplements, and special care should be taken in these instances to supply a plentiful source of low-salt water.

Water is measured in total soluble salts, and this is probably the best overall indication of water quality. Water will be reported in total ppm of salt. This means there is one pound of salt per million pounds of water.

Water that analyzes less than 1000 ppm should be excellent for all classes of livestock. From 1000 to 3000 ppm water is satisfactory for most classes of livestock with the possible exception of poultry. Water quality ranging between 3000 and 5000 ppm is satisfactory for most livestock. If animals are not accustomed to it, they may refuse to drink it for a few days, but in time will usually adapt to it. From 5000 to 7000 ppm water is considered questionable for livestock, especially for pregnant or lactating animals, although steers or open (non-pregnant) cattle may adjust to it without serious effects to their health or productivity. Seven thousand to 10,000 ppm is a poor livestock water that should not be used at all for swine. It can be used for older, low-producing ruminants or for horses that are not pregnant or lactating. Water is considered unsatisfactory for all classes of livestock when it contains over 10,000 ppm of total salts.

Occasionally, a livestock producer will be concerned with nitrates, alkalinity, dissolved toxic metals, and bacterial contamination. These conditions are very rare and should not concern the average stockman. The tests for these contaminants are also much more complicated, and common sense would indicate that the best preventive of disease from poor quality water is to use only free-running or clean-appearing sources of water. Occasionally, heavy algal growths occur in stagnant or slow-flowing bodies of water. A few of these algae can become toxic. Although there are no tests for these toxins at present, we can only recommend avoiding using any stagnant source of water for livestock. A reasonable effort should always be made to provide the animal with a clean, sanitary supply of water.

The function of water is to regulate body temperature, to dissolve the other nutrients and act as a medium in which to carry them, and to serve as a pathway for waste elimination. Water provides for 80% of the makeup of the body itself. Water circulating throughout the body carries the dissolved nutrients to the cellular level; so a lack of total water or a contaminated source may prove disastrous to the animal.

About the only precaution that need be taken with water is to make sure that water troughs are cleaned and kept relatively free of sand, silt, and contaminants. It is especially advisable to make sure that chemical residues are not accidentally dumped into your stream, tanks, lakes, or other sources of supply. A sharp lookout should be kept for aerial drift of insecticides during the spraying season. Many chemicals are poisonous or may even block out the function of some vital nutrient so that the clinical signs may appear to be due to a nutritional deficiency or disorder.

PROTEIN

Protein is the basic structural material from which all body tissues are formed. It makes up muscles, nerves, skin, blood cells, hair, hooves, horns, and even the basic structure of the bones. It is also necessary for growth of the young animal, even before birth. It is especially required for milk production. Most enzymes and hormones that create the miraculous variety of normal body functions are made from proteins.

The protein itself is made up of many smaller units, generally referred to as the "building blocks" of protein. These building blocks are technically known as *amino acids*, which are made up of derivatives of nitrogen. Think of these building blocks or amino acids as bricks absorbed by the digestive system and transported to the cells to build a wall of protein. This wall of protein is the lean meat produced in the form of steak, roasts, etc.

Two protein feeds may look very similar, in the case of those that come from natural sources, but they may have widely differing values from the standpoint of their quality (amino acid) makeup. When two proteins have differing levels of amino acids, one may supplement the other by providing a building block in which the other is low. For example, one protein feed may have only 3 or 4 amino acids, whereas another may have 14 or 15; but together they can provide the required total quantity of amino acids.

Quality is generally not necessary in the case of ruminants. A ruminant's "motor" runs on low-quality protein supplements. Although ruminants have the same total dietary requirement for amino acids as nonruminants have, they do not have the same need for quality intake because of the bacteria and protozoa that manufacture the amino acids in the rumen or paunch. These microscopic organisms take relatively poor quality forages or concentrates and, through a "population explosion" of microbes, break them down into the necessary ingredients for their own bodies. These organisms live out their lives within the animal's digestive system; they die and are then themselves digested—thereby providing protein for the ruminant with the necessary levels of nutrition. Thus, protein quality is not usually a matter of consideration in developing rations for cattle. There are some exceptions when nutrition is so poor that a protein quality problem arises, but this is most often related to a total lack of feed intake.

There is a minimum requirement for protein in the ration of farm animals, and interestingly enough, the total amount varies very little. Depending on the class, age, and type of animal, the total protein requirement of the ration will be somewhere between 8% and 18%. *Although many other excess nutrients may be used to satisfy other functions, no other nutrient can replace protein in the ration.* For this reason, protein has probably received more attention and stimulated more research, as well as creating fear of the consequences of leaving it out of a ration, than any other nutrient. However, these fears are usually unfounded. A characteristic mistake in economics, especially of cattle, is to add more protein to a ration than is needed to make sure that this nutrient is not slighted. Actually, there are more deficiency signs brought about by a lack of total feed, or by slight starvation, than by all of the protein deficiencies lumped together.

Many cattlemen will put out expensive protein supplements while being very conservative with hay, silage, pasture rotation, or other energy feeds on the basis that although cattle may be going hungry, at least their protein requirements are filled. This is a common error. The body has first call, *on any feed substance*, to meet its *energy requirements*. Thus, the protein source is burned for energy, and a protein deficiency develops anyway. This can be a very expensive mistake.

There are occasions when another element may have what is known as a "sparing effect" in the ruminant animal. This is often diagnosed as a desire or craving for some other substance missing in the ration. A good example is the craving for sulfur, which is not needed by beef cattle or dairy cattle in any form other than as one or two of the essential amino acids that make up the total protein requirement. A protein-deficient animal may very likely exhibit an unnatural craving for sulfur. The reason for this is that the sulfur is being manufactured into a couple of essential sulfur-containing amino acids by the bacteria in the rumen. Some feed companies that produce mineral supplements will point to this craving for sulfur as positive evidence that the cattle need that element. This is incorrect. However, this is not to say that sulfur cannot be utilized by the animal and some good derived from it. Generally, though, the problem stems from a lack of proper protein supplementation management in the first place, and therefore the cheap way out of providing sulfur may lead to a very expensive disorder in protein deficiency. However, there are exceptions to almost every rule, and in the case of sulfur there are occasions when it is needed. When nonprotein nitrogen (NPN) sources such as urea or ammoniated products are used, there is not enough sulfur in the ration to produce sulfur-containing amino acids, and in this instance sulfur would be required by beef and dairy cows. This is a partially synthetic-type diet and explains the unusual circumstances. In nature, using natural substances, this situation would not occur.

A deficiency of protein is not easy to diagnose because the signs are of a very general nature; however, since this deficiency can affect so many of the external parts of cattle (hide, hair, hoof, and horns), the following outward signs might be expected to yield some clues. A general rough, dull haircoat is perhaps one of the key clinical signs in a protein deficiency. The animal will appear dull-eyed and listless and will have a characteristic "dead" look to its haircoat. Since protein deficiency seldom occurs by itself, some of these signs may also accompany other nutritional disorders. If adequate levels of feed are known to exist otherwise, a protein deficiency may be the causative factor for such characteristics.

Curing this problem is relatively simple, and a rapid return to normal can be achieved within 45 to 50 days. The most complicated part of correcting a protein deficiency is deciding on one of the myriad of choices of protein feeds available. A roughage form or a concentrate form will do equally well. Sources of many protein-containing feeds available throughout the world are shown in Table 5-1.

There may be instances when an animal will not or cannot eat, and it is necessary to provide protein nutrition through intravenous injections. Such preparations do exist and are readily available to veterinarians. However, it should be pointed out that it is virtually impossible to support an animal entirely through the veins. Oral supplementation is not only the cheapest and best form of feeding; it is a necessity. Miracles should not be expected to come from a magic tap from bottle to vein.

As previously mentioned, ruminants are able to synthesize protein through microbial action. As a result, cattle and sheep are able to manufacture a certain amount of protein from nonprotein sources. These sources must contain the basic element of the essential amino acids, which is nitrogen. One such source is urea. A couple of precautions must be taken in using urea or any other similar substance such as ammoniated rice hulls, etc. The major precaution is to be aware that urea and other nitrogen-containing synthetic products are toxic in amounts of more than about one-third of the total protein requirement. Actual useful levels will vary with the circumstances. Ammoniated products are very high in equivalent protein and may have to be thought of on an artificial basis as containing as much as 262% equivalent protein or more. Actually, the majority of feed-grade urea now on the market is 281% crude protein-equivalent. Using the generalized rule of one-third of the total requirement as the absolute maximum, it does not take very much to get close to the toxicity level. For example, if a cow's requirement is calculated to be 13% crude protein, no more than 4 percent should come from the artificial source. Follow the manufacturer's instructions exactly to prevent toxicity. The reason for the toxicity of this material is that urea or any ammoniated products are broken down by the bacteria to produce ammonia (see Chapter 6). Although ammonia is normally handled by the system at low levels, an overabundance can cause a condition known as *alkalosis*.

Excess urea produces too much ammonia, actually causing poisoning by ammonia toxicity. The antidote to counteract this is vinegar (acetic acid): one pint to one quart of household vinegar diluted in one-half to one gallon of ice water should be given by stomach tube. The cold water is used to help stop bacterial action on the urea, reducing the production of more ammonia.*

---

*W. E. Lloyd, "The Mechanism of Urea Toxicity," Iowa State University Library, Ames Iowa, Ph.D. Thesis, 1977.

Table 5.1. Feeds Listed and Grouped According to Their Percentage
of Crude Protein—as Fed Basis

GROUP A—*Mostly the Meat and Poultry Byproduct Meals, Fish Meal, the Oil-Seed Meals, the Oil Seeds, and the Dried Milks*

Feather meal	87.4%	41% cottonseed meal	41.4%
Blood meal	80.2	Safflower meal without hulls	40.4
Fish meal	60.4	Corn gluten meal	39.0
Digester tankage	59.2	Soybean seed	37.9
Poultry byproduct meal	55.4	36% cottonseed meal	35.9
Meat scrap	54.9	Linseed meal	35.9
49% soybean oil meal	50.8	Dried skimmed milk	34.0
Meat and bone meal	49.5	Peanut kernels	28.4
Peanut oil meal	47.4	Distillers dried grains	27.4
Tankage with bone	47.1	Brewers dried grains	25.8
Sunflower meal	46.8	Dried whole milk	25.5
44% soybean oil meal	45.8	Ground cottonseed	23.1
Sesame oil meal	44.3	Copra meal	22.7
41% solvent-extracted cottonseed meal	41.9		

GROUP B—*Consists for the Most Part of the Legume Hays and Meals, Barley, Oats, Rye, Wheat, and the Wheat Byproducts, and Most of the Grain Sorghums*

Dehydrated alfalfa leaf meal	20.8%	Rice bran	13.0%
Dehydrated alfalfa meal	17.9	Lespedeza hay	12.7
Oat groats	16.5	Sericea hay	12.6
Cowpea hay	16.0	Dehydrated alfalfa stem meal	12.5
Wheat shorts	15.8	Alsike-clover hay	12.4
Wheat bran	15.7	Wheat grain	11.9
Alfalfa hay	15.5	Kafir grain	11.8
Kudzu hay	15.5	Oats grain	11.7
Wheat middlings	15.5	Barley grain	11.6
Dehydrated coastal Bermuda-grass meal	15.1	Rye grain	11.3
Sweet clover hay	15.0	Soybean hulls	11.3
Dried whey	14.9	Milo grain	10.9
Red-clover hay	13.2	Dried bakery product	10.9
Soybean hay	13.1	Hominy feed	10.6
		Peanut hay	10.6

Table 5.1. (Continued)

85
PROTEIN

GROUP C—*Made Up Primarily of the Nonlegume Hays; Snapped, Ear, and Shelled Corn; and Certain Grain Sorghums*

Brome-grass hay	10.5%	Ground ear corn	8.0%
Reed canary-grass hay	10.2	Meadow hay	7.8
Orchard-grass hay	9.8	Ground snapped corn	7.7
Potato meal	9.7	Oat hay	7.7
Hegari grain	9.6	Redtop hay	7.4
Kentucky bluegrass hay	9.1	Bermuda-grass hay	7.2
Coastal Bermuda-grass hay	9.0	Steamed bone meal	7.1
Dried beet pulp/molasses	9.0	Johnson-grass hay	6.9
Grain sorghum grain	8.9	Beet molasses	6.6
Yellow shelled corn	8.8	Peanut hulls	6.6
Dried beet pulp	8.7	Dallis-grass hay	6.5
Sudan-grass hay	8.7	Dried citrus pulp	6.4
Millet hay	8.5	Timothy hay	6.3
Tall fescue hay	8.2	Citrus pulp/molasses, dried	6.2
Corn bran	8.0		

GROUP D—*For the Most Part High-Moisture Feeds, Mineral Feeds, Certain Low-Quality Roughage, the Pure Fats, Cornstarch, and Molasses*

Fresh brome-grass forage	6.1%	Fresh skimmed milk	3.3%
Prairie hay	5.8	Wheat straw	3.2
Citrus molasses	5.7	Fresh crimson-clover forage	3.0
Corn stover	5.7	Fresh Dallis-grass forage	3.0
Fresh alfalfa forage	5.7	Grain sorghum silage	3.0
Wet brewers grains	5.5	Fresh Sudan-grass forage	2.9
Fresh white-clover forage	5.0	Ground corn cob	2.8
Sweet-potato meal	4.9	Rice hulls	2.8
Cane molasses	4.5	Corn-stover silage	2.6
Fresh Kentucky bluegrass		Corn (fodder) silage	2.2
forage	4.5	White potatoes	2.2
Fresh ladino clover forage	4.5	Cabbage heads	2.0
Bahia-grass hay	4.3	Sorgo silage	1.9
Fresh coastal Bermuda grass	4.3	Sweet potatoes	1.7
Fresh rye forage	4.3	Carrots	1.3
Fresh red-clover forage	4.2	Wet beet pulp	1.3
Restaurant garbage	4.2	Fresh citrus pulp	1.2
Cottonseed hulls	4.0	Turnips	1.1
Fresh ryegrass forage	3.9	Oyster-shell flour	1.0
Corn-ear silage	3.8	Corn starch	0.6
Fresh orchard-grass forage	3.8	Wood molasses	0.6
Oat straw	3.8	Animal fat, feed grade	***
Barley straw	3.6	Corn oil	***
Oat hulls	3.6	Defluorinated phosphate	***
Fresh cow's milk	3.5	Ground limestone	***
Fresh fescue forage	3.5		

***Very little, if any.

Reprinted from *Feeds and Feeding*, Arthur Cullison. Reston, Va.: Reston Publishing Co., 1975, pp. 78–80.

The second precaution in using nonprotein nitrogen sources is to be aware of the limitations in regards to other nutrients. The bacteria in the paunch are the key to converting a synthetic form of protein into a biological one. This requires energy, or carbohydrates, for the bacteria to live on while they do the work of breaking down the artificial source to convert it into natural proteins and amino acids. Therefore, when urea is used, there must be sufficient levels of energy to produce the reaction. Many farmers and ranchers have used urea with a very poor-quality forage, thinking that sufficient feed was supplied in the forage, and that the artificial protein was handling that department in a very cheap way. Disappointments inevitably follow because the animal is worse off under these conditions than before. The key is to provide energy in the form of palatable forages or concentrates, or a liquid source of carbohydrates such as molasses.

As noted above, although protein has received a great amount of attention, it probably is not the most often deficient ingredient or nutrient in a feeding program. Many times people pay high prices to insure that their cattle are receiving sufficient protein, and instead the cattle wind up with a simple deficiency of carbohydrates due to the lack of bulky items. These bulky feeds (carbohydrates) are the ingredients most often found to be deficient in a ration.

CARBOHYDRATES

Carbohydrates generally provide the bulk of the feed to the ruminant animal, and for all practical purposes they can be thought of as hay or grain. Carbohydrates are divided into two sources: (1) *roughages*, supplied from a variety of plants harvested for that purpose, and (2) *concentrates*, supplied by a great many grains and similar products (see groups B, C, D, and E in Table 5-2).

The building blocks of carbohydrates are sugars, which provide most of the animal's energy requirements. These sugars are available in a variety of feeds, but the end result is the same in most animals. Just as the sugar in a candy bar gives quick energy to a human, the energy locked up in roughage and concentrates is made available to drive the major reactions of maintenance, growth, fattening, reproduction, and lactation in animals. Carbohydrates may be thought of as the fuel that maintains the fire of life.

The sugars produced from feeds are broken down by the microbes in the paunch in a manner similar to the way proteins are broken down. However, the end product here is glucose, or blood sugar, which is used to provide all of the energy reactions within the cells of animals. Sugars are found in many natural forms, the most common of which are fiber and cellulose. These two forms make up the bulk of hay and other roughage-type material. So a bale of hay made up of fiber and cellulose is eaten by an animal and is then broken down by the microbes, converted into sugars, and absorbed as glucose. Glucose is the log thrown in the fireplace to provide the heat to produce steam to turn the wheels of growth, reproduction, fattening, and lactation.

Table 5-2.   Feeds Listed and Grouped According to Their Percentage of
TDN for Cattle—as Fed Basis

GROUP A—*Primarily the Pure Fats and Other High-Fat Feeds plus Certain
Other Feeds of Generally High Digestibility*

Animal fat, feed grade	175.2%	Ground cottonseed	86.6%
Corn oil	172.8	Cornstarch	85.8
Peanut kernels	131.1	Hominy feed	84.9
Dried whole milk	110.1	Soybean seed	83.1
Oat groats	90.5	Dried bakery product	82.7

GROUP B—*Mostly Low-Fiber Grains and Grain Byproducts and Low Fiber-
and Low Bone-Containing Protein Feeds, plus Dried Citrus Pulp
and Cane Molasses*

Wheat grain	78.3%	Copra meal	73.7%
Wheat middlings	78.3	41% cottonseed meal	73.6
Yellow shelled corn	78.0	Linseed meal	73.6
Dried whey	77.8	Poultry byproduct meal	73.0
Dried skimmed milk	77.4	Wheat shorts	72.7
Citrus pulp/molasses, dried	77.0	Sweet-potato meal	72.7
Dried citrus pulp	76.6	Ground ear corn	72.6
Distillers dried grains	76.4	Sesame oil meal	72.6
49% soybean oil meal	76.3	Hegari grain	72.0
Corn gluten meal	75.4	44% soybean oil meal	72.0
Cane molasses	73.9	Barley grain	71.9
Potato meal	71.7	Milo grain	71.3
Rye grain	71.4	Peanut oil meal	70.3
Grain sorghum grain	71.3		

GROUP C—*Largely the More Fibrous Grains and Byproduct Concentrates and
the High Bone-Containing Protein Feeds, plus Beet Molasses*

Safflower meal without hulls	69.5%	Kafir grain	65.0%
41% solvent-extracted			
cottonseed meal	68.5	Tankage with bone	62.7
Corn bran	68.1	Wheat bran	62.7
Fish meal	67.8	Feather meal	62.2
Dried beet pulp/molasses	67.7	Meat scraps	62.0
36% cottonseed meal	67.1	Beet molasses	61.1
Ground snapped corn	66.7	Meat and bone meal	60.6
Oat grains	66.3	Sunflower meal	60.6
Digester tankage	65.5	Brewers dried grains	60.3
Dried beet pulp	65.2		

Table 5-2. (*Continued*)

GROUP D—*Predominantly the Hays, the Hay Meals, the Straws, and the Hulls (except Peanut and Rice Hulls), plus Corn Cobs, Corn Stover, Citrus and Wood Molasses, and Blood Meal*

Dehydrated alfalfa leaf meal	59.6%	Citrus molasses	52.5%
Rice bran	58.9	Alsike-clover hay	52.4
Blood meal	58.8	Corn stover	51.4
Soybean hulls	58.8	Kudzu hay	51.0
Peanut hay	58.3	Bahia-grass hay	50.8
Redtop hay	57.0	Brome-grass hay	49.8
Dehydrated alfalfa meal	56.7	Alfalfa hay	49.1
Meadow hay	56.1	Coastal Bermuda-grass hay	49.1
Kentucky-bluegrass hay	56.0	Millet hay	49.0
Dehydrated coastal Bermuda-		Timothy hay	48.8
grass meal	54.6	Dehydrated alfalfa stem meal	48.2
Oat hay	54.4	Prairie hay	48.1
Johnson-grass hay	53.8	Reed canary-grass hay	46.9
Sweet-clover hay	53.5	Cottonseed hulls	46.5
Wood molasses	53.4	Oat straw	46.5
Cowpea hay	53.3	Soybean hay	45.8
Sudan-grass hay	53.1	Ground corn cob	44.8
Lespedeza hay	53.0	Bermuda-grass hay	44.7
Dallis-grass hay	52.9	Wheat straw	42.8
Orchard-grass hay	52.9	Sericea hay	40.5
Red-clover hay	52.7	Barley straw	38.2
Tall fescue hay	52.6	Oat hulls	32.2

GROUP E—*For the Most Part High-Moisture and High-Mineral Feeds, plus Peanut and Rice Hulls*

Corn ear silage	31.0%	Fresh Dallis-grass forage	15.2%
Sweet potatoes	25.4	Steamed bone meal	15.0
Restaurant garbage	22.4	Fresh rye forage	14.8
Fresh brome-grass forage	21.4	Fresh ryegrass forage	14.8
Corn-stover silage	20.2	Fresh red-clover forage	14.6
Corn (fodder) silage	19.7	Fresh Sudan-grass forage	14.3
Fresh coastal Bermuda grass	19.4	Fresh ladino-clover forage	13.5
Fresh Kentucky-bluegrass		Fresh crimson-clover forage	11.8
forage	18.6	Fresh white-clover forage	11.8
White potatoes	18.5	Carrots	10.6
Fresh fescue forage	18.4	Rice hulls	10.0
Fresh orchard-grass forage	17.6	Fresh skimmed milk	8.5
Grain sorghum silage	17.6	Cabbage heads	8.3
Fresh alfalfa forage	16.8	Turnips	8.3
Peanut hulls	16.7	Wet beet pulp	7.2
Fresh cow's milk	16.1	Defluorinated phosphate	***
Sorgo silage	16.1	Ground limestone	***
Wet brewers grains	15.9	Oyster-shell flour	***
Fresh citrus pulp	15.2		

***Very little, if any.

Note: TDN stands for total digestible nutrients.

Reprinted from *Feeds and Feeding*, Arthur Cullison. Reston, Va.: Reston Publishing Co., Inc., 1975, pp. 48–50.

The difference between concentrated sources of carbohydrates and roughages is that concentrates are made up of starch, not fiber and cellulose. Starch is actually many molecules of glucose and is the principal form of stored energy in grain. This might explain more readily why the value of grain as an energy producer is higher than that of forage. The starch molecules require very little digestion to be converted directly into glucose, either by action of the microbes or through natural action by the stomach acids.

It should be noted here that feed-tag information rarely ever discusses or mentions the word *carbohydrates*, or even refers to *energy* per se. This is unfortunate for the layman because he does not know how to interpret for energy, the most important piece of information available to him on the feed tag. There is a term, however, that is available on the feed tag that can give an estimate of the energy level contained in the feed. That term is *NFE*, which stands for "nitrogen free extract," and represents the more soluble form of carbohydrates. Other energy estimates are *TDN*, "total digestible nutrients" (see Table 5-2), and *DE*, "digestible energy." Sometimes other terms such as *ME*, "metabolizable energy," or *NE*, "net energy," are used. But these, with the exception of TDN, are generally not noted on a feed tag.

Signs of carbohydrate deficiency are related to starvation or to a lack of adequate growth and are easily corrected by the addition of all the roughage an animal wishes plus a fixed amount of concentrates. Tables 5-3 and 5-4, at the end of this chapter, give recommended levels.

FATS

Generally, fats are not of importance in cattle rations. When they are included purposely, they are used to increase the energy value of the feed. Since fats contain $2\frac{1}{4}$ times as much energy as carbohydrates, it stands to reason that this nutrient is a high source of energy.

Furthermore, fats are generally not used in cattle rations as much as they are for the more simple-stomached animals because cattle are able to economically utilize energy from high-roughage sources. Therefore, it is not recommended that fat be added to the cattle ration unless it is for the general purposes that the feed industry uses it—that is, to keep down dust, to improve palatability of some coarse feeds, and to grease the normal mixing machinery in order to keep it in good working order with a slight film of oily substance over it. In addition to the above reasons, the feed industry usually uses fat at a level of 3 to 5% to create a uniform texture and color in the feed. When a cattleman opens a bag of feed, he wants it to look like and feel like the last bag of feed that was sold to him under the same label. Therefore fat is most often used to satisfy this consumer demand for uniformity, although in reality many different feeds are bought and mixed in the ration by feed companies to come up with the same level of nutrition.

Choices of fat fall almost entirely in the concentrate category, such as byproducts of the oil seed crops and rendered animal fats. Any vegetable oil would fall in this category. The industry generally uses fats that have been recovered from slaughter and then processes these into a stabilized product known as *rendered animal fat*. If you should need a little fat for some reason in a ration, a good source for a mixture of small amounts would be the common vegetable oils found in any grocery store. Also see Group A in Table 5-2.

MINERALS

Probably the best way to visualize minerals is to imagine the burning of a tree or other living matter until only ashes remain. These ashes represent the indestructible or inorganic content of that once-living matter. Everything else was consumed by the fire. The total mineral content of a feed, or for that matter of an animal, is generally referred to as *ash*. This is the term often seen on feed tags and represents the sum total of all the minerals contained in that sample. Ash contains 15 specific minerals that are necessary for normal functions. A deficiency of one or more can cause mild to serious disorders. The function of each mineral, its deficiency signs, and a readily available source for that mineral are described below.

Salt

Salt is actually two minerals, sodium and chlorine. The common table salt found in every home is the same type of salt that could be utilized. The chief function of salt is to maintain the water balance in the body, and it is used in the manufacture by the body of gastric juices.

The deficiency signs of the lack of salt are a coarse haircoat and a general lack of appetite. These signs are not very obvious and could be confused with a disease or many other disorders.

The best way to prevent a deficiency of salt is simply to put out salt blocks or loose salt free-choice (uncontrolled access) for an animal to consume. There are several types of salt on the market. Some contain sulfur, iodine, and various other mineral elements. Any of these are suitable; however, except for areas where known micromineral deficiencies exist, a plain salt block or one with iodine in it is generally recommended. Sulfur salt blocks do not have an advantage since cattle have little or no requirement for sulfur. You may recall from the discussion on protein that sulfur can be utilized by bacteria to form some of the "building blocks" of protein called *amino acids*, but this is generally not necessary if cattle are receiving sufficient feed in the first place. If they are not receiving an adequate ration, the sulfur will do very little good in elevating protein levels. However, because there are those who believe it does do some good, some manufacturers market a sulfur-containing salt block.

Calcium

Calcium is needed for bone formation and is particularly essential in young growing animals to provide adequate skeletal development and other vital functions. It also has a role in blood coagulation.

Deficiency signs in young animals show up as rickets. This is a condition involving bowed legs, crooked bones, fragile bones, and enlarged knee joints. The chief sign of a young animal with rickets is distorted bone development so that it appears to be deformed. If caught early enough, this disorder is reversible simply by the addition of adequate calcium in the diet.

In the mature animal, a lack of calcium does not cause rickets but causes a condition known as *osteomalacia*. This involves a stiffness of the legs and enlarged joints. However, since the animal is already grown, the condition more often results in broken bones or a crippling of the animal without deformation.

A simple source of calcium is steamed bone meal. Since this is a rather palatable feed, it should not be put out free-choice, especially if animals are hungry, as they are during the winter; they will consume more than needed to meet their minimum requirements. A good mixture of steamed bone meal and salt will prevent overeating the bone meal.

Another often used source of calcium that will also supply phosphorus is dicalcium phosphate. A mixture of one-third salt, one-third dicalcium phosphate, and one-third steamed bone meal is often provided free-choice to supply the animal's requirements for calcium, salt, and phosphorus.

Calcium carbonate (limestone) is the most common ingredient used to supply calcium in feed-lot rations where high levels of grain are being fed. Most grains are adequate in phosphorus but very low in calcium, so that a calcium-phosphorus ratio correction is necessary to provide a balanced diet. Calcium carbonate is added in this instance to bring the ratio into proper proportions.

Phosphorus

Phosphorus is very closely associated with calcium. It also aids in the formation of bones and is involved in absorption of the end products of carbohydrates and fats.

The lack of this element produces classical deficiency signs, although a deficiency of phosphorus may also cause rickets and frequently does. The classical sign of phosphorus deficiency is a depraved appetite. Animals very often will chew old bones, rags, and wood in an effort to get the phosphorus that their body craves.

A good source of phosphorus is steamed bone meal, monosodium phosphate, or dicalcium phosphate. The same mixture recommended for calcium will apply equally well here.

Potassium

Potassium is another mineral element necessary in bone formation, but its lack does not produce the characteristic signs that calcium and phosphorus do. Potassium is involved in muscle control in cattle and is very necessary for strength and normal function of the muscular system. Deficiency signs are vague and seldom seen. However, since the element is involved in muscle control, it is believed to cause a general weakness, perhaps even an uncontrollable shaking of muscles in severe deficiency cases.

Potassium is generally abundant in the United States. Good quality roughages, especially those that have been well fertilized, have sufficient potassium in them to meet most animals' needs. Another source of potassium is edible potassium chloride, but this is not readily available. It is recommended that fertilizers containing potassium be used on pastures in order to insure that no deficiency will develop.

Some rocky-based soils in Texas, New Mexico, and the Rocky Mountain states have very high potassium levels, producing "strong" grass and heavy-boned cattle. In the belief that there is some connection, some ranches have started "charging" their water supply to provide high levels of potassium.

Magnesium

The bones as well as the teeth and muscles require an adequate amount of magnesium. A classic deficiency sign exists when magnesium is in short supply. It is called *grass tetany*, often referred to as *grass staggers*. Since magnesium is used in muscle coordination, a deficiency of this element could affect the muscles of animals. Grass staggers is most often seen on lush, spring pastures when young growing plants outstrip their uptake of minerals through rapid growth. An animal consumes a great deal of this lush forage in the early spring because of its high palatability and thus creates the condition of grass tetany, which is characterized by an intoxicated appearance, a staggering gait, convulsions, and in many cases death.

A layman's antidote is a subcutaneous injection of a saturated solution of magnesium sulfate (Epsom salt), to be used when veterinary help is not quickly available. A saturated solution is created by dissolving Epsom salt in water until no more will go into solution. The liquid portion is then used to make the subcutaneous injection.

Adequate commercial preparations are available to supply magnesium. If these are not available, use Epsom salt, which you can purchase in the local grocery store.

Sulfur

Cattle do not need sulfur except as it is found in a couple of the sulfur-containing amino acids or "building blocks" found in protein. Since the microorganisms in the rumen can synthesize proteins, a deficiency of sulfur is generally not a condition to be concerned with. However, when NPN is used, cattle must have sulfur to "construct" these sulfur-containing amino acids.

There are no outward signs of a sulfur deficiency. Good quality roughages contain sufficient sulfur to meet the requirements of the bacteria in the rumen.

The thyroid gland uses iodine in the formation of a hormone needed to regulate body metabolism. For this reason it is advisable to make sure adequate iodine is available. Most land areas near the sea contain adequate iodine in the soil due to contamination thousands of years ago from sea water that contained high levels of iodine. However, iodine is very cheap and very little is needed to insure peace of mind.

A deficiency of iodine shows up as an enlargement of the thyroid gland located in the neck. This enlargement is called *goiter* and results in an oversized gland, nature's way of trying to compensate for low production by enlarging the manufacturing organ. Poor growth and a lazy appearance are characteristic of this deficiency. Iodized salt is recommended to prevent a deficiency.

Cobalt

Bacteria that manufacture so many of the needed nutrients in the paunch of the rumen need cobalt to synthesize vitamin B_{12} for cattle. When cobalt is missing from the ration and vitamin B_{12} is not being synthesized in the rumen, a condition develops in which cattle actually appear to be starving to death in grass up to their bellies. Appetite is also dulled, and it appears that affected animals care very little about eating anything.

This is a fairly well-documented condition seen around the world when cobalt is lacking in the soil or in the feeds. The condition exists, in mild form, in many parts of the United States. The general signs are weakness and a failure to eat. Cobalt has some influence on appetite and is often used on show animals to stimulate their appetites.

The source of cobalt is not as easy to find as other elements, but it is found in mixtures such as cobalt sulfate. It is also available in some areas in the form of a cobalt bolus that is given forcibly to the animal, then lies in the bottom of its digestive system, failing to move through the intestines, and thus releases its cobalt very slowly over a long period of time. These boluses last from six months to one year and provide needed cobalt to cattle and sheep in areas where it is necessary.

A trace mineral-salt block usually has cobalt, and it is unlikely that a deficiency would arise with regular use.

Copper

Copper is needed for proper hair development and for hemoglobin in the blood. Hemoglobin is the substance that carries oxygen from the lungs through the blood system to the cells.

Deficiencies of copper result in severe diarrhea; weight loss; lack of appetite; anemia; and a rough, coarse, haircoat that is often discolored. For example, a Hereford cow afflicted with a copper deficiency will appear to have a bleached reddish color rather than the normally dark pigment in its haircoat.

Copper sulfate is a common source of supply. It is also referred to as "bluestone" or blue vitriol. However, the best source of copper is probably a trace mineralized salt.

Manganese

Manganese is needed in bone formation. A deficiency does not exist very often, but it has been noted in the United States. Deformed or "crooked calves" are signs of a lack of manganese. These signs are seldom seen in mature cattle. Good-quality roughages or a trace mineral salt is the best source of supply.

Iron

Iron is necessary as a part of the hemoglobin molecule that carries oxygen through the blood. A deficiency of iron shows up in cattle as listlessness and anemia. The best way to tell if an animal is anemic is to look at the blood vessels on the inner surface of the eyelids. A very pale appearance indicates anemia. One type of anemia is caused by the lack of iron.

Good-quality roughages usually supply adequate levels of iron. Iron phosphate has been used with success, although it is not readily available in some areas. A good trace mineral salt will supply adequate levels of iron.

Zinc

Zinc is necessary for normal skin and hair development. A deficiency in cattle is not very likely and may be very difficult to see unless an extreme deficiency exists. The characteristic sign is a rough skin, sometimes with small cracks in it. It may take on the appearance of a "chapped" skin.

Quality roughages will supply adequate levels of zinc except in specific areas of the United States such as Florida where zinc deficiencies are known to exist. In this case, zinc sulphate or a trace mineral salt can be used.

Selenium

Selenium is associated with vitamin E. A deficiency in young calves results in a type of muscular dystrophy known as *white muscle disease*. Calves with this disease are uncoordinated, weak, and in severe cases unable to stand. There is labored breathing and, eventually, death.

The disease or disorder is not completely understood and fortunately is not widespread. It is a rare occurrence that is mentioned here only for the sake of general information. Linseed oil meal has levels of selenium that are adequate to correct most deficiencies. It is unlikely that the average stockman will ever see this disorder. In fact, some soils in the United States have such high levels of selenium that the exact opposite of a deficiency occurs; that is, a poisoning develops. This poisoning is called *alkali disease*.

Selenium is associated with vitamin E, which has long been suspected as having some influence on reproductive efficiency in animals. Selenium is getting much more attention lately, as it is thought to be a limiting factor in the reproductive performance of cows in selenium-deficient areas. Some attempts have been made to get selenium cleared for use in cattle feeds as it has been for hogs.

Molybdenum

Molybdenum stimulates fiber digestion by the bacteria in the paunch. Very rarely is a deficiency ever reported, and the signs are vague.

When feeds are grown on average soil with adequate fertilization, these feeds will supply sufficient mineral elements. Some deficiencies do exist, however. Therefore these mineral requirements have been briefly discussed in order to point out some of the possibilities that may exist in some areas of the United States or the world. It is recommended that a preventive program be utilized so that these conditions will probably never be seen, rather than to wait until the problem occurs and then try to correct it. A very simple supplement of one part trace mineralized salt and two parts dicalcium phosphate, or one part trace mineralized salt and two parts bone meal, will insure against the more common deficiencies occurring nearly anywhere in the world. This should be offered free-choice to cattle near a source of water. The salt controls the intake, and adequate supplies of water assure that other problems do not develop and that minerals are quickly dissolved and enter the system.

There is a cafeteria-style method of providing mineral supplementation to cattle, with compartments containing most or all of the required minerals in a special feeder. The theory is that cattle will crave and consume the right product. This has never been proven to be superior to the more simple and much less expensive mixtures. Taking the time and trouble to fill and maintain the compartments is also a major disadvantage.

VITAMINS

There are two divisions of vitamins that are important to domestic animals—fat-soluble and water-soluble. The fat-soluble vitamins are A, D, E, and K. The water-soluble vitamins are normally referred to as the *B-complex vitamins*. Because of the unusual nature of the ruminant digestive system, virtually all of the B-complex vitamins are synthesized by the rumen micro-organisms, assuming that adequate levels of raw materials are available in the form of pasture, natural roughages, and whatever supplementary grain may be needed for normal requirements. Therefore, in general, we need only be concerned with the fat-soluble vitamins.

There is one other class of vitamins called the *citrate-soluble vitamins*, which includes vitamin C. This is not required by domestic animals and is used in animal feed preparations only for purposes of preventing oxidation or breakdown of certain ingredients. It is required only by man, monkeys, and guinea pigs, and should not be of concern for cattle.

The function of vitamins is to act as a catalyst, something to speed up or slow down the natural body functions. Vitamins might be thought of as a transmission, providing a shift of gears for the correct speed for body functions to operate. Although they are needed in very small quantities, they are vital to life. The name itself comes from the French, who originally thought these small quantities of nutrients were amines. They referred to this substance as *vital amines*, and this term was later reduced to the word we know today—*vitamin*. As little as one gram per ton of feed in some instances is sufficient to cover the vitamin requirements of most animals. Although vitamins are only needed in very small quantities, some vitamin deficiencies do exist, and they occur on a regular and widespread basis.

The fat-soluble vitamins are called *fat soluble* because they are found in association with fat and the normal way in which it is metabolized. Researchers have found that any solvent that will dissolve fat will also dissolve these vitamins. Although there are four of them, actually only vitamins A and D are of much concern in cattle feeding.

Vitamin A

The most commonly deficient vitamin in cattle is vitamin A. Its function is involved with the normal vision of cattle, natural joint movements of the limbs, and some not yet completely understood function involving the birth of calves.

Deficiency signs are quite common throughout the United States and the world. One of the most common signs of vitamin deficiency in feed-lot cattle is a swelling of the joints of the legs and the brisket, known as *anasarca*. It is not an obvious swelling, just a matter of slight fluid retention in comparison to normal animals.

Another characteristic sign of vitamin A deficiency is night blindness. Normally, most cattle are able to see quite well in the dark, but if vitamin A is deficient, they will have almost no night vision. One of the early research techniques for determining vitamin A deficiency was to place oil drums or other obstacles in an alleyway and drive cattle individually through at night. Normal cattle were able to weave around the obstacles without knocking them over. Deficient cattle had no such warning and knocked over everything in their path.

Excluding night blindness, mature pregnant females do not have obvious range signs of vitamin A deficiency until the birth of their calves. The calves are born very weak, and the disorder may be diagnosed as some other problem. These calves may die, but the condition is very easy to correct and if caught before a severe prolonged deficiency, it is reversible.

The best source of vitamin A is any fresh green leafy hay. Alfalfa or alfalfa leaf meal is especially high in vitamin A. In extreme cases where vitamin A is needed rapidly, such as in the case of very weak newborn calves, vitamin A injections such as vitamin A palmitate, etc., may be given. One-half to 1 cc of material containing 500,000 I.U. injected intramuscularly at birth is thought to help prevent the development of calf scours and pneumonia, and to provide an immediate high level of vitamin A in the liver.

A much better plan is to give vitamin A injections to the gestating cows and in this way take care of the problem before a deficiency develops in the unborn calf.

Injectable vitamin A provides economic insurance against marginal or outright vitamin A deficiencies and is a valuable support to good nutrition according to many authorities. When it is used in the feed-lot, levels of 1 to 2 cc are recommended at the beginning of the feed-lot period. This dosage is normally repeated 90 days later. One or 2 cc of a high-quality product will provide 500,000 to 1,000,000 I.U. of vitamin A. The theory is that this added level of vitamin A aids animals in overcoming shipping stresses, and there is some indication that it prevents ringworm, foot rot, and pinkeye.

In the case of beef-breeding stock, injections of 1 to 3 million I.U. of vitamin A every six months is reported to improve bull fertility and to insure adequate vitamin A levels in the livers of herd animals during periods of dry range.

Vitamin D

Vitamin D is often called the *sunshine vitamin* because any animal that is in the sunlight, even for short periods of time, absorbs enough rays from the sun to convert a substance in its skin into vitamin D. It is very rare to have a vitamin D deficiency occur in cattle unless they have been housed inside, such as on the show circuit for very long periods of time.

The function of vitamin D is involved with the metabolism of calcium and phosphorus. Deficiency signs of vitamin D are the same as those shown for deficiencies of the minerals calcium and phosphorus, that is, rickets.

A natural source of vitamin D is any sun-cured hay. An injectable synthetic vitamin D preparation may also be given to prevent or treat rickets.

Vitamin E

The function of vitamin E is not clearly understood, but it is thought to be associated in some way with reproduction. There are a number of vitamin preparations on the market that claim reproductive efficiency will be improved through the use of a vitamin E supplement. This is speculation based on research mainly with rats. Vitamin E is associated with selenium in that availability of one is sparing of the other.

It is rare for a vitamin E deficiency to occur, but when it does, the signs are similar to those shown for a deficiency of selenium—one example is muscular dystrophy of calves, referred to as *white muscle disease*.

A source of vitamin E is any feed containing natural oil such as soybeans. There is also a synthetic vitamin E preparation that may be added to the feed. Some manufacturers' research has indicated an improvement in animal reproductive performance by the use of this product.

Vitamin K

Blood clotting is necessary in the animal to prevent cuts, bruises, and scrapes from causing excessive external or internal bleeding. If an animal did not have a mechanism to produce clotting, it would soon bleed to death even from such a minor operation as dehorning. Vitamin K is a part of that mechanism.

Vitamin K deficiency is not very common, but it does occur around the world. It is almost always brought on by the consumption of some particular substance that destroys the blood's ability to clot. One common cause for this problem is the consumption by cattle of moldy sweet-clover hay. A substance called *dicumarol* is contained in the moldy hay, and this interferes with the action of vitamin K and thus the blood's ability to clot. Dicumarol is a substance used often in human medicine for pharmaceuticals that prevent blood clots in stroke victims. If you should have an animal that bleeds profusely from a small scratch or cut, this could be the reason. However, the more common observation of this problem in an animal is when it gets a severe bruise or when a hematoma or large blood blister develops under the skin. This is a form of internal bleeding.

Quality forages will normally supply all of the vitamin K needed, except in those rare occasions when moldy sweet-clover hay causes problems. In this case an injectable form of synthetic vitamin K is available to correct the condition. Vitamin K_1, a human product, is 75 times more active than vitamin K_3, veterinary label. The relative price should be considered when vitamin K products are being purchased.

Again, it should be emphasized that vitamin C is not needed by domestic animals, and in the case of cattle, the B-complex vitamins are all synthesized by rumen organisms if the raw materials such as cobalt are available. The only vitamin deficiencies that we need be concerned with are vitamin A, vitamin D, and vitamin K, and it is doubtful whether vitamin E has any place in the average cattleman's operation.

RATIONS

Any feed or combination of feeds is a ration, but a balanced ration contains sufficient amounts of nutrients to meet the animal's requirements so that no disorders result from a lack of some nutrient in the feed.

It is the intention of this book to give you a few "rules of thumb" that are relatively easy to understand and apply.

First, let's suppose that you are not inclined to balance a ration at all, but would simply like a few good examples. Tables 5-3 and 5-4 will give the stockman some sample rations that will generally meet an animal's needs.

The ration developed will depend on the goal intended. Fattening a steer, wintering a cow, or feeding for maximum milk production makes for a variety of ration ingredients. However, an excellent idea to keep in mind in feeding is to observe the animals and adjust the ration depending on their performance. "The eye of the master fattens his cattle," the Bible tells us, and this is a good rule of thumb to keep in mind even today. Even though a ration may work out fine on paper, if it does not produce the desired performance, some changes should be made. The beginning point, however, is based on certain guidelines. The following guidelines should be kept in mind in deciding amounts of materials to be used in a ration.

1. Two % of the body weight of cattle may be fed daily as hay (roughage).

2. Three times this amount is used in a ration using silage.

3. Generally, $1\frac{1}{2}$ to 2 lb of oil meals are used to satisfy protein requirements, unless the ration is to be otherwise scientifically balanced.

Table 5-3. Suggested Rations for Beef Cattle

		SUPPLEMENTING A 1000-LB COW, DRY, PREGNANT (LB PER DAY)	FATTENING A 600-LB CALF (LB PER DAY)
1.	Nonlegume hay	20	10
	Oil meal	2	2
	Grain (shelled corn or ground grain sorghum)	—	6
2.	Silage	60	20
	Oil meal	2	1.5
	Grain (shelled corn or ground grain sorghum)	—	6
	Nonlegume hay	—	3
3.	Nonlegume hay	16	8
	Legume hay	6	2
	Grain (shelled corn or ground grain sorghum)	—	6
	Oil meal	—	1.5
4.	Silage	48	—
	Legume hay	6	10
	Oil meal	—	1
	Grain (shelled corn or ground grain sorghum)	—	7

Reprinted from *The Science of Animal Husbandry*, James Blakely and David Bade. Reston, Va: Reston Publishing Co, Inc., 1976, p. 83.

Note: With any ration, provide suitable mineral supplements.

Table 5-4. Rations for Fattening Cattle—(Choice of any one of six rations—read down)

When barley is fed, it should not make up over one third of the grain ration

Calves—initial weight 400 pounds

	First 30 days						Second 30 days						Third 30 days					
	1	2	3	4	5	6	1	2	3	4	5	6	1	2	3	4	5	6
Ground: shelled corn, grain, sorghum grain, or barley	5		5	4	6		7		7	5	7		8		8	6	9	
Ground: ear corn or grain sorghum heads		6				6		8				7		9				9
Hay: prairie, sorghum, ground grain sorghum fodder, etc.	7	5	2				5	4	2	2			4	3	2	2		
Cottonseed meal or cake	1.5	1.5	1.5	1.5	1	1	2	2	2	2	1	1	2	2	2	2	1	1
Alfalfa hay	1			2	7	7	1			2	6	6	1				5	5
Cottonseed hulls				6		7				6		6				6		5
Silage: corn or sorghum			14						12						11			
Limestone or oyster shell flour	.1		.1	.1		.1	.1		.1	.1	.1	.1	.1		.1	.1		.1

Yearlings—initial weight 600 pounds

	First 30 days						Second 30 days						Third 30 days					
	1	2	3	4	5	6	1	2	3	4	5	6	1	2	3	4	5	6
Ground: shelled corn, grain, sorghum grain, or barley	7		6	6	7		9		9	8	9		11		12	10	11	
Ground: ear corn or grain sorghum heads		8				8		10				10		12				12
Hay: prairie, sorghum, ground grain sorghum fodder, etc.	11	10	3				9	7	3				7	5	3			
Cottonseed meal or cake	1.5	1.5	1.5	1.5	1	1	1.5	2	1.5	2	2	2	2	2	2	2	2	2
Alfalfa hay	2	2		2			2	2		2			2	2		2		
Cottonseed hulls				8		10				15		9				12	7	8
Silage: corn or sorghum			20						15	15					12			
Limestone or oyster shell flour	.1		.1	.1		.1	.1		.1	.1	.1	.1	.1		.1	.1	.1	.1

Two-year-olds—initial weight 800 pounds

	First 30 days						Second 30 days						Third 30 days					
	1	2	3	4	5	6	1	2	3	4	5	6	1	2	3	4	5	6
Ground: shelled corn, grain, sorghum, grain, or barley	8		8	8	10		10		10	10	12		13		12	12	14	
Ground: ear corn or grain sorghum heads		9				10		11				14		14				16
Hay: prairie, sorghum, ground grain sorghum fodder, etc.	12	12	4	2			10	10	4				9	8	4		3	3
Cottonseed meal or cake	2	2	2.5	1	3	1.5	2	2.5	2.5	2	3	3	2.5	2.5	3	3	2.5	2.5
Alfalfa hay	1	1	1	12			1	1	1	11			1	1	1	10		
Cottonseed hulls				12	12						11	9				8	10	8
Silage: corn or sorghum			25						20						20			
Limestone or oyster shell flour	.1		.1	.1		.1	.1		.1	.1	.1	.1	.1		.1	.1		.1

Table 5-4. (Continued)

When barley is fed, it should not make up over one third of the grain ration	Fourth 30 days						Fifth 30 days						Sixth 30 days					
	1	2	3	4	5	6	1	2	3	4	5	6	1	2	3	4	5	6
Calves—initial weight 400 pounds																		
Ground: shelled corn, grain, sorghum grain, or barley	10	11	9	8	10		11	12	12	10	12		13	14	14	12	14	
Ground: ear corn or grain sorghum heads						11						12						15
Hay: prairie, sorghum, ground grain sorghum fodder, etc.	4	3	2				4	3	2				4	3	2			
Cottonseed meal or cake	2.5	2.5	2.5	2.5	2	2	2.5	2.5	2.5	2.5	2	2	3	3	3	3	2	2
Alfalfa hay	1	1					1	1					1	1				
Cottonseed hulls					5	5					5	5					5	5
Silage: corn or sorghum				10						8						6		
Limestone or oyster shell flour	.1	.1	.1	.1	.1	.1	.1	.1	.1	.1	.1	.1	.1	.1	.1	.1	.1	.1
Yearlings—initial weight 600 pounds																		
Ground: shelled corn, grain, sorghum grain, or barley	13	14	14	12	13		15	16	16	14	14							
Ground: ear corn or grain sorghum heads						14						16						
Hay: prairie, sorghum, ground grain sorghum fodder, etc.	6	5	3				5	4	3									
Cottonseed meal or cake	2.5	2.5	2.5	2.5	2	2	2.5	3	3	2.5	2	2						
Alfalfa hay	2	1					2	1										
Cottonseed hulls					7	7					7	7						
Silage: corn or sorghum				10						8								
Limestone or oyster shell flour	.1	.1	.1	.1	.1	.1	.1	.1	.1	.1	.1	.1						
Two-year-olds—initial weight 800 pounds																		
Ground: shelled corn, grain, sorghum grain, or barley	15	16	14	14	16													
Ground: ear corn or grain sorghum heads						18												
Hay: prairie, sorghum, ground grain sorghum fodder, etc.	8	5	3															
Cottonseed meal or cake	2.5	3	3	3	2.5	2.5												
Alfalfa hay	1	1	1															
Cottonseed hulls					9	8												
Silage: corn or sorghum				15														
Limestone or oyster shell flour	.1	.1	.1	.1														

Source: Courtesy of Texas A & M Agricultural Extension Service.

4. Four and one-half to 6 lb of alfalfa or other legume hay will meet this requirement.

5. In fattening cattle, figure 3% of the body weight as a guideline for total feed needed per day.

6. A ration generally should contain no more than 60% concentrates (grains) and 40% roughage (hay or silage). The more normal situation is to reverse this and set the roughage at 60% or higher and work from there.

The exception to rule 6 has been the professional feed-lot finishing rations containing 85 to 100% grain. Leave those kinds of rations to the professionals. They are experienced at coping with the accompanying problems of bloat and a host of other digestive disorders.

The scope of ration balancing is simply too broad to be covered in this short chapter on feeding. If you are interested in studying the science of feed formulation and nutrient requirements, an excellent source of information in outline easy-to-read form, is Arthur Cullison's *Feeds and Feeding* (Reston, Va.: Reston Publishing Company, Inc., 1975).

In the event you would like to avail yourself of expert nutrition and ration formulation but are not inclined to do the work yourself, many companies now offer a ration-balancing service done by computer. A few forms are filled out listing the ingredients you have available to you and those you wish to purchase and the company develops a ration to your specifications, charging a reasonable fee for this service. Of course, these companies are also in the business of selling certain supplements to the ration, and you should be aware that federal regulations govern their action concerning ingredient claims and contents. The companies do an excellent job of balancing rations in this way, and the computer service is fast, taking the drudgery out of ration balancing. It will become a more and more usable tool in the future. Consult your local extension agent for an area representative nearest you. Some states also have computer service available through county extension offices where no products are for sale. The fees for this service are very reasonable.

6

Diseases of Cattle

HOW TO IDENTIFY A SICK ANIMAL

A nasal discharge or any sign of respiratory problem such as coughing is an indication of impending problems. Vomiting by cattle should also be taken as a very serious sign of difficult illness because this is an unusual condition to see in any ruminant. Spasms, convulsions, and drooling are characteristic signs of many types of poisonings, either by natural plant or man-made substances.

Lack of appetite in cattle may go unnoticed by all but the most observant cattlemen. However, many minor disturbances such as a cobalt deficiency make themselves known in this relatively unnoticed manner. Scours should always be taken as a positive sign of digestive disturbances, parasitism, or infection.

Temperature elevation or depression can be measured readily with a rectal thermometer and can be compared to the normal levels for healthy animals (see section on vital signs in Chapter 1). The vital signs are the earliest clue to a condition deviating from normal health.

Discolored urine is a sign of infection or of severe problems in the metabolism of an animal and should be treated immediately by a professional.

In short, any deviation from normal activity, or any changes in appetite, or in urine or fecal excretions, along with the simple observation of vital signs, can determine whether or not an animal is sick.

Some of the signs of illnesses that many stockmen look for are: an elevated body temperature (103.5° F or higher), drooping of one or both ears, a drooping head carried in an abnormal position, reluctance to rise, reluctance to move, failure to come to the feed bunk, a gaunt appearance, a stiff gait, dragging of the hind feet when walking, abnormal discharges from the eyes or nose, dull or sunken eyes, a dry crusted muzzle, pus discharging from the nose, a harsh dry cough, rapid or labored breathing, scours, dehydration, and a rough haircoat. Many calves will exhibit one or perhaps most of these symptoms in extreme cases.

RESPIRATORY DISEASES

It is the herdsman's responsibility to assess the cause of the disease and to decide whether or not to seek professional help. Respiratory diseases are relatively easy to spot even in the early stages. The primary signs of all respiratory diseases are difficult breathing and a runny nose. The various respiratory disorders that normally occur with cattle are listed below.

Nosebleed (Epistaxis). The prevailing sign of epistaxis is blood running from the nose.

Cause. A nosebleed may be due to an ulcerative infection, cancer (neoplasm), a heavy blow to the nasal area, or a fractured facial bone leading to ruptured blood vessels. Except for cancer, this is normally not a condition to create panic and may cure itself without treatment if it is due to some minor injury.

Treatment. Time is the number one cure. Given time the nosebleed will probably stop, but a veterinarian should be called if the condition persists for more than 24 hours.

Bronchial Asthma. Asthma in cattle is rare, but dust, mold, and other allergy reactions create a condition that is quite similar and should receive attention.

Signs. Signs of asthma are an attack lasting 1 to 2 hours, which consists of difficult, wheezing respiration due to spasmodic contractions of the circular muscles along the air passages to and through the lung tissue.

Treatment. Steroids and antihistamines are often used as supportive treatment along with epinephrine or antispasmodics.

Pneumonia. Pneumonia is an inflammatory disease of the lungs that usually involves the upper respiratory tract. Our discussion will divide the subject into chronic and acute cases.

Signs. Chronic or prolonged pneumonia is characterized by an animal with a hollow, "tucked up" appearance, rough haircoat, difficult and rapid breathing, possibly pus draining from the nose, and salivation. The prolonged stage is usually a case in which the affected animal has never completely recovered from acute pneumonia.

Acute pneumonia is characterized by rapid onset of a lack of appetite and labored respiration.

Treatment. Chronic pneumonia is usually treated unsuccessfully; however, ultra-high levels of antibiotics may be tried. Removal of the initial cause of the problem, such as dust, parasites, etc., would prevent many of the cases and certainly would aid in treatment.

Treatment of acute pneumonia consists of broad-spectrum antibiotics (these are substances that cover a large number of different bacteria). Examples of broad-spectrum antibiotics are penicillin, tetracyclines, etc. Other treatment is isolation and prevention of undue stress. If a chemical or dust problem is thought to be precipitating the disease, a steroid drug may be used.

Choking

Signs. Bloat and salivation are primary signs of choking. Cows may go through chewing motions, show protrusion of the tongue and extension of the head and neck, and experience difficulty in breathing. Grunting and coughing are also seen.

Cause. An obstruction in the esophagus by foreign objects is the main cause of choking. In cattle, choking is usually caused by solid objects such as apples, pears, beets, potatoes, turnips, and occasionally ears of corn. On rare occasions cattle can choke on some foreign object found in the feed.

Prevention. If local crops such as apples or potatoes are used for feeds, these materials should be mechanically reduced to smaller size before using in cattle rations.

Treatment. If the choking is noticed very early, there is a good possibility that the object may be massaged upward and removed through the mouth. Occasionally a steel wire may be made into a loop, then passed through the mouth and beyond the object, slowly withdrawing it. The object may also be pushed on into the stomach with a flexible rubber hose (use a soft tip on the hose to avoid injury to the throat). The problem with choking is that if it persists for more than a half-hour, a severe bloat may develop, which places more pressure on the diaphragm and lungs, creating even more difficulty in breathing. A veterinarian should be called immediately upon seeing these severe signs of distress. A puncture of the rumen with a trocar (stylet) and cannula (tube) to relieve the rumen pressure is usually a part of the treatment, and the esophagus may also have to be surgically opened to release pressure and to facilitate breathing. The foreign matter is then removed and the necessary steps taken to close the incision.

IBR (Infectious Bovine Rhinotracheitis or Red Nose) and IPV(Infectious Pustular Vulvovaginitis).

IBR is a disease caused by a virus normally thought of as a respiratory disease in cattle. However, this virus also causes an inflammation of the vulva and vagina, and abortion (IPV). Abortion usually occurs about 20 to 35 days after infection. IBR is highly contagious. It was first observed in Colorado but now is distributed throughout most of the United States and Canada. It has been reported on every continent except South America. Only cattle are susceptible to this virus. IBR is most prevalent in large concentrations of cattle such as feed-lot and large dairy operations.

Signs. With IBR, temperatures will range between 104° F and 108° F, and there will be profuse nasal discharges (sometimes containing flecks of blood), depression, rapid breathing, and an encrustation on the muzzle by exudates. When these encrustations are removed, the underlying tissues appear bright red, hence the term *Red Nose.*

The acute part of the disease takes about one week to run its course. Uncomplicated cases make a rapid and uneventful recovery, with death losses rarely exceeding 5%.

The IPV form may be difficult to detect. The most obvious sign is swelling of the vulva with a small amount of sticky discharge. Pain is obvious to the close observer because cattle show a reluctance to allow the tail to rest on the vulva. Even though abortion does occur, permanent infertility does not result.

Prevention. A modified live virus vaccine is available commercially for the various syndromes caused by the virus. Pregnant cows should not be vaccinated since the vaccine can also cause abortion.

Treatment. There is no specific treatment for IBR or IPV; however, antibiotics may be extremely helpful in combating secondary bacterial infections that often lead to bronchial pneumonia.

Hemophilus Somnus. Hemophilus somnus is a relatively new disease that occurs in feed lots. It is a stubborn situation that has not responded well to therapy—therapy that usually has shown a good response in shipping fever outbreaks.

Signs. A dry, hacking cough, depression, heavily congested lungs, and pneumonias that don't respond to treatment are characteristic signs. In some groups, animals also become lame and stiff. As many as 90% of the cattle may be affected, and sudden death is not uncommon. Death is usually caused by a brain abscess.

Cause. The organism *H. somnus* is the cause.

Prevention. The disease is often spread by mixing two different groups of cattle. Incoming groups should be isolated for 30 days to minimize the disease spread. A vaccine is now available (Philips Roxane) that will protect most cattle. It is reported to be an immunizing agent that will not produce the disease.

Treatment. There is no treatment except for supportive treatment through the use of antibiotics to control secondary bacterial infection.

REPRODUCTIVE DISEASES

A high level of reproduction is the goal of every cattleman. There are so many problems affecting reproduction that it is tempting to classify every disorder in this category as a disease. The truth is that many abnormalities occur for developmental reasons; the fetus just doesn't develop normally.

The cause of abortion, when known, varies in different parts of the country. For instance, in California abortions in beef herds are often due to foothill abortion (EBA—Epizootic Bovine Abortion), a disease shown to be spread to the pregnant cow by the bite of the pajaroello (*Ornithodoras coriaceus*) tick. This tick is commonly found in the foothills where cattle and deer bed down.

The more common reproductive diseases causing abortion are covered in Table 6-1. In the event an abortion does occur and you suspect a disease, the fetus and fresh placenta (afterbirth) should be saved by refrigerating it at 3-5°C (38 to 45°F). Avoid freezing if possible, so that your local veterinarian may determine the exact cause. If a transmittable disease is diagnosed, then you will want to consider a vaccination program for replacement heifers. Some very common abortive diseases spread throughout the United States and most countries are brucellosis, Vibriosis, Red Nose (IBR), and leptospirosis. A program of annual booster vaccinations may be necessary for some or all of these diseases and can best be worked out by a local veterinarian.

Occasionally, abortions may be caused from factors other than disease, such as moldy, spoiled, or poisonous feeds; feeds high in nitrate; consumption of pine needles when eaten during a susceptible stage of gestation; toxic substances such as lupines and acorns; and vitamin A deficiency.

The first step in solving any problem is to determine what kind of a problem you have. If the field can be narrowed down to a few possibilities, then more detailed information can be sought and appropriate action taken. A discussion of the more common reproductive problems follows.

Brucellosis (Bang's Disease)

Signs. The key sign of brucellosis is abortion after the fifth month of pregnancy and poor or irregular calving records afterward. Occasionally the fetus is carried to full term, but a retained placenta (the bag surrounding the calf) is sometimes seen along with metritis (inflammation of the uterus), which develops sometimes after calving. Normally, when the disease strikes, a cow or heifer aborts once or twice and then calves normally. The cow becomes immune but remains a "spreader" of the disease for life.

Bulls are also affected with a condition known as orchitis (swollen testicles). The scrotum appears swollen and reddish. The bull is in obvious discomfort, and the scrotum is painful to the touch. Brucellosis can result in sterility in bulls.

Cause. A microscopic bacterial organism, *Brucella abortus*, is the cause.

Prevention. A government program consists of:

1. A vaccination program in young heifers to create immunity. *Strain 19* vaccine is the only approved vaccine in the United States. The vaccine

Table 6-1. Diseases Causing Abortions in Cattle

Disease	Organism	How Spread	Stage of Gestation at Abortion	Samples Needed for Diagnosis	Vaccination	Remarks
Vibriosis	Bacteria (*Vibrio fetus venerealis*)	Venereal disease spread by infected bulls.	Early abortion (sporatic)	Vaginal mucus from cow; fetus; washing from bull.	Killed vaccine 30–60 days before breeding.	High incidence of repeat breeding and open cows.
Trichomoniasis	Protozoa	Venereal disease spread by infected bulls.	2–4 mo.	Preputial washings from bulls; uterus from cull cow; fetus.	None	Treatment: sexual rest for 60–90 days; AI; cull infected bulls.
Leptospirosis	Bacteria (at least 5 serotypes)	Infected urine or aborted fetus.	Any stage, usually 6–9 mo.	Blood sample 10% of herd.	Annually—more often if needed.	Laboratory should determine serotype.
Brucellosis	Bacteria (*Brucella abortus*)	Aborted fetus.	6–9 mo.	Blood sample from cow; fetus; placenta.	Dairy heifers: 3–6 mo. Beef: 3–10 mo.	Infected animals are culled.
Foothill abortion (EBA)	Unknown	Suspect spread by tick.	6–9 mo.	Fetus; blood sample; placenta.	None	Aborting animals usually immune.
Red Nose (IBR)	Virus	Infectious from cow to cow.	6–9 mo.	Fetus; placenta; blood samples.	Live vaccine.	Abortion may or may not occur.
Virus diarrhea (BVD)	Virus	Contagious from cow to cow.	Variable, usually early in gestation	Two blood samples, 3 weeks apart.	Vaccinate animal after 8 mo. of age.	Calves may be born with brain damage.
Listeriosis (circling disease)	Bacteria	Other animals; rats; moldy feed.	Variable	Fetus; placenta; blood from cow.	None	Uterine infection; illness in cattle.

AI-Artificial Insemination

Serotype—there are several types of Lepto organisms. They can be differentiated through serology.

must be given between 2 and 10 months of age for beef replacement heifers (2 to 6 months for dairy). There has been controversy over this program because even though immunity develops from this vaccination, the testing program often indicates a reactor, and cattlemen have become skeptical of needlessly slaughtering animals that are reactors but never abort. Supplemental tests have been developed to differentiate between a true carrier of the disease and one that merely reacted positively to testing but is free of the actual disease. Serum samples are submitted to state labs for final analysis.

Heifers that are vaccinated receive a tattoo in the ear with the date of the vaccination. They are also identified with an ear tag or a brand for follow-up observation.

2. A testing program for individual herds as well as cattle passing through regular market channels. Any animal changing owners or sold for any purpose other than slaughter must be tested in endemic areas. Testing involves taking a blood sample and analyzing by a simple card test or the plate agglutination test. The most widely used is the card test, which is quick, accurate, easy to perform, and definitely the most recommended. Positive reactors are branded with a B on the left jaw and must be slaughtered. Although the disease may be spread through a cow licking the aborted fetus of another, there is no transmission through the marketing of the dressed carcass or byproducts. All animals known to be in contact with this reactor are quarantined and must be tested at 30-day intervals for two negative tests at least 120 days after the last reactor is found. If no reactors are found after this quarantine, and two negative tests, the herd may be certified clean.

The market cattle testing program identifies reactors going through auctions and other outlets. Through a trace-back program to the place of origin the herd is quarantined until the herd can be certified clean.

Government regulations cannot enforce every compliance with the program. Many cattlemen are tempted to ignore the regulation because of the expense and trouble involved. But replacement heifers definitely should have had negative tests within the last 30 days prior to herd entry. This is a must if the disease is ever to be completely eradicated.

Transmission.   Brucellosis can be spread to man through contact with unpasteurized milk, causing a condition known as *Undulant fever*. It can be spread to animals through direct contact with carrier cattle. Spreading from cow to cow is quite common because the organism is present in the placenta (afterbirth) and may contaminate grass, ground, and the haircoat of the calf. Since every stockman has seen cows eating the placenta or licking the dead fetus, it is easy to understand how serious a problem transmission to others can be.

Treatment.   There is no known treatment. Government regulations are now in effect to control and eradicate the disease. During the late 1930s the government estimated that up to 50% of the cattle herds in the United States were infected. Strict enforcement of a clean-up program has reduced this figure to less than 2% of the herds, with many states certified as free of the disease. However, this 2% has been a nagging thorn in the side of government officials for many years. Some animals carry the disease and spread it to others without showing signs. Also, at times there has been a lack of cooperation between cattlemen and government officials in testing programs.

Vibriosis

Signs. It is difficult to detect vibriosis, but the first hint of the problem is a breakdown of a definite calving season to one of unmanageable order. Calves may be dropped every month of the year. This is caused by undetected abortions at gestations of less than 5 months. An aborted fetus may be too small to be seen, or may be eaten by scavengers. You may think that your problem is a weak bull or a nutrition disorder, but what causes the staggered calf birth is a cow or heifer aborting once or twice, becoming immune, then breeding normally but spreading the disease to others. The disease may delay calving 10 to 12 months, causing tremendous economic loss and throwing the planned calving season out of sequence. The disease is very hard even for a veterinarian to prove through lab methods. Stomach contents of the aborted calf and uterine scrapings or discharges are examined, but in reality probably the best way to check for the disease is to vaccinate and see if calving dates can be routinely managed afterwards. If so, the culprit could be vibriosis.

Cause. The cause is a microscopic organism, *Vibrio fetus*, or *Campylobacter fetus*.

Prevention. It is recommended in areas where vibriosis is a known problem that cows and heifers be vaccinated annually with a good quality vaccine about two months before turning in the bulls. Vaccination of the bulls is debatable in the United States, but research in Europe indicates that bull vaccination is to be highly recommended in controlling vibriosis.

Transmission. Vibriosis is a venereal disease that is spread mechanically by the bull from female to female through the normal act of breeding.

Treatment. There is no effective treatment, although a new technique is being researched in which multiple vaccinations of the bull around certain lymph nodes is being tried in order to stop the spread of the disease. It is a true venereal condition spread from cow to cow through the natural reproductive process involving mechanical transmission by the bull. However, vaccination of the bull is questionable at present. Some authorities say it has no effect because the bulls spread the disease mechanically; others claim the organism actually grows on the penis and therefore treatment could be effective.

Leptospirosis

Signs. In leptospirosis, basically the kidney is affected, but in such a variety of ways that many conditions are exhibited. The following conditions may occur either singularly or in combination: abortion, mastitis (resulting in blood-tinged milk from a noninflamed udder), high temperature, icterus (a jaundice or yellowing of the pink membranes especially around the eye, vulva, penis, and gum), wine-colored urine, and anemia. Death is common in very young animals. Older cattle have a mortality rate of about 5%. An autopsy reveals gray to white lesions on the liver. A definite diagnosis is made through a culture of the tissues of the infected animal. Recovered animals appear dull and unhealthy.

Cause. A spirochete bacterial microorganism is the cause. There are three major strains—*L. pomona*, *L. grippotyphosa*, and *L. hardjo*. The *L. pomona* strain was previously thought to be the chief infecting agent, but the other two are also prevalent now, so most vaccines cover all three types. Look carefully at the vaccine you buy to see that all three strains are covered. A cheaper vaccine may only cover the more common *L. pomona* strain, and your cattle could still come down with the disease.

Prevention. It is recommended that all cattle be vaccinated regardless of location or the prevalence of the disease. The leptospiral vaccines, including various strains, are widely available and can be combined with other vaccines for a one-shot treatment. Since deer carry the disease and cannot be vaccinated, it is very important to immunize cattle. Definitely use the three-strain vaccine.

Transmission. Leptospirosis is a very highly contagious disease that can be spread not only to other animals but also to man. The chief carrier is water. Infected animals may urinate in streams or in low-lying areas that are drained by streams. Since the organism passes through the kidney, it is easy to understand how it can spread to others who drink the water or who stand in water where entry is gained through cuts or abrasions. Wildlife carry and spread the disease also. Bulls can spread the organism through semen in the normal reproductive process, and it can also be transmitted through artificial insemination.

Treatment. Antibiotics (tetracycline, streptomycin, penicillin) have been of some assistance, although the recovered animals may remain carriers; so the best treatment is prevention. Any suspect should immediately be isolated from the herd.

Trichomoniasis

Signs. Abortion in heifers or cows at very early stages (2 to 4 months) of gestation is the key sign, and an infected uterus often follows abortion to keep cows from coming back into heat. Trichomoniasis is one of the true venereal diseases of cattle.

Cause. A protozoal microorganism, *Trichomonas fetus*, is the cause.

Prevention. Normally trichomoniasis is a very rare disease and few stockmen will ever need to be concerned with it; however, if an outbreak is suspected or cases nearby are confirmed, close observation of the herd and careful checking of replacements, especially bulls, are in order. The bull spreads the disease.

Transmission. The organism is passed from cow to cow by bulls that are infected with it. An inflamed prepuce on the bull is exhibited in fully developed stages of the disease. Artificial insemination also serves to transmit the disease. However, any commercial semen is treated with antibiotics and poses no threat of infection.

Treatment. The disease is arrested by administering broad-spectrum antibiotics to both males and females. Carriers should be isolated or culled completely, and a period of sexual inactivity is also helpful.

Listeriosis (Circling Disease). Cattle are most susceptible to this disease. It affects the brain of cattle through a form of meningitis or encephalitis (inflammation of the brain). The disease is most prevalent in cold weather and seldom occurs in warm climates or during summer months. Almost invariably, outbreaks occur 2 to 4 days after there is a severe drop in temperature.

Signs. Animals of all ages may be affected and signs may last from 4 to 14 days. At the onset of the disease, affected animals separate themselves from the rest of the herd, crowd into a corner, or lean against stationary objects. When walking, they often move in a circle. Circling is by no means a definite clinical sign, but when present it is always in one direction. Many cows display a paralysis of the facial and neck muscles, making it difficult if not impossible for them to eat or drink.

Cattle abortions occur between the fourth and seventh months of gestation.

In order to get a definite clinical diagnosis, the aborted fetus, placenta (afterbirth), or blood from the affected cow must be analyzed.

Cause. The bacteria *Listeria monocytogenes*, which gain entrance probably through the upper respiratory tract or the eye, are the cause. The disease is associated with moldy feeds, especially silage. The condition is so common in Iceland that it is not known as circling disease but as *silage disease*. The connection between the bacteria and silage is not clearly understood.

Prevention. No vaccine is available. The only precaution that can be taken is to separate and isolate suspected victims during an outbreak.

Treatment. Although no treatment is effective, sulfonamides and penicillin are recommended as supportive treatment until the infection is cleared up. Cattle that are affected by listeriosis may succumb again to the disease at a later date.

BVD (Bovine Viral Diarrhea). BVD is discussed in more detail under systemic diseases. In the abortive form it is contagious to cows, spread from one to another through simple contact. The effects are variable, but abortion usually occurs early in the gestation period.

If BVD is suspected, two blood samples taken three weeks apart are needed for a definite clinical diagnosis.

Cattle may be vaccinated after 8 months of age to protect against both the diarrhea and the abortive nature of the disease.

IBR (Red Nose) (Infectious Bovine Rhinotracheitis). IBR has an abortive form as well as a respiratory effect. Both situations are more thoroughly discussed under the previous section on respiratory diseases. The abortive form is much less common than the respiratory type.

Effect of Nutrition on Reproduction. Several nutritional problems are associated with failure to reproduce and abortion.

Heifers on inadequate levels of energy (poorly fed) often come into heat irregularly or late, or may not settle if they breed.

Inadequate levels of protein over an extended period of time may decrease breeding efficiency, particularly in developing heifers.

A deficiency of essential minerals may also affect reproduction adversely. A classic example accounting for the failure to reproduce due to a lack of mineral supplementation is a phosphorus deficiency. Calcium and salt may be involved to a lesser degree, but invariably phosphorus is the key element in reproduction for cattle.

A deficiency of vitamin A brings about the most common known abortion due to nutritional causes. Vitamin A is needed for proper implantation of the fertilized egg in the uterus and also for the maintenance of the developing fetus. Vitamin A deficiencies are usually characterized by extremely weak calves that die soon after birth, or by an abortion or stillbirth in the last few days of gestation.

Other nutritional problems include high nitrate levels in some feeds and grasses, which has been known to cause abortions, and excessive fatness, which has been indicated as causing infertility. However, the exact role of these factors has not yet been defined.

Retained Placenta. Normally, cows and heifers expel the placenta (afterbirth) within 6 hours after calving. Numerous conditions prevent this expulsion, such as brucellosis, leptospirosis, and Vibriosis. Nutritional deficiencies or metabolic diseases may also increase the incidence of retained placentas.

Cattlemen should wait 72 hours before taking action. Many cows will expel the placenta several hours later than normal without incident. Removal is more likely to be successful after 72 hours anyway; so don't press the situation. Removal is best accomplished by applying tension to the membrane and running the hand between the membrane and the maternal tissues, thus separating the "buttons." If separation cannot be performed easily and rapidly, the uterus should be medicated with antibiotics or other drugs and the membrane left in place until a later time. Some veterinarians do not recommend manual removal of the placenta at all, relying on infusion of the uterus with one or more broad-spectrum antibiotics and using hormones to expel the afterbirth.

Cleanliness and complete removal of the afterbirth are essential to prevent metritis (an inflammation of the uterus). Metritis symptoms are the production of a grayish-white or yellow-white discharge from the vulva following calving and a retained placenta. However, some cows show no evidence of a discharge, so you should watch out for signs of toxicity or sickness. Metritis is also treated with antibiotics, hormones, and other types of drugs depending on the type of infection and the bacteria involved.

Many veterinarians report that improved nutrition results in fewer retained placentas; so it is especially important that cows and heifers receive adequate nutrition to meet their minimum daily requirements not only to ward off disease but also to prevent other nondisease-associated problems that may precipitate a disease.

Prolapse of the Uterus. An eversion of the uterus, or the "calf bed," is fairly common in cattle. The displaced organ protrudes through the vulva and is usually a complete reversal of the entire uterus (womb).

The causes may involve a diseased uterus, unusual straining at calving time, or the condition commonly called *fat cow syndrome*. In almost every case the prolapse is precipitated by calving. It may occur at the time of calving or shortly thereafter.

The signs are obvious. The animal is usually lying down when it occurs, but upon standing, the uterus hangs from the vulva to the hocks in a massive display of flesh. The uterus is usually enlarged and may be covered with dirt and debris if the condition has existed for any length of time. It is not uncommon for other abdominal organs to be within the prolapse.

Treatment should be undertaken by a veterinarian, but you can assist greatly by wrapping the uterus in a wet towel or sheet to prevent further contamination. The uterus should be washed thoroughly with normal warm saline solutions, and fetal membranes should be removed if excessive bleeding does not occur.

Treatment is usually effective if the prolapse is a normal part of calving, and if professional assistance is promptly available. Future occurrences of the condition may develop, but not always. The method used by the veterinarian is to replace the uterus by starting with the portion nearest the vulva and alternate replacing upper and lower surfaces. A mild pistonlike motion with a clenched fist may aid in getting the entire uterus through the cervix.

After it is replaced, a hormone injection is given to restore the muscle tone to the uterus. Antibiotics are recommended to control secondary infection. Usually the vulva is sutured to contain the uterus, or a truss may be applied.

In extreme cases, to save the life of the dam or when replacement is impossible, surgical amputation may be the only answer.

Cystic Ovaries. Cystic ovaries occur more often in heifers than in cows, although the condition can occur in any female. The cause of cystic ovaries is not completely understood, but it is thought to be related to nutrition, hormone imbalances, and inherited characteristics. The condition causes nymphomania (continuous heat) in cows or heifers and is related to a follicle (egg) that develops on the ovary but is not shed in the normal manner.

If a heifer is observed to be in heat constantly, the veterinarian may be able to correct the condition through rectal palpation and a gentle massage of the cystic follicle. This is usually followed up with an injection of a luteinizing hormone given intravenously, repeated in 5 to 7 days, to stimulate the release of the egg and subsequent normal reproductive activity.

Oral organic iodides are sometimes recommended through this treatment period. The grain ration should be evaluated because many nutritionists and reproductive specialists feel that an unbalanced vitamin and/or mineral ration can inhibit the correction of the condition once it has developed.

VIRAL AND BACTERIAL SYSTEMIC DISEASES

Systemic diseases are so named because they usually attack the entire animal, not just one system.

Diseases Produced by the Clostridial Organisms

Blackleg and Blackleg-Type Diseases. Blackleg and Blackleg-type diseases are grouped together because they are caused by similar organisms and produce similar clinical signs.

Blackleg may be caused by one of several clostridial organisms. Depending on the organism, the disease may be called Blackleg, malignant edema, enterotoxemia, etc. True Blackleg is caused by *Clostridium chauvoei*; malignant edema is caused by *Clostridium septicum*; enterotoxemia is caused by *Clostridium perfringens*. However, the three are often grouped together and referred to simply as Blackleg. We will treat them separately first for purposes of distinction between specific causes, and collectively later for purposes of general treatment or prevention of any Blackleg-type clostridial disease.

Signs. The signs are an acute, infectious disease characterized by inflamed muscles, severe toxemia (poisoning), and a high death rate —approximately 100%. Usually the young, fastest growing animals between 6 months and 2 years are affected first. The highest rate of outbreaks occurs in the warmer months between spring and autumn.

The first sign of a problem is usually a dead calf. This disease is fatal within 24 hours of onset of clinical signs; so an unexpected death of the fattest, most healthy calf in the herd for no obvious reason could mean an outbreak. Since it occurs so quickly, it is difficult to see the signs; but close observation of younger cattle in those first 24 hours of infection should reveal some telltale signs. There may be an obvious lameness, a swelling of upper parts of the leg, and a slight "dragging" of hind feet in a tired walk. Swellings that feel hot and look painful are obvious. Later, these same swellings will be cold and painless. Appetite will be depressed, and the temperature will be high, between 105 and 106°F.

There is often a gassy discolored swelling under the skin in the upper part of the leg. These swellings have a dry, crackling, tissue-paper feeling if touched. The skin will be dry and cracked. Occasionally, lesions show up at strange locations such as the base of the tongue, heart muscle, diaphragm, brisket, or udder.

However, this disease is so acute that even the best of cattlemen may fail to recognize the signs, and the first indication of impending trouble may be a dead calf. Even so, fast action may prevent other animals from developing Blackleg if immediate treatment and vaccination are started and if those showing obvious signs are isolated.

Specifically, true Blackleg is caused by only one microorganism, *Clostridium chauvoei*, but there are six other strains that cause a Blackleg-type disease. They should receive equal attention because it is important to know what to look for when reading the label on a vaccine bottle. The organisms, in order of greatest danger, are *Cl. chauvoei*, *Cl. septicum*, *Cl. novyi*, *Cl. sordellii*, and *Cl. perfringens* (types B, C, and D).

Malignant edema, similar to Blackleg, is caused by a deep puncture wound; so vaccination needles should be kept sterilized and old nails and other sharp objects should be removed from pastures and facilities. Malignant edema is caused by *Clostridium septicum*.

Blackleg and malignant edema are contagious; that is, they are spread by direct contact from one animal to another.

Prevention. Vaccination is the only reliable means of control for both Blackleg and malignant edema. All calves 4 to 6 months of age should be vaccinated. In some herds where losses occur at younger ages, vaccination may be done earlier. Revaccination is recommended at 6 months of age to get lasting immunity. Check with your local veterinarian to determine the need. A combination Blackleg–malignant edema bacterin produces a high degree of immunity in 10 to 12 days. Immunity lasts from 9 to 12 months or longer.

Treatment. Little or no value comes of treatment when animals are sick, but a few early cases may respond successfully to antibiotics such as tetracyclines or penicillin.

Enterotoxemia (Overeating Disease). Enterotoxemia is another Blackleg-like disease often associated with other clostridial infections. It is discussed separately from true Blackleg and malignant edema because of its common observation in the feeding industry. It is an unpredictable disease, associated mostly with feed-lot cattle on full feed or with a minimum of roughage, or those cattle turned to the self-feeder without previous exposure. The sudden ingestion of high-energy feeds may cause illness, and frequently deaths, resulting in 3 to 5% head losses.

Cause. The disease is caused by *Clostridium perfringens*. Toxins are also released in the intestine that may produce hemorrhages. These toxins flow throughout the bloodstream causing death sometimes in a matter of a few hours.

Treatment. In the case of feed-lot animals where enterotoxemia is the only concern, it is recommended that grain rations be reduced immediately and roughage given free-choice. The use of antibiotics in the feed for 5 to 7 days may also help. Vaccination before the animals start on full feed, followed by a booster injection in 90 days, will give added protection during the feeding period at the end of the fattening period, when concentrate intake is at its highest and immunity is at its lowest.

General Treatment for All Blackleg-Like Clostridial Diseases. Very large doses of penicillin (5000 to 10,000 units per pound of body weight) are recommended when an outbreak is definitely confirmed and "suspects" are noted by observation. It is not likely that observation will be early enough to do much good, but it is worth trying. If an outbreak occurs, you can vaccinate animals from two years old all the way down to three weeks of age. Younger animals should be revaccinated at about 4 to 6 months of age. Immunity does not build up for about 10 to 14 days, so deaths may continue to occur.

An antiserum is available, but it is very expensive. In the case of a very valuable animal, the antiserum may be advisable, but there is some doubt as to its effectiveness.

The best way to fight the condition is through prevention.

General Prevention for All Blackleg-Like Clostridial Diseases. Annual vaccination with a good quality vaccine is recommended. Vaccines may be different prices, and you might think you are getting by with a cheap vaccine; but it is advisable to look closely at the organisms covered on the label. A one-way vaccine covers *Cl. chauvoei*, a two-way covers additionally *Cl. septicum*, and the three-way adds *Cl. novyi* to the first two. A seven-way vaccine covers all of those organisms previously discussed. It is recommended that you spare no expense here and buy at least a three-way vaccine. A seven-way vaccine covers all of the Blackleg-like diseases (Blackleg, malignant edema, enterotoxemia). Vaccinate all animals between the ages of 4 months and 2 years of age.

Redwater (Bacillary Hemoglobinuria)

Signs. Redwater is an acute, highly fatal disease. It usually occurs in the spring of the year and is characterized by high fever and a breakdown of hemoglobin in the blood, which travels through the kidneys to cause a port wine-colored, blood-tinged urine (hemoglobinuria). The blood-tinged urine is the key sign to watch for in this disease. In addition, jaundice or icterus (a yellow coloring of the pink membranes) is usually seen. You have to be looking closely for the jaundiced condition to notice it, but examination of normal pink parts around the eye and vulva, or the prepuce in males, will show a slight yellowish tinge instead of a healthy pink color.

This is a rapidly fatal disease (about 12 hours from the onset of signs) with almost 100% mortality. If you should find an animal with the disease before it dies, the signs will usually be labored breathing and grunting, an arched back indicating abdominal pains, a weak and rapid pulse, temperature elevation, and a swollen brisket. The manure of an affected animal is very dark, and of course wine-colored urine should be looked for as a positive conclusion.

Cause.   The cause is a bacterium, *Clostridium hemolyticum.*

Prevention.   A Redwater vaccine is available for herds in areas of high risk. Vaccination is recommended every 6 months, but if you want to be more liberal and take a chance on vaccinating only once per year, it is recommended to do so in the spring when the disease is most prevalent. Adequate drainage of pasture to control flooding and snails, thought to be "spreaders," is another method of control.

Transmission.   Redwater is most commonly spread by flooding from an infected area to a clean one. There have been reports of spreading through hay grown in low-lying infected areas and by scavengers, especially dogs or wolves, carrying bones and carcass residue of animals into an uninfected grazing area. It is also thought to be associated with liver flukes, which are known to be spread by snails, and the disease may very likely be spread at the same time by this same carrier.

Treatment.   Very high doses of tetracycline with very high levels of dextrose and electrolyte solutions given intravenously may occasionally save an animal, but the outcome of treatment is doubtful. The most important measure is control through prevention.

Botulism

Signs.   Botulism is a rapidly fatal clostridial disease that causes paralysis of muscles, especially of the legs, jaw, and throat. These signs appear within 3 to 7 days of ingestion of decomposing plant or animal material—in experimental animals. Muscle weakness starts in the hindquarters and progresses forward to the neck. An animal will appear restless, lack coordination, stumble, and will eventually fall and be unable to raise its head and neck. This is due to total paralysis in the later stages of development. Some animals will have normal skin reactions, and will respond to pinpricks with a natural pain reflex.

The tongue and jaw become paralyzed, and the animal drools saliva uncontrollably. Constipation, as opposed to diarrhea in many other diseases, is common. Death occurs due to paralysis of respiratory muscles.

Cause.   The cause of botulism is the organism *Clostridium botulinum.*

Prevention.   The only control of botulism is to keep pastures free and clean of decaying plant or animal matter. The botulism organism is a naturally occurring microorganism that has a good place in nature for decomposing materials in a natural way, but it can cause disaster if consumed by animals.

A mixture of one-third salt, one-third steamed bone meal, and one-third oil seed meal (cottonseed, soybean, etc.) will prevent a general craving for phosphorus or protein. This mixture should be offered free-choice if there is a lot of decaying residue around, to reduce the temptation of cattle to eat decomposing materials.

Transmission.   Botulism is mainly transmitted through decomposed material that an animal may eat. The disease is noted to be common in areas where protein- or phosphorus-deficient cattle crave these nutrients and eat strange residues in an effort to get them. Outbreaks are most common during drought, when cattle are more likely to eat dead, decomposing material, or to chew on old bones that contain the organism. Removal or burning of dead plant and animal remains is highly recommended, especially during times of poor nutrition under dry pasture conditions.

Treatment.   Treatment is usually ineffective, but two methods are commonly attempted. An antitoxin is given by some veterinarians, whereas others prescribe various types of enemas to try to flush the toxins from the digestive system. Since the disease takes 3 to 7 days to incubate, but is rapidly fatal once signs are seen, the treatment is usually a disappointment.

Tetanus

Signs.   Tetanus is a highly fatal, infectious disease of all domestic animals characterized by hyperextension ("sawhorse" posture, stiff joints), tetany (an uncontrollable stiffness), and convulsions. These signs are produced because of a neurotoxin (nerve poison), which varies in its effect on different species of animals. Horses are most susceptible, cattle the least.

The toxin ascends through the nerve tissue to cause a constant tightness of muscles. The animal can't relax, and the muscles will feel unusually hard to the touch. The first sign is a stiffness that gets progressively worse, then a muscular tremor. The jaw appears restricted in movement, making eating difficult. A consistent clue is the third eyelid, which prolapses (slides over a portion of the eyeball). Look closely at the eye of a normal animal, then look at the eye of a "suspect." If tetanus is the problem, the difference will be obvious.

The victim appears very alert, the ears are erect, the nostrils flared, and it generally overreacts to stimulation. A loud clap of the hands may cause an explosion of activity rather than normal movement.

Temperature and pulse will be near normal, although they may rise during later stages due to involuntary muscle activity. Constipation and urine retention are common, due to inability to position the body for these functions. Younger animals may develop a minor bloat at the onset of the symptoms. The duration of the fatal illness is usually 5 to 10 days, although occasionally a mild case may recover completely. In this case the stiffness gradually decreases over a period of weeks or even months.

Cause.   The cause is the toxin of *Clostridium tetani*. The organism forms spores that live in the soil and are extremely difficult to kill with disinfectants or even steam heat.

Prevention.   Injecting a vaccine in cattle is usually not necessary or recommended routinely, unless you are in a known problem area. Any animal that has been wounded, especially with a puncture, should have the wound flushed out so the organism is not harbored in a closed-type wound. Antibiotics should be administered and/or a tetanus vaccine given to produce immunity.

Calves born in confinement or on a pasture with a heavy animal population should have their navel cord dipped in a mild disinfectant such as tamed iodine as soon as possible after birth.

Transmission. The organism that causes tetanus is present in the manure of all grass-consuming animals. Any soil with a high concentration of animal population is likely to be a source of contamination. The organism persists indefinitely in the soil and is most often transmitted through an open wound such as those produced in castration and dehorning. A puncture wound is especially dangerous. Newborn calves are very susceptible through the navel cord. The spores lie dormant in the body until clinical symptoms start to be evident.

The spores remain at the site of entry, and a poisonous substance (neurotoxin) is produced through growth by the organism. This neurotoxin affects the nerves and makes muscular activity more and more difficult for the animal to control.

The normal incubation period varies from one to three weeks.

Treatment. Although a veterinarian will need to supervise treatment with specific recommendations, the procedure is normally handled by the cattleman because of the excessive amount of time required on a regularly scheduled basis throughout a 24-hour period. Treatment is usually divided into three steps. The first step is removal of the organism itself by the use of antibiotics. Second, the muscle contractions are relaxed by the use of muscle relaxants such as tranquilizers or chloral hydrates. Third, very high doses of tetanus antitoxin (up to 300,000 units every 12 hours) are recommended. Some local injection of the same antitoxin around the wound is also advisable.

Of all the animals affected, cattle are given more of a chance to recover than any other species. Cattle should be kept in a dark, quiet area during treatment, and excess exertion or noise should be avoided.

Anthrax

Signs. Anthrax is a very acute disease characterized by a reaction of the entire body (septicemia) and sudden death. Usually there is no warning; an animal just drops dead for no apparent reason. Telltale signs are a carcass that bloats very quickly and bloody discharges the color of tar coming from the rectum, nose, and other body openings. The classic signs are a "sawhorse on its side" appearance, a failure of the blood to clot, and a failure of rigor mortis to set in as quickly as normally expected. If anthrax is suspected, an autopsy is usually not done because the organism that causes the disease is extremely contagious to man as well as to animals. Blood samples can be taken with extreme care for submission to a laboratory for culture and identification under a microscope. If this is done, precautions should be taken to label the package plainly. If anthrax is confirmed or highly suspected, the carcass along with any contaminated bedding should be burned or buried at least 6 feet deep with adequate quicklime spread on top before covering.

Two forms exist: acute and peracute (very acute). The peracute is the most common. The disease is so rapid that only 1 to 2 hours elapse from infection to death. Should you happen to be observing the animal, at the onset, you would see muscle tremors, difficult breathing, a total collapse, and convulsions ending in death. The discharges mentioned above will then begin at the same time that bloat begins to develop.

The acute form is slower, running its course in about 48 hours. Signs exhibited are: obvious depression, a reluctance to move alternating with short periods of excitement, an elevated temperature up to 107° F, rapid breathing, membranes that are congested (possibly bleeding), no appetite, and the possible abortion of pregnant cows. Milk production drops to almost nothing, and the milk may be blood-tinged or deep yellow in color. There may be a swelling around the throat and tongue. Death in the peracute form is almost 100%; in the acute form it generally exceeds 90%, even with treatment.

There are some other conditions that you might confuse with anthrax such as cattle struck by lightning, Redwater, several types of poisoning, and acute bloat. If there is any doubt, use extreme caution because of the highly contagious nature of the anthrax organism to both man and animals.

Cause. The cause is a microorganism, *Bacillus anthracis*. When exposed to the air this organism forms a spore called *Anthrax bacillus*. This spore has been known to exist in the soil in a viable condition for over 60 years.

Prevention. Annual vaccination with anthrax gives good protection. However, it is recommended only in areas where the disease is known to be a problem.

Transmission. The organism may be eaten or inhaled, or it may enter the body through breaks in the skin. It is quite often associated with rough, stemmy feeds that have been grown in an area where anthrax is known to exist. The coarse feeds irritate the inner linings of the digestive system, creating a minor wound and allowing absorption of the spore and onset of the disease.

Treatment. Antibiotics such as penicillin and antiserums are used but with poor success. The only real defense is prevention through vaccination.

Mastitis

Signs. The disease is an inflammation of the mammary gland. One or all four quarters of the udder may be affected. The bag may become swollen, reddish, hard, hot; and painful to the touch. Some discoloration is common, varying from red to deep purple or even black when gangrenous mastitis develops.

The key early sign is a change in density and color of the milk, which may be blood-tinged, yellow, thick, and ropy. If not treated, gangrene could develop and prove fatal, although treatment is simple and generally effective. This disease is more common with dairy cows but can occur in any mammal. A more complete, detailed discussion is given in Chapter 12.

Note: Edema in the udder of first-calf heifers and occasionally in older cows is often seen and has an appearance similar to mastitis. However, this condition is much less serious than regular mastitis. Fluid accumulates along the underline about 10 days to 2 weeks just before or just after calving. Unless this swelling or edema is severe, it is nothing to worry about, but if it is severe and there is obvious discomfort, diuretics are recommended to reduce swelling.

Cause. Many organisms can cause the onset of mastitis. Normally, in beef cattle a bacterium creates the disease when the udder is damaged by injury, chilling, or any type of trauma. Improper sanitation in dairy milk parlors is a common cause of spread of the bacterium from one cow to another. However, an injury is generally required to create the condition.

Prevention. The best precaution is to reduce injury through less "cowboying" and rough treatment.

Transmission. Mastitis is not highly transmittable in beef cattle without an injury taking place first; however, never use the same injectable syringe without sterilizing between cows, and use common-sense sanitary procedures after working with an infected cow.

Treatment. At the first sign of mastitis, the cow should be milked thoroughly and "stripped" clean. Systemic antibiotics are helpful and specially prepared broad-spectrum antibiotics are available in throw-away sterile syringes for injection through the teat canal directly into the infected quarter. This injection should be given very slowly while the thumb and index finger gently pinch off the end of the teat to ensure that all medication goes up into the infected glandular tissue. By gentle "reverse milking" procedure, the antibiotics should be forced up thoroughly into the infected quarter.

Response to treatment is generally good, but it works better in dry cows than lactating cattle. Treatment should begin immediately after signs are seen and should continue until the signs are gone. If the condition has not cleared up within 5 days, a sample of milk should be taken and should be sent to a laboratory for cultural growth to identify specific antibiotics that will control the organism; the animal should then be treated with that specific antibiotic.

Occasionally, a case can be so severe as to cause gangrenous mastitis. The gland becomes acutely affected, persists for several days, changes color to black or purple, and the affected quarter eventually loses blood circulation. That quarter will feel cold to the touch. If not treated, it could be fatal or the quarter could slough off. Amputation of the quarter is usually advisable as the only effective treatment. Usually only one quarter is lost and the other three have a tendency to compensate, continuing to produce the same amount of milk in beef cattle.

If the cow has raised good calves in the past, her total milk production will not be noticeably impaired through the loss of one quarter, and similar results can be expected in future calf crops.

Actinomycosis (Lumpy Jaw) and Actinobacillosis (Wooden Tongue)

Signs. Actinomycosis is a disease characterized by a very hard swelling of the bony tissue about the head, usually the jaw. An infection of the bone develops gradually (osteomyelitis). It starts out as a painless swelling of the jaw, upper or lower. By the time the swelling is large enough to notice, it is difficult to treat. The swelling may break through the skin, discharging pus and a sticky honeylike fluid containing little white granules. The eruption actually forms a sinus tract, spreading the organism back into the surrounding area.

Actinobacillosis is characterized by an attack on the tissues of the throat and tongue. This is an infectious disease that causes inflammation of the tongue, usually the inability to eat, excessive salivation, and a chewing motion of the tongue. The tongue will feel hard and swollen, especially around the base; ulcers may appear along the edge; and movement of the tongue from side to side by the observer causes pain. Later the tongue becomes shrunken and immobile. There may be swelling of the lymph nodes around the area. These nodes may rupture and exude pus.

Cause. *Actinomycosis bovis* is the microorganism that causes actinomycosis (lumpy jaw). *Actinobacillus* is the microorganism that causes actinobacillosis (wooden tongue).

Prevention. The best preventative is to eliminate rough, coarse feeds or any other objects that cattle might pick up, and, by chewing, injure the lining of their mouths. And remove infected animals from the herd as soon as possible.

Transmission. The organism is allowed entry into the body because of wounds to the lining of the mouth caused by eating sharp objects such as rough hay or feeds containing awns, trash, or wire. The organism is actually injected through the damaged area around the gums and teeth to create the condition.

Treatment. Iodides are used as a treatment for both actinomycosis and actinobacillosis. Usually, sodium iodide is used at the rate of 1 gram per 25 to 30 lb of body weight given intravenously as a 10% solution. The solution is repeated in 10 to 14 days. Actinomycosis will usually only be arrested; that is, the disease is stopped, but the permanent disfigurement always remains in the form of bony swellings.

Some antibiotics such as tetracyclines may be helpful as a treatment.

Shipping Fever Complex (Hemorrhagic Septicemia)

Signs. If an animal has just undergone the stress of castration, vaccination, dehorning, weaning, working, perhaps has been chilled or wet, or especially if it has been moved a considerable distance to a new location, this animal is most likely to develop Shipping Fever. A sudden high temperature of 104 to 106° F, depression, going off feed, difficult breathing, coughing, runny nose and eyes, unthrifty appearance, and diarrhea characterize the disease. The animal is the picture of what a sick animal is expected to look like. It may die within three weeks or may recover, but it never does well in a feed-lot situation.

Cause. Stress along with an overriding effect from bacterial infection, especially the *Pasteurella multocida* organism, causes the disease, but there may be a multitude of organisms involved in this complex disorder generally brought on by rough handling and shipping long distances.

Prevention. A preconditioning program has been developed through research that has been fairly effective. Since it is known that stress is the major contributing factor, this part of the complex is reduced by not doing all of the jobs such as weaning, dehorning, castration, etc., at one time. The cattle are worked moderately and with as little jousting around as possible through a series of jobs that need to be done over a period of time. The animals are thus given time to adjust, thereby reducing the shock to the system that apparently allows the organisms to gain a foothold.

Transmission. The mode of transmission is not fully understood, but the disease is thought to be transmittable from one animal to another through contact, feed, or drinking water. However, it should be emphasized again that stress is the precipitating factor.

Treatment. High levels of antibiotics such as penicillin, streptomycin, tetracycline, and tylocin, combined with steroid therapy, are most often used. Vitamin injections are also used as a supportive therapy.

Sick animals should be isolated from the herd, kept warm and dry if possible, and treated the same as if they had pneumonia.

Eye Problems

Pinkeye (Infectious Keratitis)

Signs. General signs are a reddening of the membranes of the eye with excessive tears, pain when exposed to light, and a clouding of the cornea. The cornea may be ulcerated and sometimes covered with a cloudy, whitish film that has a perforation in it. This may lead to temporary or permanent blindness or loss of the eyeball. The course of the infection may run from 4 to 8 weeks or longer.

Pinkeye rarely causes death in cattle; however, the loss of weight due to reluctance to forage for feed in the bright sunlight results in losses of $25 to $50 per calf in many instances and up to a 50% decrease in milk production in dairy cows. The disease appears suddenly and spreads rapidly. Young animals are more susceptible than older ones. Large numbers of flies are almost always associated with the disease.

Cause. At one time it was believed that the bacterium *Morexella bovis* was the sole cause of pinkeye. However it is now known that the disease is a complex situation involving several factors in addition to the bacterial organism.

The most frequently involved causes are:

1. *Morexella bovis*, plus an irritation such as bright sunlight, dust, wind, flies, or weed seed. The National Animal Disease Center at Ames, Iowa, has reproduced pinkeye experimentally in calves with a combination of ultraviolet light and the *Morexella bovis* organism. This work demonstrates the importance of the role of light and also proves that not only white-faced cattle but others as well are susceptible to the disease. The disease is more common in Hereford cattle because the reflection of light from the white unpigmented face produces more irritation and increases susceptibility to pinkeye.

2. IBR Virus—This virus is now known to be one of the contributing factors in some forms of pinkeye development. When IBR has been found to be involved, it has been more common in the fall and winter than in the summer. It is not as frequently involved as ultraviolet light and other irritations to the eye.

3. Ultraviolet light is more involved than previously thought. It is now known that this light irritation, along with a virus or bacterium, is the major factor involved in precipitating pinkeye.

4. Phenothiazine, a worming compound that sometimes in an overdose creates sensitivity to light. Photosensitization results, thus lowering the resistance to pinkeye.

5. Marginal amounts of vitamin A—Since this vitamin is involved in eyesight, it is easy to see how a deficiency of vitamin A could be a contributing factor to a lower resistance.

Prevention. Management must be directed toward influencing the means of transmission, mainly flies, including face flies. The control of flies, insects, dust, and the clipping of pastures to reduce irritation from grass and weed seed are important. Providing shaded areas to reduce irritation from ultraviolet light is also extremely helpful.

Vaccines to prevent pinkeye have little effectiveness. Management is the only major preventive. Supportive treatment may be in the form of vitamin A injections at the rate of 3 to 6 cc injected twice a year and vaccination on a 6 to 12 month schedule for IBR to reduce the possibility of inflammation of the eye from the virus that causes IBR.

Transmission. Dry, dusty conditions, bright sunlight, and feeding in tall grass are common in many of the outbreaks. It is known that flies most probably are the carriers, transmitting the disease from one cow to another.

Treatment. Treatment is difficult but recent developments have proven to be very effective. The various treatments being used follow:

1. Ophthalmic sprays—An anesthetic plus a dye to act as a filter for some of the sun's rays is sprayed directly into the eye. Most of these products come in self-contained and pressurized cans. They are most effective if applied daily.

2. Ophthalmic ointment and drops—A 5% solution of boric acid as an eyewash and a 2% solution of mercurochrome ointment can be used with good results. Ophthalmic ointments also are available, providing relief from pain and a soothing lubrication.

3. Cauterization—Silver nitrate used in a $1\frac{1}{2}$% aqueous solution, 5 to 10 drops in each eye, two treatments given 4 days apart, has proven effective. In more advanced cases, a 5% solution, 3 to 5 drops in the affected eye, once daily for 3 to 5 days, has been beneficial.

4. Suturing of eyelids—In severe cases the eyelids are sutured together. This should only be done by professionals. The technique keeps the eyes closed, bathed in tears, and shuts out irritants and sunlight. Tears have some antibacterial action to hasten healing. Frequently an antibiotic steroid injection is also employed at this time to promote healing and reduce inflammation.

5. Eye patches—Affected eyes may be covered by a patch that is kept in place by an adhesive for 1 to 3 weeks before falling off. The type of adhesive used will determine the length of time the eyes may be kept sealed. This shuts out sunlight and other irritants and allows for faster healing.

Although only one eye may be affected, it is recommended that both eyes be treated because it is known that both eyes usually contain the *Morexella bovis* organism. Of course, a patch or suturing should be used only on the clinically infected eye.

Cancer Eye

Signs. Cancer eye is a chronic eye problem most commonly encountered in Herefords. The white hair and light-colored pigment around the eye lead to an irritation in that area and a chronic sunburn. These factors may not be directly related to cancer eye, but the irritation is very commonly noted prior to the development of cancer eye. A small, wartlike growth on the eyelid, third eyelid, and eyeball is often seen. The growth may get as large as a softball, and any injury often produces bleeding. It can progress to involve the whole eye or the bones around the eye. Usually tears will be discharged and there will be considerable drainage. The cancer can spread to the lungs and other parts of the body, eventually causing death.

Cause. The cause is thought to be a virus.

Transmission. Cancer eye is transmitted in unknown ways. The condition is also possibly abetted by sunlight irritation.

Treatment. If caught early in its development, cancer eye can be treated by freezing and removing the affected area or surgically excising the area. This operation is sometimes successful in eliminating the growth, but the cancer very often returns no matter how it is removed. At times the whole eye may have to be removed. After the cancer invades the bony tissue and spreads to the lungs, no treatment will be effective, and the animal will probably be condemned on the slaughter floor. For this reason, unless the animal is very valuable, it is generally best to mark it for slaughter at early stages rather than risk the low percentage of success in surgical treatment.

Foreign Bodies, Ulceration, Keratitis

Signs. The signs include red, swollen, and irritated eyes. Tears are discharged. A severe mechanical injury may cause ulcerations in the eye or an actual puncture of eye tissue.

Cause. Causes are dust, sticks, nails, wire, and any foreign matter that irritates. Some actual punctures may occur, leading to ulceration.

Prevention. Prevention involves proper cleanliness and ventilation.

Transmission. Transmission is strictly mechanical.

Treatment. Remove any foreign body from the eye, being careful to get all of it. You can flush out the eye with plain water, but boric acid eyewash is preferred. If there is an ulcer or puncture in the eye, a systemic antibiotic should be given and treatment continued periodically with an ophthalmic ointment until the condition is eliminated. If the problem is just an irritation from small matter like dust, just an eyewash should be sufficient without further treatment.

BVD (Bovine Virus Diarrhea)

Signs. Signs are diarrhea, high temperature, tear discharges from the eye, and nasal discharge. Erosions or sores in the mouth occur in about 80% of the cases. This disease occurs mostly in the winter, and range or housed cattle are affected equally. Three forms are recognized:

1. Acute form—The acute form is characterized by high fever, sudden diarrhea, decreased milk production, and dehydration. Usually about the third day the diarrhea becomes profuse, watery, and foul-smelling. About the fourth day, lesions appear in the mouth, which may develop into ulcers, producing a stringy salivation. There is a hacking, dry, nonproductive cough and heavy difficult breathing. The muzzle may be crusty and the eyes may discharge tears. The cornea may appear gray or clouded.

This disease is characterized by a "mummy-dummy" syndrome. A pregnant cow that is affected early in her gestation may give birth to a mummified fetus (mummy). In later stages of gestation, the fetus may be stillborn or muscularly uncoordinated (dummy). The calf often remains unhealthy, rough-haired, lame with dermatitis (lesions) between the toes, and exhibits signs of damage to the central nervous system.

The acute form affects nearly 100% of all cattle exposed but is fatal in only 4 to 8% of the cases. There is an incubation period of 1 to 3 weeks from exposure to outbreak.

2. Mild form—The mild form has a low infection rate of 2 to 5% but is fatal in 90% of the cases. Diarrhea lasts 15 to 20 days, causes severe dehydration, secondary infections, and death.

3. Chronic form—The chronic form applies to survivors of the acute form that remain "poor doers" over a long period of time. Animals 8 months to 2 years are characteristically affected. There may be some lameness along with unthriftiness. These signs are quite similar and may be confused with some of the following conditions: Rinderpest (not found in the United States), Vesicular stomatitis (causes lesions on lips but occurs mostly in insect seasons rather than the winter as BVD does), blue tongue, malignant catarrhal fever, salmonella, and several acute poisoning cases that cause similar reactions.

Diagnosis to distinguish for sure what disease you are dealing with is done through serology: taking paired blood samples 2 to 3 weeks apart and comparing the titer change (measurement of immune response to a particular disease organism by a particular individual animal). The titer usually increases after exposure to an organism.

Cause. The cause is a virus that affects mostly cattle, sporadic in occurrence.

Prevention. Vaccination can be given in endemic areas, although several precautions should be taken: pregnant animals should not be vaccinated; bulls should not be vaccinated normally, although it is sometimes recommended in severe outbreaks; the vaccine should not be given to nursing calves until after 4 months of age; calves vaccinated at less than 8 months of age should be revaccinated at 14 to 16 months.

Transmission. Transmission is directly from one animal to another.

Treatment. Broad-spectrum antibiotics, astringents, and electrolytes to combat dehydration, and kaolin or pectin solutions to coat the stomach are recommended.

Tuberculosis

Signs. Animals usually appear normal but start losing weight and get progressively weaker. The pulmonary type of disease produces a cough that may be heard by squeezing on the throat. There may also be wheezing. The lungs in a post-mortem inspection may show nodules (little lumps) throughout.

Mastitis is commonly associated with tuberculosis, but the milk in this case looks normal, although the bag is swollen and hard. Cattle should be tested before milking.

Many types of tuberculosis affect cattle. Although the pulmonary type is most commonly recognized by the layman, the reproductive organs, uterus, lymph nodes, liver, tonsils, and intestines are also often affected.

Cause. The cause is a bacterium, *Mycobacterium bovis*.

Prevention. There is no prevention, except to test and destroy. This disease used to be very prevalent in the 1930s in the United States. Interstate or foreign markets have now made it mandatory for negative tests to be verified before shipping, and these regulations have almost eradicated the disease from this country.

Transmission. Inhalation is the most common method of transmitting the highly contagious organism, which is passed on in manure and may remain viable for 6 to 8 weeks. Urine, milk, and stagnant water may also harbor the organism. Cases have been reported of the bacterium remaining viable in the water source for up to 18 days after an infected animal drank from it.

Milking machines were also formerly a common means of transmitting tuberculosis in the milking shed.

Treatment. There is no prescribed treatment. Government regulations require that the tuberculin test be given. Tuberculin is a substance taken from the cultured preparation of *M. bovis*. This tuberculin is injected intradermally into the fold of the tail, and 72 hours later the area of the injection is palpated for any enlargement. All positive reactors are condemned by the government and are destroyed.

Cancer (Neoplasia Malignant Lymphoma)

Signs. Most people don't think about cancer in cattle until they see the classical form. The most common description by the layman to the veterinarian is, "Doc, she's got lumps all over her." These lumps will be around the throat, the flank area, on the back legs just above the knee on the outer side, and at the point of the shoulder. These lumps are the lymph glands that are affected and swollen due to cancer. The animal will also be emaciated and unthrifty. If only one node or lump is seen, this may be just an abscess and is relatively unimportant. If lumps are seen all over, and they persist, it is probably cancer.

The external type is the only one that you can see. However, a more sinister type lurks unseen and may be characterized by degeneration or a "wasting disease" and is difficult to diagnose even by a veterinarian, except in a post-mortem inspection. This inner cancer may affect the intestinal tract, produce a persistent cough, and it may also affect the liver, spleen, or heart muscle. The uterus or ovaries can also become cancerous, causing a failure to conceive.

Cause. Cause is unknown. Thought to be caused by a virus.

Prevention. There is no known means of prevention.

Transmission. Method of transmission is unknown.

Treatment.   Most forms are not treatable and there is no known cure. However, certain forms of skin cancer can be removed surgically. There is a tumorous growth in the form of a big knot on the skin known as a *neurofibroma*, which is generally not dangerous to the patient. Although it may be scraped and bleeding, quite often it is benign (nonmalignant) and can be surgically removed without too much concern.

Salmonellosis (Paratyphoid)

Signs.   There are three syndromes (types) of salmonellosis.

1. Septicemia—This infection is basically seen in newborn calves. They exhibit depression, appear dull and uncoordinated, and will run a high fever. Death generally occurs within 24 hours.

2. Acute intestinal form—This form occurs mostly in adults. Symptoms include fever and watery diarrhea. The fever disappears with the onset of diarrhea. Strings of mucus appear in the fecal matter, caused by a sloughing of the lining of the intestine. Affected animals don't eat but drink lots of water. There is an obvious abdominal pain, creating a "tucked up" position. There is generally dehydration, debilitation, and "dying with diarrhea." Pregnant animals abort, and mortality in general is about 75% for all victims.

3. Chronic intestinal form—This form affects adults also. The main symptom is a wasting away with uncontrollable diarrhea.

Cause.   Microscopic organisms are the cause. Several species of *Salmonella* organisms are the invading factor.

Prevention.   Isolation is the key. "Carriers" are often found in a herd that is affected by the disease; they get over it but remain spreaders of the organism thereafter. Prolonged treatment with neomycin or nitrofurazone is required to get rid of the bug from affected cattle. A vaccine is available but is not recommended as routine procedure. There is some question as to the effectiveness of the vaccine. The cheapest way is simply to cull out affected animals.

Transmission.   The main route of transmission of the infection is through wild animals or birds, which cannot be controlled, and "carriers" (those animals that recover develop immunity, but spread the organism to nonimmune cattle) that can be controlled. The carriers remain active as a potential hazard of spreading the organism for 3 to 4 months. The organism is transmitted mainly by ingestion of organic materials. In the past, when this country imported large quantities of unsteamed bone meal, it was found that almost 70% of this feed stuff was contaminated with the organism. Since then, laws have been passed requiring steaming of the bone meal to kill the organism. Wildlife remains the chief problem today, as uncontrolled carriers.

Treatment.   Sulfa drugs or antibiotics such as streptomycin, tetracycline, or neomycin are recommended. Supportive treatment for dehydration is given intraperitoneally or intravenously, along with vitamin therapy. Kaolin and pectin should be given to coat the intestines for relief.

Warts

Signs. Any solid growth from the skin having a horny appearance, or any flat dry or cauliflower-shaped protuberance with no hair-growth, is generally classified as a wart. There may be from 1 to 1000 such growths on affected animals.

Cause. A virus is the cause.

Prevention. Avoid direct contact between animals affected with warts and those unaffected.

Transmission. The virus invades the skin through small breaks. It has been spread experimentally by making injections from wart cultures to prove that the disease can be spread.

Treatment. There is a commercial vaccine that can be given as an initial injection for an animal exhibiting warts. A period of 2 to 3 weeks is allowed to lapse after the first injection, and then the injection is repeated. Recovery requires 3 to 6 weeks or longer.

Anaplasmosis

Anaplasmosis is a protozoan disease of cattle that destroys red blood cells and causes anemia and death.

Signs. The most common form of anaplasmosis is a subacute form, which means that the disease does not develop very quickly. The body temperature rises slowly, a poor appetite is exhibited, and the emaciation progresses. There is a slight jaundice or a yellowing of the pink membranes, creating a very pale, anemic victim. Anemia is one of the main clinical diagnostic characteristics of anaplasmosis. The disease may progress to a conclusion anywhere from 2 days to 2 weeks. Calves undergo mild discomfort with few or no deaths occurring. Yearling cattle usually appear sicker but recover. Cattle over 2 years of age are most severely affected, with 20 to 50% death losses. Pregnant cows will abort. All affected cattle will exhibit signs of hyperexcitability and may attack their attendants just before they die. Some cattle do recover, but they will experience bouts of anemia off and on for several months.

The acute or peracute form is characterized by high temperature, anemia, difficult calving, and death within 24 hours. A "jugular pulse" is very common. The anemia makes the heart beat so hard that the pulse can be seen at the jugular vein area of the throat.

Cause. The cause is a small protozoan, *Anaplasma marginale*. This microscopic organism attaches itself to the red blood cells, causing their rupture. Therefore oxygen is not carried sufficiently through the bloodstream, and death occurs through internal suffocation. This has been characterized as "bleeding to death without bleeding."

Prevention.   Back rubbers and spray to keep down infestation of ticks, flies, and insects are methods of prevention. It is also important that the vaccinating needles be sterilized between each use to prevent spread of the disease.

Vaccination has been recommended in the past, which gives good immunity against the disease; but it is not always recommended because of a curious and distressing situation that sometimes arises the year following an outbreak of anaplasmosis and immunization for it. Some immunized cows that were protected against anaplasmosis give birth to healthy calves. These calves then die suddenly within days of birth, although the cow is not affected. The problem, called *neonatal isoerythrolysis*, has been defined as a genetic rarity. Anaplasmosis vaccine is made from the red blood cells of donor animals. The problem starts if there is a factor in the genetic makeup of the vaccinated cow that causes her to produce antibodies in reaction to the red blood cells of the vaccine. After the birth of a calf, these antibodies are found in the colostrum milk. If the calf is genetically sensitive to the antibodies when it nurses, the antibodies that are consumed destroy the calf's red blood cells, causing jaundice and death.

The problem almost always appears to affect the most vigorous and healthy calves because they nurse so rapidly after birth and thus consume the antibodies at the most potent level. If the cow is milked completely of the colostrum milk soon after birth and before the calf nurses, the level of antibodies will be sufficiently reduced and will possibly help prevent a reaction in the calf.

In vaccinated cattle, a calf mortality rate as high as 30% might be anticipated. Because the condition involves genetics, changing bulls after an outbreak of anaplasmosis and vaccination has been found to be somewhat effective due to dilution of the genetic makeup that apparently lowers the sensitivity of antibody reaction.

The condition appears worse in Charolais cattle due to closer inbreeding practices, because of fewer animals available as compared to other breeds. However, the situation has occurred in all breeds and in crossbreeds.

For these reasons, field evidence suggests that vaccinating brood cows for anaplasmosis can be a calculated risk. Protective benefits must be weighed against this risk. As always, a veterinarian should be consulted before a final decision is made.

Transmission.   Insect vectors or dirty needles and dehorning instruments are the primary causes of transmission. These instruments should be disinfected between use on each animal. Insects should be controlled.

Treatment.   Broad-spectrum antibiotics such as tetracycline are recommended. Three to 5 mg per pound of body weight are given daily for 3 days. For a very valuable animal, massive blood transfusions may be advisable.

The affected cattle should be handled with care so as to create as little stress as possible because extra excitement aggravates the condition. Treatment of the whole herd with injections of tetracycline has eliminated the disease from the herd. Tetracycline has also been added to the feed for 30 days, and this has proved quite effective.

Ringworm

A fungus causes ringworm in cattle, and although ringworm is more common in calves, all ages of cattle may be affected. The hair in the infected area breaks off, falls out, and by 2 to 3 months after infection, round, thickened circles are observed, with the hair generally denuded inside the ring. The disease is more commonly seen during the winter months in stabled animals; however, it can occur at any time of the year.

To treat ringworm the crusts must be removed first. This is easily done with a brush and mild soap. The condition responds well to local applications of any fungicidal material, but treatment for about 2 weeks on a daily basis is generally required to clear up the condition. Daily applications of a mixture of equal parts tincture of iodine and glycerin make a good fungicide treatment. Ringworm is contagious for the human being, and rubber gloves should be worn when treating affected animals.

Foot Rot (Infectious Pododermatitis, "Foul Claw")

Dairymen, cattlemen, and feed-lot operators are aware of the problem of foot rot. This disease causes a great economic loss because of reduced weight-gaining ability and a lowering of milk production. Only one animal may be affected or as many as 80% of the herd can be afflicted.

Signs. Inflammation of the foot brought about by an injury produces severe swelling and extreme pain of the feet. This disease is probably responsible for 40 to 60% of all the diseases of the bovine foot. Over 60% of the problems in the hind feet are foot rot. The reddened swelling between the toes and at the bulb of the heel sometimes extends up the legs. In more chronic cases, a smelly discharge may occur. Cattle appear lame in one, two, three, or all four feet; they hold up or raise a foot often, are reluctant to move, have a hobbling gait, loss of appetite, and decrease in milk production. Severe illness or death can occur in prolonged cases, although this is very rare.

Cause. Recent research from the University of Missouri indicates that *Spherophorous necrophorous* and *Bacteroides melaninogenicus* are the predominant bacteria that cause foot rot. However, it is known that many other organisms are probably involved, including viruses.

In most cases these organisms are only a secondary infection brought about by a traumatic injury to the foot from impact with stones, frozen mud, and foreign bodies such as nails, wire, etc.

In some cases, the organisms progress from the foot into the veins and directly to the lungs and liver, where they may cause abscesses.

Prevention. A high incidence of foot rot occurs in muddy, filthy lots, particularly where the foot can be easily injured. Reducing excessive moisture by good drainage is a good start in preventive management. Lime or phosphate fertilizer on the area where animals stand also promotes drying of the feet and serves to prevent the condition.

In the case of dairy cattle, foot baths are often used containing copper sulfate solution, formaldehyde solution, or air-slaked lime. An old standard treatment of 1 lb of copper sulfate to a gallon of water placed in a foot bath is still considered adequate. Many feeders have modified this system by placing kerosene on top to prevent freezing and sand on the bottom to prevent slipping.

In feed-lot operations, this treatment is not practical; so preventive measures include the feeding of 50 mg of organic iodine compounds per head per day in the feed or salt, fed continuously. Feeding 500 mg in the feed per head per day for 8 to 10 days has also been thought to be effective.

Treatment. Lame animals should have their feet examined for foreign particles first. Provided no wires, nails, etc., are found, the drugs of choice are penicillin, penicillin dihydrostreptomycin combinations, or the oxytetracyclines. Sulfonamides, at one grain per pound of body weight, have also been used successfully. Chlortetracycline (Aureomycin) as a feed additive may be used for treatment on a herd basis. To be effective, the minimum dose for calves should be at least 1 gm per animal per day, and more than that for larger animals. All treatments should be under the direction of a veterinarian.

Rabies

Rabies is a worldwide problem except for special places like Australia and New Zealand where it has never existed. Sweden, Norway, France, Switzerland, Great Britain, Japan, and a few other nations have eliminated the disease through systematic eradication of carriers.

In other countries of the world, rabies is still a very real problem and is not restricted to dogs and cats. In nature, it is transmitted from animal to animal by means of a bite introducing a virus carried in the saliva.

Signs. In cattle the disease takes on the nature of the "furious rabies" form, which is an excitative phase. Cattle become irrational and aggressively vicious. They appear very alert or anxious, and have dilated pupils. A slight noise or any movement invites attack and the instinctive desire to charge. Cattle rarely live beyond 10 days after the initial signs appear.

Cause. The cause is a virus bringing on an acute encephalomyelitis (an attack on the central nervous system), which affects the brain. Rabid foxes and skunks are responsible for most pasture cattle losses. Skunks are the most dangerous carriers for dairy cattle. They have been known to attack dairy cows in barns. A typical clinical sign in cattle is bellowing of a nature that is not soon forgotten once it is experienced.

In South America, Trinidad, Central America, and Mexico, the vampire bat is a serious threat to the spread of rabies to cattle. These bats live solely off the blood of warmblooded mammals, and cattle are the most frequent victims.

Prevention.   Prevention methods involve controlling the population of wildlife carriers, including foxes, skunks, and bats, by an official trapping and poisoning program. There are vaccines available for cattle in areas where outbreaks are known to be imminent because of an outbreak of rabies among the wildlife population.

Treatment.   There is no known treatment.

Pseudorabies (Aujeszky's Disease, "Mad Itch")

Pseudorabies is a frequently fatal disease affecting most species of domestic and wild animals. In cattle, severe itching and self-mutilation are seen. The disease is transmitted mostly through swine, but the itching and self-mutilation are rarely seen in hogs.

The disease was first recognized as a disease in cattle and dogs in Hungary by Aujeszky in 1902. It soon became evident, however, that swine were the natural hosts of the virus, and that the condition caused fatalities also in young pigs (see swine section).

Signs.   Pseudorabies in cattle is quite different from the disease in swine. Affected animals (cattle) lick the hair on some part of their body, and a few hours later begin violent rubbing against any solid objects. The skin becomes raw and swollen, producing an exudate. The animal frantically bites and gnaws at the skin lesions, thus exhibiting the signs of a "mad itch." Cattle become progressively weak, lapse into a coma, and die 18 to 36 hours after the first evidence of the disease.

Cause.   A virus of the herpes group is the cause. The disease is widely prevalent in swine, where it often goes unnoticed until it spreads to cattle. In most instances mature swine show only a mild elevation in temperature when infected with the virus and develop an immunity, but thereafter serve as a host to spread the disease to cattle and other animals (see swine section). Sheep, cats, dogs, skunks, foxes, raccoons, opossums, and possibly rodents also are infected in outbreaks. Humans are not affected by the virus but can physically carry it from one farm or livestock facility to another.

Prevention.   The practice of running cattle with pigs should be avoided, particularly in those areas where outbreaks have occurred. Disposal of young pigs suspected of dying of the disease should be by deep burial and lime coverage or by cremation. Check with your local veterinarian or state or federal officials to determine if pseudorabies has been diagnosed in the area. If it has, protect your cattle from stray dogs, keep cats off premises, and be on the lookout for wildlife carriers.

A licensed pseudorabies vaccine is available through veterinarians for use on swine only. Under no circumstances is it to be used on cattle.

Treatment. There is no treatment. Prevention through proper control of animal hosts, especially swine, appears to be the best hope for controlling the disease in cattle.

DIGESTIVE DISORDERS

Digestive disorders will be discussed in the following manner: rumenstasus and rumenitis will be grouped together since they are quite similar digestive disorders, but will be separated to identify the differences between the two. Other disorders caused by twisting of the intestinal tract, ingestion of foreign objects, or natural chemical reactions will include displaced abomasum, hardware disease, and bloat. The opposite reactions of constipation and scours will also be discussed. Scours are so important that distinctions are made among the several types of digestive disorders that can cause them. These disorders are Johne's disease, parasitism, and food-induced scours. In addition, a general discussion summarizing the scour problem, regardless of cause, will be included. Finally, a related problem often associated with severe digestive disorders—prolapsed rectum—will be discussed.

Rumenstasis and Rumenitis

Signs. Rumenstasis and rumenitis are both characterized by a general overall distressed appearance. There is usually abdominal cramping, arched back, abdominal pain, a "tucked up" appearance, kicking at the abdomen, and bellowing.

If bloat accompanies the disorder, there could also be respiratory problems. Bloat commonly accompanies both rumenstasis and rumenitis.

Cause. Rumenstasis is due to an overloading of the digestive system, particularly the rumen. This is caused by a severe impaction from heavy, dry roughage, weeds, and hard-to-digest materials. (See explanation concerning the rumen outlined in Chapter 4.)

This impaction may build up very slowly. At first there will be no sign other than a loss of weight. The key point to remember in this disorder is that the rumen muscle completely ceases to function, so that there are no contractions of this compartment to allow passage of food on through to the abomasum, or true stomach.

Another cause of this condition could be a killing off of the microflora in the rumen. If these microflora, or rumen bacteria, have died off, the normal function of the rumen could cease, bringing on the condition. This occasionally happens for unknown reasons, but is suspected to occur more often due to prolonged antibiotic therapy. A lack of bacteria adds to the dryness. The condition compounds due to a lack of storage capacity, and the rumen is filled to the point that it ceases its normal function.

Treatment. The first step is to determine if the cause is from the feed ingested or the microflora being killed out. If feed problems exist, some ration modification is in order. If microflora are dead, the source of the killing agent should be traced and adjustments made. In either case, the compaction should be relieved as soon as possible by cleaning out the material by forcing the animal to drink lots of fluids. Plain water can be used to drench the animal and get the material moving. Mineral oil has been given also in combination with water therapy to make a slicker material allowing easier passage. If the condition has been caused simply by feed conditions, this will be all that is necessary in the way of treatment.

However, if the bacteria have been killed, or if that possibility is suspected, the second step is to replace the bacteria with materials such as Lactinex, which can be purchased at any drugstore. This is used in human nutrition for replacing bacteria needed by babies. Another source of bacteria is simply to pick up a gallon or two of rumen material from a local slaughterhouse, just as it comes from the slaughtered animal. Use a stomach tube to drench the sick animal with these rumen bacteria in order to reinoculate the rumen.

If antibiotic therapy was not responsible for the lack of bacteria, the third step is to make use of broad-spectrum antibiotics during or shortly after the therapy begins. The reason for this is that the impacted material probably has produced some toxic substance that could cause infections elsewhere. This is just a precautionary measure.

Rumenitis. Rumenitis, or ulceration of the rumen wall, affects young calves that have come off of a pasture directly to the feed lot to high-concentrate rations. There are no specific symptoms, although the calves exhibit poor conversion and never appear to do very well on their feed. Rumenitis is a very common condition. The disorder is an erosion of the lining of the rumen with an ulceration surrounding the eroded area. The cause is excessive ingestion of feeds rich in starch or sugars, primarily grains or high-concentrate rations. This condition usually is seen only on the slaughterhouse floor in the form of ulcerated areas of the rumen and occasionally liver abscesses. However, evidence found when tracing back the history of calves coming from pasture to feed lot has indicated that the condition is quite common, even though few outward signs exist.

Prevention of both Rumenstasis and Rumenitis. Addition of roughage to the ration is extremely valuable in restoring proper rumen condition. In the event this is not practical in certain feed-lot operations, low-level antibiotics should be fed throughout the course of the feeding period.

Displaced Abomasum

Signs. (See Chapter 4 for a thorough discussion on location and function of the abomasum.) As the name of the disorder implies, the abomasum or true stomach is displaced from its regular position. Normally, the abomasum is located in the lower-right abdominal wall. Some peculiar condition may cause it to shift to the left side. It "flips" under the rumen, resulting in a twist that impedes the passage of food through the digestive system. This happens occasionally after parturition. It is more common in dairy cattle that are fed heavy grain in late stages of pregnancy, than in beef cattle.

The key signs are a decrease in appetite, abdominal pain, and distension of the abdominal cavity. The temperature is elevated to 103 to 104° F. There is a rapid heartbeat; after the acute form passes, the heartbeat returns to normal. Cattle may become very particular as to what they eat, refusing everything but dry hay. Milk production is decreased and body-weight losses occur.

Prevention. There really is no way to prevent this condition. Perhaps the best precaution is not to feed cattle too heavily just before parturition.

Treatment. When this condition is suspected by experienced stockmen or veterinarians, the best technique is usually to starve the animal for a couple of days and then possibly try something like a "rolling technique." The animal is cast on its side, rolled quickly to the right, and then stopped in an abrupt motion, to hopefully "untwist" the abomasum.

Several other "old farmers'" remedies have been tried such as getting cattle to jump ditches and other types of acrobatics. However, the rolling technique appears to have the best possibilities. If these techniques fail, surgical correction is required.

Hardware Disease

Signs. The condition known as *hardware disease* involves the reticulum (second stomach, see Chapter 4) and a foreign body. Generally, the reticulum acts as a trap for foreign objects, but occasionally a problem arises that cannot be handled successfully. A sharp metallic object, for instance, could cause irritation and could even perforate the reticulum. Either of these conditions can create hardware disease.

The diaphragm is a thin muscle sheath that separates the abdominal cavity from the thoracic cavity in the immediate vicinity of the reticulum. The heart lies just in front of the reticulum. A metallic object that is causing irritation in the reticulum can create a condition that irritates the membrane, or sac, of the heart. If this situation becomes worse, a perforation can occur, creating inflammation of the sac surrounding the heart (pericarditis) and congestive heart failure, resulting in death.

In the event the perforating agent does not go into the heart, it could go into the abdominal cavity, creating a leakage of rumen fluids and bringing on a fatally severe inflammation of a thin membrane surrounding the stomachs (peritonitis), or simply leaking toxic materials into the abdominal cavity, which can also cause death.

A sharp object in the reticulum can also travel toward the lung cavity. In this case, it creates a condition almost identical with pneumonia.

It can readily be seen that the lungs, abdominal cavity, or heart, all vital areas, could be severely affected by this disorder.

The outward signs are many and varied. An animal suddenly develops a lack of appetite, a drop in milk production, abdominal pain, and/or a slowness in movement. A characteristic symptom is that when animals walk downhill, they tend to grunt because of the pressure applied on the heart. They prefer to stand still, have a "tucked up" appearance, urinate frequently, and their normal body functions may be impaired. They show obvious pain on occasions, and the grunting sound may accompany the pain symptom. The temperature is slightly elevated, there may be shallow breathing, the pulse is increased, and often an animal kicks at its belly to indicate some type of pain.

Cause. The cause of hardware disease is debris such as nails, screws, wire, and many other forms of trash often found in a pasture. This type of debris quite often appears because the hay has been baled along highways, railroads, etc. Occasionally, metallic objects will fall into the feed and create the problem. Cattle are not selective as to what they eat; so this condition is a very real threat whenever poor management practices permit the existence of such objects in hay operations and feed mills.

Prevention. In the case of the average farmer and rancher, good housekeeping methods are in order to assure a lack of temptation for cattle to eat wire, nails, and other trash.

Feed mills have installed magnets to remove the contaminants from feeds and have done an excellent job in keeping the problem to a minimum.

Treatment. This disorder can possibly heal of its own accord. Mild cases have been known to be corrected simply by immobilization, letting the animal remain still so that the ingested object "quits working," allowing the body to build up natural defenses around it. The front feet may be elevated on a platform on occasions to allow some relief and better healing. The main method is to reduce feed intake for at least 2 weeks and to force the animal to swallow a commercially available magnet, which will fall into the reticulum and attract the object to reverse its path. Recovery occasionally is so dramatic that the cattleman is tempted to stop treatment in less than 2 weeks. This should not be done. Keep the feed intake reduced for a full 2 weeks, and administer antibiotics during this period of time to control possible infection.

Occasionally, surgical removal of the object is justified in the case of a very valuable animal. It might be noted that surgical removal has a much higher percentage of recovery than the other methods discussed.

Bloat

Signs. The rumen and reticulum are both overdistended in this disorder because of gas created internally due to fermentation that occurs rapidly in some incompletely understood way involving the digestive process. This gas may be mixed with, or separated from, the fluid contents. The gas that is mixed with the fluid contents is trapped in tiny bubbles and is referred to as the "frothy" type. This is the most dangerous kind because the individual bubbles must be burst to relieve the stress. Pressure from the other kind, the "gaseous" type, is much easier to reduce. In either case, there is a tremendous rapid distension. All of this occurs on the left side of the animal in the early stages of bloat. In the later stages, the bloat will be so thorough that it will be difficult to tell which side is bloated. But generally, looking from the rear, the left side will show much more than the right. This bloat may occur within 10 to 15 minutes. Cattle move about, kick, roll, breathe heavily, salivate, vomit, have their tongue hanging out, exhibit diarrhea, often collapse, and often die.

Cause. Certain feeds or an interruption of the natural digestive process brings on the condition. In general, there is a frothing or foaming of digestive contents. A variation in saliva, gastric juices, or bacterial content changes the viscosity of rumen fluids, creating the condition.

There are some animals known as *chronic bloaters* that do not die from bloat but contract it so often as to be a worry to the owner. These animals generally are "poor doers"; they cannot be permanently cured and should be culled.

There is an acute form of bloat that causes great distress to the animal and difficult breathing; it brings pressure on the heart and lungs, causing suffocation. The animal dies simply from a lack of oxygen. This disease is very often brought on by grazing on legume and wheat pastures and is very common in alfalfa and clover pasturage, particularly during the succulent rapid growth that occurs in the early spring. It is also associated with high-nitrogen fertilization of pastures. There is some evidence that genetic susceptibility is a factor in animals that bloat.

There is also a condition known as *secondary bloat*, caused by something that blocks the esophagus. This could be a growth or it could be a foreign object. This type of bloat usually occurs in young animals and is very complicated. It can be a real mystery sometimes because nothing shows up in the autopsy.

Prevention. Protein blocks with the antifermenting agents mixed in them are commercially available and do seem to be of some help. It is also recommended that cattle be fed large quantities of dry hay before they are turned on to lush spring pastures, especially legumes. And in the springtime, short periods of grazing or strip-grazing have been found to be effective in "working up" the animals to the new type of feed. There is also a commercially available form of penicillin that is used to "charge" the water troughs. In areas with a history of bloat-producing forages, this drug has been very effective in preventing bloat by apparently controlling some types of organisms responsible for producing excessive gas.

Treatment. A rubber hose can often be passed down into the rumen, twisting the curved end so that it is above the level of fluid in the rumen. If the animal has a simple, gaseous type of bloat, the pressure will be relieved in this manner. If the bloat is a "frothy" type, it is doubtful that this technique will do much good, and antifermenting agents should be used to reduce the surface tension of the frothy bubbles, allowing the gas to be released and eructated. There are several antifermenting agents on the market that generally go under such names as "bloat guard." In acute bloat, medication is given by tube or dose gun.

A severe bloat condition might be helped through the use of a trocar and cannula. This is a device used to puncture the wall of the rumen from the outside, to relieve the pressure. A small pipelike object remains in the wall of the rumen for removal later. If the condition is a frothy bloat, it is doubtful that this technique will be of any aid. The trocar and cannula is really a last-resort method.

Certain first-aid methods should be attempted while waiting for the outcome of the condition or the arrival of a veterinarian. A stick can be tied in the mouth of cattle much like a bit in a horse's mouth, to allow some gas to escape. A 6 to 8 ounce bottle of mineral oil or vegetable oil may be given to help reduce the surface tension of the trapped bubbles. The animal should be walked or moved around if that is possible; however, common sense would indicate that if the animal is having severe difficulty in breathing or standing, the movement should not be excessive.

Constipation

Signs. Any reduction of the flow of feed material through the lower bowel as compared to normal is considered constipation. Sometimes this reduction will be almost complete and in the case of penned animals should not be difficult to diagnose.

Cause. Certain animals have tendencies to develop this disorder, but digestive disorders more commonly cause it. Conditions such as a fractured pelvis can also create it.

Treatment. The use of oils or emulsifying agents are normally recommended as treatment. A laxative also may be given in the form of such natural feeds as wheat bran.

Scours (Diarrhea)

Calf scours or diarrhea is one of the least understood diseases of cattle. It has been "cussed and discussed" over corral fences and in educational institutions for many years. It is estimated that 10 to 12% of all calves born, otherwise alive and healthy, will die from calf scours in the first 30 days of their lives. Calves less than 10 days old are especially vulnerable, and newborn animals often die within 12 to 96 hours. Death rates commonly exceed 50% in some beef and dairy herds. Those animals that do recover often are stunted and remain "poor doers" for the rest of their lives.

An outbreak of scours is generally thought to be a problem of bacterial or viral invasion. However, research has revealed this disease to be much more complex than that, with many known causes, and undoubtedly many more yet to be discovered.

A brief discussion of general causes could be divided into the following three groups:

1. Bacterial scours caused by *Escherichia coli*, *Salmonella*, and *Clostridium perfringens* type C.

2. Viral causes—*Rotavirus* (formerly called *Reovirus*), *Coronavirus*, BVD, and IBR.

3. Environmental causes—High concentrations of cattle, lack of colostrum, overfeeding, vitamin A deficiency, and parasitism.

Because of the wide variety of causes it is easy to visualize that the first step in treating scours is to determine specifically the reason for it. This often necessitates the use of a veterinarian and a diagnostic laboratory to isolate the specific organism or other causes. Once the reason for the scours has been determined, vaccinations may be given to prevent future outbreaks, and treatment may be started to control the current situation.

In the case of any outbreak of scours, it is best to know what to do immediately while you are waiting for the answer to the specific reason for the outbreak. It is important to understand just what causes the unnatural, watery discharge of fecal matter. This is the key to successfully treating scours. Read this carefully, two or three times if necessary. It will tell you how to reduce losses and gain rapid recovery in outbreaks of scours.

The principal damage caused by scours is not due to the invasion of bacteria or viruses; it is the loss of water, bicarbonate, sodium, and potassium from the blood and body fluids. A parasite causes irritation to the intestines, and the calf's body reacts by trying to neutralize this agent, to destroy it and flush it out. This simply means that instead of fluids and nutrients being absorbed from the intestine as nature intended, the reverse happens—water, sodium, potassium, and bicarbonate ions leave the body fluids and escape into the intestinal contents. This is why the calf passes watery feces and loses weight. The calf dies within a few hours not because of infection, generally, but because of dehydration. A calf that loses 5% of its body weight because of dehydration may not show any clinical signs. A 10% loss, however, results in severe depression, sunken eyes, dry skin, and usually the inability to stand. Treatment must commence rapidly if this animal is to be saved. If a 15% body-weight loss results from dehydration, the calf goes into a coma, and is considered a "goner."

The key to treating the sick animal is to treat dehydration, to replace the fluids lost from the body. This can be done simply through *electrolyte therapy*.

Table 6-2 gives several mixtures designed to replace the lost ions, energy, and liquids brought about by the dehydration. The calf can be orally drenched with this material at the rates recommended while you are waiting for an analysis of the specific organisms that may have precipitated the diarrhea. These ingredients work somewhat like Gator Aide, which professional athletes drink on the sidelines in order to rehydrate their bodies after dehydration and loss of electrolytes (ions) caused from excessive exercise.

Table 6-2. Recommended Electrolyte Mixes for Fluid Therapy

MIXES THAT CAN BE MADE FROM HOUSEHOLD INGREDIENTS	

Formula #1 (to be given orally)

White corn syrup (dextrose)	8 tbsp
Salt (sodium chloride)	2 tsp
Baking soda (sodium bicarbonate)	1 tsp
Warm water	1 gal

Feed $2\frac{1}{2}$ pints to a 90 lb calf four times/day (total of $1\frac{1}{4}$ gal).

Formula #2 (to be given orally)

Condensed beef consommé	1 can
Warm water	3 cans
Baking soda	1 tbsp

Feed this to calf twice a day.

MIXES THAT CAN BE MADE FROM DRUGSTORE INGREDIENTS	

Formula #3 (to be given orally)

Sodium chloride	4 oz
Potassium chloride	5 oz
Sodium bicarbonate	$5\frac{1}{2}$ oz
Potassium monobasic phosphate	$4\frac{1}{2}$ oz

Add 1 oz of above mix plus $\frac{1}{2}$ lb of dextrose to 1 gal warm water. Feed 2–3 qt of this solution four times/day (total of 2–3 gal).

Formula #4 (to be given either orally or intravenously)

Sodium bicarbonate	1 tbsp
50% dextrose solution	100 cc
Warm water	900 cc

Give 1 to 2 liters (quarts) four times/day (total of 1–2 gal).

MIXES THAT CAN BE MADE FROM GROCERY STORE INGREDIENTS	

Formula #5

MCP Pectin	1 pkg.
Low-sodium salt	1 tsp
Baking soda	2 tsp
Beef consommé	1 can
Plus water sufficient to make 2 quarts	

Feed this mixture 3 times per day, or more if dehydration is severe, in place of milk. After 1 or 2 days, gradually introduce milk, i.e., 1/3 milk, 2/3 formula #5, etc. (*Source*: Dr. R. D. Phillips, Colorado State University)

Source: Michigan State University.

Both Gator Aide and the mixtures in Table 6-2 are designed to be absorbed without delay and to be carried directly to the cells of animal tissues.

Calves will respond best to treatment if you begin early in the course of an outbreak. Sick calves should be isolated in a warm, dry pen or stall. It is also a good idea to reduce or completely eliminate milk consumption for one or more feedings in order to stop the growth of any bacteria in the intestine. For nursing calves this is easily done by removing the calf from the cow, skipping one feeding, and slowly bringing it back to feed allowing it to nurse two or three times a day for 5 minutes or less.

You can often treat mild cases orally with antibiotics and sulfanomides. However, in more severe cases injections of antibiotics are recommended. The specific type of antibiotic will depend on the results of the diagnostic tests to determine the type of organism causing the scours. If bacteria are involved, antibiotics may be effective. If viruses are present, treatment may also include antibiotics because they are effective against the secondary bacteria.

In general, if calves respond to antibiotics, do not discontinue the treatment too quickly. Most injectable antibiotics are effective for only about 12 hours; so daily injections will be needed. Scours often seem to improve with only one treatment, but then recur a few days later. A good rule of thumb is to continue treatment for 1 to 2 days after the scours have cleared up.

In general, prevention can be in the form of vaccinations for identified organisms that are troublesome in a particular area. Research has revealed several specific organisms that infect the gut. Rotavirus, corona (2 strains), and parvo are names of new viruses. The longer known BVD and IBR viruses have also been linked with calf scours. Vaccines recently developed by the University of Nebraska are available for these viruses.

Other preventive measures are:

1. Provide adequate amounts of vitamins A and D for cows before calving.

2. Provide sufficient mineral nutrition for cows.

3. Be sure calves are born on clean pastures or in a clean well-bedded pen.

4. Clean old calf pens using high water pressure and effective disinfectants (see Chapter 2).

5. Isolate infected calves.

6. Dip the calf's navel with tincture of iodine immediately after birth to prevent entrance of organisms into the bloodstream.

7. Make sure the calf receives a full feed (about 2 quarts) of colostrum milk within the first hour after birth.

8. Do not overfeed a calf or allow it to gorge itself, thus creating a food-induced diarrhea.

In general, all of the above methods work quite well on any type of scours. The following specific situations indicate a particular type of scours and give recommendations in addition to the fluid therapy previously discussed.

Johne's Disease.   Johne's disease produces one of the more serious forms of diarrhea. This disease is an infectious intestinal disorder, creating conditions of emaciation, thickening or folding of the intestinal wall, edema (the characteristic "bottle jaw"), a particularly abnormal offensive odor of the diarrhea but with no blood, and a general weakened condition. The animals never do well and the condition may keep recurring. The development of the disease is very slow. Most affected animals are 2 to 6 years of age before they develop any signs.

Cause.   A small bacterial organism, *Mycobacterium paratuberculosis*, causes the tuberculosislike disease.

Treatment.   Treatment is not very successful. There are vaccines available, but normally they are not recommended, and it is generally thought that culling the affected animals is the only practical recommendation.

There are two types of tests that should be mentioned here to identify animals that are suffering from Johne's disease. The *intradermal test* is done in the early stages before clinical signs occur. It is a good herd test, and if caught at the right stage, can be used to cull infected animals from the herd before an outbreak occurs. The *serological test* is of little value until an outbreak has already occurred. It is used to determine what types of organism may have caused the diarrhea problem.

Colibacillosis (Calf Scours)

Signs.   Colibacillosis is a digestive disorder that causes diarrhea in very young calves, generally within the first two weeks of life.

Cause.   *E. coli* is the cause. Research by the University of Nebraska has proven the theory that a virus infection first occurs, allowing the *E. coli* bacteria to act. The university has developed a vaccine to prevent this most common problem, now available through Norden Laboratories. The *E. coli* organism is found worldwide, but was not determined to be harmful until the last decade or so. The affected calf may suddenly collapse, have a subnormal temperature, cold clammy skin, occasional convulsions, and may die within 3 to 4 days or less. The disease is characterized most often by a liquid yellow feces, occasionally tinged with blood, most often occurring during the first 3 weeks of life (frequently in the first week).

Prevention. It is extremely important that baby calves receive sufficient colostrum (mother's milk) during the first 12 hours of life. The natural antibodies that exist in the mother's milk pass through the epithelial lining of the bowel during the first 12 hours of a calf's life. After about 36 hours there is almost no passage; so this natural immunity has to be absorbed very rapidly. Therefore the best preventive of the disease is the management of the newborn. There should not be overcrowding or allowing calves to be born in areas where there has been a high concentration of cattle and therefore poor sanitation. Individual pens are recommended if cattle are being housed. Also make sure calves nurse soon after birth.

Treatment. High levels of antibiotics are recommended, especially the newer synthetic forms of penicillin. No whole milk should be fed. A mixture of one-third milk and two-thirds water and oral electrolytes is generally recommended along with lots of tender loving care.

Parasitism. A severe infestation of parasites can also create scours. Antibiotics and fluid therapy will be of only temporary value in alleviating the condition. If parasites are found to be the problem, the only solution is to treat for removal by chemical means (see internal parasites, discussed later in this chapter).

Viral-Induced Scours. Numerous viruses such as BVD, IBR, reovirus, etc., are known to be primary causes of baby-calf scours. If viruses are found to be the causative agent, a vaccine may be recommended as an annual injection for baby calves. As noted earlier, the University of Nebraska has pioneered recent research in the area of viral-induced scours and has developed vaccines to prevent it.

Food-Induced Scours. Overeating by young calves can produce a less serious form of scours. Too large a volume of milk at a single feeding appears to cause more problems than smaller, more frequent feedings or than milk replacer, which is more concentrated. A cow giving excessive milk may need to be milked out on occasion until the calf adjusts to the oversupply of milk. This type of scours usually can be treated simply by management, without antibiotic, and normally without fluid therapy.

Summary—Scours (general remarks on any diarrhea). Treatment of diarrhea in general should be handled in the following way:

Consider first the source of the disorder, whether it is food or toxic material. Once the source has been detected, it can be removed.

If the source cannot be found, you should immediately reduce the feed intake of the affected animal and begin water and electrolyte therapy.

Antibiotics should be given as soon as the condition is noticed. Probably the cheapest broad-spectrum antibiotics should be used in this case. A combination of penicillin and streptomycin is excellent for aiding the body in responding to the condition imposed on it. Neomycin, astringents, and intestinal coatings should also be considered as an alternate or in combination with the antibiotics.

Several home-remedy paregoric preparations have been concocted, and almost any paregoric preparation will be of aid. Paregoric can be purchased at your local drugstore by prescription.

There are also a number of commercially available preparations or one can be prescribed by your veterinarian to add to the drinking water, which will reduce the intensity of the diarrhea.

There are sulfa drugs on the market in bolus form, which can be administered orally to the affected animal.

Large amounts of fluid are always necessary in treating any condition involving diarrhea. To keep the animal hydrated and to keep its energy levels high, electrolytes plus dextrose are needed. This may have to be given parenterally (other than orally) but should be given orally if possible.

In summary, any treatment of diarrhea will necessitate the use of both fluids and antibiotics.

Prolapsed Rectum

Signs. The rectum simply turns inside out, and you will see a red, pendulous, fleshy protrusion about the rectal area.

Cause. The condition is generally caused by straining of an unnatural nature or by calving. Diarrhea and constipation have also been known to create this condition.

Treatment. Remove the cause and the treatment will be initiated. The condition can be aided by replacing the prolapse and putting a few sutures to hold it in place. A loose purse-string suture can be used to secure the rectum (Figure 6-1). This suture merely holds the prolapse in place until healing can occur. The stitches are normally not removed but are simply absorbed by the body.

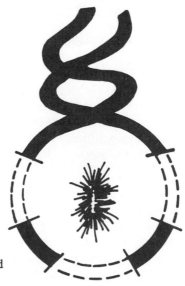

Figure 6-1. A rectal prolapse may be secured through the use of a simple purse-string suture.

POISONS

The Heavy Metals

Lead. Lead is the most common poisoning agent in cattle because it is used in such a variety of materials (car batteries, leaded windows, linoleum, putty, oil filters, many varieties of paint, some agricultural sprays and oil-field materials). Lead has even been inhaled under certain conditions, such as around smelters.

Signs. There are two syndromes of lead poisoning—acute and sub-acute. The acute syndrome causes death within 12 to 24 hours. This is mainly a disease of baby calves. The signs of lead poisoning include the following: staggering, muscle tremors, head and neck convulsions, and collapse. In the adult animal the sign is a general blindness. A cow may charge fences or even humans when under the influence of this poison because of its failure to see. Cattle will show unsteady coordination and move in a very jerky fashion. Adult animals generally die from respiratory failure.

The subacute syndrome runs its course in a matter of 3 to 4 days. Cattle will be very dull and have no appetite; they may show a blind, staggering gait, muscle tremors, grinding of teeth, and salivation; and they may kick at their belly because of abdominal pain. Generally the subacute form causes death by some means other than poisoning, such as falling into a water hole and drowning. On a few occasions, affected cattle are observed to die quietly but generally there is a more violent reaction.

Prevention. The only sensible course to follow is to keep animals away from the sources of lead.

Treatment. Try to control the convulsions and use chelating agents to trap the lead. These agents are used by veterinarians but often with little success.

Mercury Poisoning

Signs. Mercury poisoning brings on gastroenteritis (inflammation of the stomach and intestine), diarrhea, uremia (a form of blood poisoning due to failure of the kidney to remove impurities from the body), and a very nervous condition. The damage to the intestine is often so severe that its function is permanently impaired.

Cause. The chief sources of mercury contamination are an accidental injection of medication containing this compound by unknowledgeable stock-men, or an animal's licking wound dressings that contain this compound. In other instances, seed grain that has been treated with mercuric compounds may be a source of poisoning. Although small quantities of mercury-treated grains can be detoxified by the animal's body, larger portions can cause kidney failure and death.

Treatment. Large amounts of protein are helpful in alleviating this condition. Raw eggs given by mouth in large quantities (1 to 2 dozen) plus a laxative are often used as a treatment.

Arsenic Poisoning

Signs. Clinical signs include severe upset stomach, diarrhea, restlessness, groaning, rapid breathing, salivation, grinding of teeth, even vomiting, and a cessation of rumen activity. This condition develops very suddenly. Within 10 to 15 hours after ingestion the signs of poisoning begin to occur. A profuse watery diarrhea is always one of the first indications of this type of poisoning. Animals have no appetite but develop a severe thirst. They show signs of abdominal pain, are stiff, mildly uncoordinated, and in most fatal cases exhibit convulsions followed by coma and death within 3 to 4 hours after the diarrhea begins.

Cause. Arsenic is a very common type of poisoning because so many arsenic compounds are employed in weed killers, cattle dips, and other chemical preparations used for both crops and animals.

Prevention No one would knowingly keep arsenic in a pasture or barn where cattle could consume it; however, the most common case in which poisoning occurs is a can of arsenic stored on the second floor of a barn. The years go by, rust takes its toll on the can, and the arsenic slowly drips or drains onto feed and/or hay stored below. This could cause either chronic arsenic poisoning or in the case of a large lump, a very rapid fatality. In other instances, arsenic has been buried, and later this material gets turned up by plow, dogs, erosion, or some other means and cattle get access to it. Prevention, therefore, is a matter of proper, safe storage or disposal.

Treatment. It is very unlikely that you will suspect arsenic poisoning early enough to administer effective treatment. However, if the animal is observed eating a product known to contain arsenic, some immediate attention is recommended. Any oily purgative or other medication that would increase motility in order to keep the digestive system functioning normally may be of assistance. Iron hydrate is a medication that has been used with mild success. In any condition causing diarrhea, it is always a good idea to begin rehydration therapy. One of the great dangers to life is losing fluids so rapidly that cellular dehydration produces convulsions and collapse. Therefore it is recommended that electrolytes be given to make it possible for the body cells to retain fluids.

BAL (British anti-Lewisite) is a product that is effective as a treatment for organic arsenic poisoning; however, it does not work on inorganic arsenic poisoning, and the dosage is extremely critical and must be given by an experienced veterinarian because this product itself is toxic. It is very expensive and generally is not justified except in the case of valuable animals.

Phosphorus Poisoning.
Phosphorus poisoning is a relatively rare type of poisoning, but it has the potential of being a problem everywhere because

it is an ingredient used in rat bait and other products that are found on the average farm and ranch.

Signs.   There is severe gastrointestinal upset as is the case in so many other poisonings. The clinical signs that veterinarians look for are the same as those that show up in liver-damaged cattle. There is severe diarrhea, tremendous abdominal pain, excessive salivation, thirst, and in most cases the animal dies of acute shock. If the animal should survive the initial shock to the system, kidney-insufficiency will occur within 5 to 10 days after these first signs are seen. There will be weakness, no appetite, and blood found in the urine. These are the same signs that are observed in cattle suffering from liver damage brought on by a variety of conditions. Convulsions, coma, and a slow death follow.

Treatment.   If an animal is observed eating a substance known to contain phosphorus, treatment should be the same as in other poison cases. Try to flush the system using oils and purgatives to produce as much motility as possible in the digestive system and thus keep the material moving out of the body.

Copper Poisoning.   There are two forms of copper poisoning—acute and chronic. The acute form is very rare since it requires that large amounts of copper be eaten. This usually occurs from an accidental overdose of medicine containing copper.

The chronic form is more common and follows the ingestion of small amounts of copper over a period of time. The copper usually comes from plants that are grown in soil that is very high in copper. The effects are cumulative. This condition is most often reported in the Rocky Mountain states.

Signs.   In the acute form, there is severe gastrointestinal inflammation and vomiting (although this will vary with the species of animal affected). If vomiting does occur, the vomitus will have the characteristic green to blue-green color associated with copper that is seen on corroded copper tubing. This color is the same as that of bluestone, a mineral compound commonly used to clear up algae in stock tanks. It should be noted, however, that this use of bluestone is a very low-level, short-period treatment that should not cause concern when used according to the proper ratio.

Chronic copper poisoning is characterized by a lack of appetite, severe thirst, a brownish urine, and yellowing of the pink mucous membranes (jaundice). In the acute cases there are no gastrointentinal upsets. The animal appears very depressed and death may occur within 24 to 48 hours after the first signs are observed.

Treatment.   In the acute form, a coating material may be tried, and the animal should be treated immediately for shock with steroids and antibiotics. BAL can be given intravenously to cause the copper to be more rapidly excreted by the kidneys. Remember BAL is extremely dangerous because it is in itself a toxic material unless given in the proper dosage.

Chronic copper poisoning may be relieved if molybdenum is added to the diet. There is an interaction between most minerals with one tying up another. When copper intake is high, molybdenum intake can be increased to tie up the excess copper in a form that prevents it from being absorbed by the animal, thus preventing the poisoning.

Calcium Poisoning. Calcium is involved in many metabolic functions. It is not a problem under normal conditions, and therefore usually an excessive amount does not cause difficulty. All of the situations involving too much calcium are man-made. In treating for milk fever—a common calcium deficiency, the treatment can kill the patient unless extreme care is taken. Calcium gluconate is normally given intravenously or intraperitoneally. If the gluconate solution is not administered very slowly, especially when given intravenously, it can be toxic, bringing on a condition that resembles a heart attack. Therefore, treatment of a calcium deficiency can very quickly become a calcium toxicity unless the proper dose is given over the proper length of time. The safe dose for a 1000-lb cow is 300 grams of calcium gluconate given at body temperature intravenously over a 15-minute period.

Molybdenum Poisoning. In a few areas of the United States molybdenum occurs in the soil at potentially toxic levels. High levels in the soil have a tendency to be taken up by plants and passed on to the animal. There are some areas where soil molybdenum is very low but fertilizers containing the element are used as a top dressing, creating an amount that is capable of causing a problem. In areas where molybdenum is naturally high during the growing season, young plants, especially clover, show a dramatic increase in the uptake of molybdenum. There have also been reports of hay grown in high-molybdenum areas causing problems. Molybdenum is a peculiar element because of its reaction in the animal; that is, it interacts with two other minerals—copper and phosphorus. Therefore an excess of molybdenum generally is expressed as a deficiency of copper or phosphorus.

Signs. If the level of molybdenum is high, signs of copper deficiency, as previously discussed, will most likely occur. There may also be rickets, a condition brought on by a lack of phosphorus, and diarrhea often occurs because of the toxic effect and the interaction of these minerals with the bacteria in the rumen. There is weight loss, a dull haircoat, and a depigmentation or "fading" of the hair color. There have been some instances where severe cases have been noted that create an almost gray or white cow from a normally Black Angus. The condition is seldom fatal; however, it should be corrected to avoid the possibility of other problems such as rickets or digestive disturbances.

Treatment. Copper sulfate can be fed to animals where toxicity from molybdenum has been diagnosed. One gram of copper sulfate per day for calves and 2 grams per day for cows is recommended in the feed. Copper sulfate is used because there is an interaction between molybdenum and copper. If copper can be increased, a balance will be reached, thus alleviating the condition. Since copper is interrelated with phosphorus, phosphorus should also be made available such as in a calcium-phosphorus mineral mixture.

Selenium or Alkali Poisoning. Selenium or alkali poisoning is called *blind staggers* in most areas and generally occurs only in the northwestern part of the United States. The condition is brought about by an excessive uptake of selenium by plants that are eaten as pasture or forage. Normally plants do not take up selenium, but if there is more than one to six parts per million in the soil, the condition can occur. There are three types of plants that are involved. The first type is called *obligate*, or an *indicator plant*. This type readily takes up selenium and, in fact, only grows where selenium is in very high levels. Such plants may contain as much as 1000 to 15,000 parts per million. The second type of plant is called a *secondary plant*. This species can take up selenium if it is in excess, but normally it does not. These plants are generally unpalatable to cattle and would not be eaten anyway; however, in times of drought or overgrazing, cattle may be forced to eat them, and blind staggers is the result. The third type of plant is called a *nonaccumulator*, which does not take up much selenium; but it does return it to the soil and releases it in a form where it may be taken up by the crop that follows it, such as wheat. Thus, this type of poisoning often occurs in wheat pastures.

Signs. There are two forms—acute and chronic. In the acute form, a large amount of selenium is ingested at one feeding. The signs are rapid and weak pulse, difficult breathing, bloat, frequent urination, a "blue" cast to the gums (caused by a failure of oxygen to be circulated through the system), collapse, respiratory failure, and death within a few hours.

The chronic form, which is more common, and has been recognized for many years by stockmen in the northwestern states, is *blind staggers* or *alkali disease*. The plants that are the cause of this disease have relatively low levels of selenium, but the cumulative effect of ingesting this substance over a period of 7 to 8 weeks can be fatal. The signs include weight loss and unthrifty haircoat. The cattle tend to wander off from the herd and develop a staggering gait, their eyesight is impaired, they often walk in circles, they salivate excessively, tears are discharged from the eyes, evidence of abdominal pain is seen, and the cattle have difficulty swallowing. They finally collapse and die of respiratory failure. Although the condition may develop over a long period of time, the signs do not show up for many weeks. Once these signs do appear, death may occur within a few days.

Prevention. You should know the area where selenium toxicity problems have historically been noted. Learn to recognize indicator plants, which grow only where selenium will most likely be a problem. Don't overgraze pastures, forcing cattle to eat the secondary, unpalatable plants that they would not normally eat.

Treatment. There is no known treatment.

Thallium Poisoning. Thallium is a common type of poisoning because of its use in rat poisons around the world. It is a potent poison and can be harmful to domestic animals just as it is to rats. It has caused many deaths of sheep and cattle in all parts of the world. Sheep are most susceptible to it, followed by cattle.

Signs. There is an obvious digestive upset. Ulcerations usually occur, first around the mouth and later may spread anywhere on the skin.

Treatment. Treatment is mostly ineffective. Only supportive treatment is used. This helps the animal to recover on its own, while giving all the aid necessary for the body to throw off the poison. Glucose, antibiotics, and vitamins are used. Treatment of the skin lesions is also advisable. These are first-aid measures but may be of value in helping the body to heal itself.

Toxic Chemical Substances

Cyanide or Prussic Acid Poisoning. Cyanide or prussic acid poisoning is a commonly occurring condition in many parts of the world where any sorghum-type plants are grown. In the southern part of the United States, Johnson grass is a sorghum-related plant and has similar tendencies. At certain times of the year, hydrocyanic acid is produced in these sorghum or sorghum-related plants. When the plants are exposed to stress, such as drought or frost, cyanide gas is produced. This is the same type of gas that has been used in the past to carry out the death penalty in those states where a gas chamber is used. It is extremely lethal and normally very rapid in its effect.

Signs. Usually this type of poisoning occurs only in certain cattle in a herd—the ones that eat very rapidly. Only one or two animals may be seen to have the condition, and they are usually the "gluttons." Signs include convulsions, a stupor, paralysis, and death within a few minutes of the onset. The animal stops breathing before the heart stops beating. If an animal consumes a lethal dose, there is little time for treatment. Borderline cases may be saved if treatment is begun immediately.

Cause. As mentioned above, cyanide or prussic acid poisoning can be the result of damage to sorghum or sorghum-related plants. Generally, this condition is related to stunting of the plants by an early frost in the fall. The hydrocyanic acid may only exist for a few hours after this frost. Once the plants are allowed to dry out thoroughly, or if they are made into hay and cured will, there is no toxic substance left, and the hay is safe to feed. Even during the critical hours after a frost or other damage by nature, cattle can quickly excrete cyanide through their lungs and urinary tract. They may ingest an amount of material that is just under a lethal dose without showing any signs at all; but if they go over a lethal amount, the reaction is extremely rapid. Cyanide actually causes asphyxiation of the tissues, causing death within seconds. In other words, the cells themselves do not receive oxygen and so they die; death of the animal follows immediately.

Prevention. The best method of preventing this problem is to use precautions any time animals graze on sorghum-type plants, especially after a frost, drought, hailstorm, or any other nature-related damage to crops. It is also recommended that cattle be given their fill of hay before being turned out to graze in "suspect" pastures.

The problem occurs occasionally in grain sorghum fields when the stalks are shredded after harvest. A heavy rain can cause quick regrowth and high prussic acid content. If cattle are turned out to graze on this unexpected "easy pickings," you should be alert for signs of cyanide poisoning.

Treatment. If borderline cases can be detected in time, the treatment involves a fixation of cyanide into a harmless form that is excreted by the kidneys. Treatment is the intravenous administration of 1 cc of 20% sodium nitrite and 3 cc of 20% sodium thiosulfate per 100 lb of body weight. Commercial solutions of this mixture are commonly available. Follow the directions on the label. Sodium thiosulfate may be given orally, in addition, to detoxify the cyanide in the rumen. Purge the animal to remove potential cyanide material.

Nitrate or Nitrite Poisoning. Nitrate or nitrite poisoning is a condition quite similar to cyanide poisoning but not quite as rapid, although it is often fatal.

During a dry period, or due to the influence of some accidental herbicide drift, certain plants may contain high levels of nitrate. The nitrate is not a problem in itself, but it does become toxic when it is converted into nitrite by bacteria in the rumen. There have also been cases where nitrate fertilizer has contaminated water supplies with subsequent conversion to nitrite at levels high enough to cause a problem.

Signs. There is abdominal pain, diarrhea, muscular weakness, and incoordination. There may be convulsions, an abnormally rapid respiration and heart beat, and a bluish color to the membranes around the mouth due to oxygen starvation. The classic sign is chocolate-colored blood that may even stain the other tissues. These signs may be followed by a coma, and in severe cases, death.

Cause. Nitrites convert the normal healthy hemoglobin in blood (which carries oxygen throughout the system) to methemoglobin (which is incapable of carrying oxygen). The animal dies due to tissue asphyxiation, as in cyanide poisoning.

Treatment. The key to treating nitrite poisoning is to convert the methemoglobin back into the normal hemoglobin, thus allowing oxygen to be transported to the body cells. This must be done as rapidly as possible. Methylene blue is used for this purpose. Two milligrams per pound of body weight in a 4% solution given intravenously is recommended as a treatment. If started in time, treatment is effective and recovery is rapid. Methylene blue solution is commercially available; follow the directions on the label.

Urea Poisoning. Urea poisoning is one of the most common forms of toxicity in today's management of cattle, sheep, or other ruminants. Urea is used to supply a portion of the animal's protein requirements, synthetically. Microorganisms break down the urea (and biuret, a similar product) to produce ammonia. Under natural feeding of nonsynthetic foodstuffs, ammonia is also produced; but the difference is that the natural system seldom produces too much ammonia to create an imbalance. With synthetic urea, however, if care is not exercised, too much can be used, resulting in poisoning.

Signs. The condition may occur as soon as 10 minutes after consumption, or within 4 hours. The attack is usually rapid and acute. Even though cattle have been consuming urea without problems, an overdose, caused by a mistake in calculations, could still precipitate the poisoning; so animals should be monitored throughout feeding.

There is usually severe abdominal pain, frothy salivation, grinding of teeth, muscle tremors, incoordination, rapid breathing, violent struggling and bellowing, convulsions, bloat, and severe twitching and tetanic ("jerking") spasms. The membranes around the mouth and other openings turn blue due to cyanosis (a lack of oxygen in the blood), and death occurs after a violent, sometimes lengthy, struggle.

Cause. Rumen microorganisms break down urea or biuret to produce ammonia. When the system is overactive, usually due to feeding too much urea to animals unaccustomed to it, too much ammonia is produced, creating acidosis and other chemical imbalances in the body.

Prevention. Be careful with urea and do not use more than is recommended—no more than 3% of the grain rations or 1% of the total ration. Biuret is recommended at no greater than 3% of the total ration.

Be sure to mix uniformly. Inadequate mixing can cause excessive consumption, depending on what portion of the feed is eaten by the individual animal.

Allow animals time to adjust slowly to urea feeds, and do not use with high-roughage rations.

Treatment. You should pump cold water (up to 5 gallons) into the rumen. Be sure it is cold because this reduces the activity of the bacteria and slows down further production of ammonia.

A layman's antidote of drenching with plain household vinegar ($\frac{1}{2}$ to 1 gallon for cattle) will also counteract the ammonia already produced and is recommended in addition to the cold water treatment. Relieve bloat if indicated. Your veterinarian can provide additional treatment through intravenous infusions. However, no treatment is highly effective in acute cases.

Fluorine Poisoning. Fluorine is present in all animal tissues, particularly in the bones and teeth. Excessive consumption of fluorine by livestock is normally due to contamination of water from industry runoff, dusts, and gases.

Signs. In the acute form there are the usual conditions of gastrointestinal upset: vomiting, diarrhea, collapse, and death.

The chronic form presents a different picture. It takes about 6 to 8 months for the signs to appear. These occur basically as a lameness. It is a shifting lameness, occurring first in one foot and then in another. The lameness stunts growth in young calves, and they never grow normally. In many cases there is an enlargement of the lower jaw that is painful when pressed with the fingers. The teeth may also be discolored, and they wear very unevenly because of varying hard and soft areas.

Chronic fluorine poisoning was a very common condition in the United States in the days when rock phosphate containing high levels of fluorine was used as a fertilizer. The same rock phosphate was also used in animal feeds, and it was then that the condition was first noticed on a wide scale. Since that time, rock phosphate has been defluorinated, and this source of fluorine poisoning has been corrected. However, there are still accidental contaminations, especially to pastures around factories that produce such products as aluminum, brick, glass, enamel, steel, and metal.

Prevention. The only solution to the problem is to switch to animals that have a shorter economic life. Since it takes 6 to 8 months for the symptoms to occur in cattle, pigs or poultry can be reared before the condition has time to develop.

Treatment. Due to the lengthy period before signs develop, treatment is generally not prescribed.

Hydrogen Sulfide Poisoning

Signs. Clinical signs are difficult breathing and cyanosis (a bluish discoloration of the normally pink membranes); the affected animals also appear very depressed. Hydrogen sulfide gas affects the oxygen-carrying capacity of the bloodstream right at the cellular level; so there is, in effect, tissue suffocation.

Cause. Hydrogen sulfide gas is a very toxic substance given off from manure pits and lagoons. Enclosed areas that utilize a lagoon system without sufficient ventilation could create this condition.

Prevention. Simple ventilation in any enclosed systems where a lagoon is used, especially in winter, can easily prevent any problems.

Treatment. Breathing a mixture of oxygen and carbon dioxide through a respiration mask has been tried with cattle with some degree of success, but generally no treatment is practical other than common-sense prevention.

Other Common Substances with Poisonous Properties

Anthelmentics. *Anthelmentics* is a general name given to any product used to rid an animal of intestinal parasites. Keep in mind that anything that will kill a parasite is also a toxic substance. If the dosage is not carefully controlled, it can kill the host animal. Do not exceed recommended levels, or the cure may be worse than the problem. Various types of anthelmentics are listed below.

1. Hexachlorophene—Used to treat flukes. It is toxic to cattle if the recommended dose is exceeded.

2. Nicotine sulfate—A general anthelmentic used for many years around the world.

3. Phenothiazine—A general anthelmentic. This is the old green drench recognized by most cattlemen. Phenothiazine is also available in granules to mix with feed and is used in salt blocks. There appears to be individual differences in susceptibility to phenothiazine poisoning, but it is still a distinct hazard. There have even been cases where an animal was given a proper dose and died. In other cases, animals have been given ten times that amount and lived. The reason is that different animals vary in their ability to withstand toxic levels of certain products. Phenothiazine is one of those products. Therefore it should always be used with caution.

The signs of an overdose of phenothiazine are more evident than the signs from an overdose of other organic compounds; these signs generally include anemia, jaundice, rapid breathing, rapid pulse, signs of colic, and an increased sensitivity to sunlight (photosensitization). The sensitivity to sunlight is the first sign to appear.

Within 12 to 36 hours after an overdose of phenothiazine, cattle may appear blind, try to seek shade, and often will get sunburn on the pink areas of the eyes, nose, and skin. Sunburn-type lesions may appear on white areas of the skin. The only treatment recommended is to keep cattle in the shade, wait, and hope for the best. If the other signs of rapid breathing, anemia, and jaundice also are evident, dextrose is recommended either intravenously or orally. If nothing else is available, try a drench of molasses dissolved in water.

More recently, phenothiazine has been combined with hexachloro-ethane to rid cattle of both worms and flukes. This is called a *two-way drench*. There can still be problems if the dosage is not carefully calculated.

4. Piperizine—An excess may cause loss of appetite and diarrhea. Calves are especially common poison victims of piperazine. It is usually not fatal, but can be.

5. Ronnel, Ruelene, Levamisole—These substances may also cause toxicity problems, and caution should be exercised in following the directions.

6. Thiabendazole (TBZ)—This is the least toxic of all the organic

compounds. It is probably the only one that can be used on weak, "downed" animals that still does the job for which it was intended.

Antiseptics, Disinfectants, Preservatives, and Cleaning Agents. Numerous deaths of cattle are reported every year from drinking of soaps, detergents, and various cleaning agents.

Phenols such as lysol, creosote, and creosol are particularly hazardous. Cattle lick posts treated with phenols or even drink from open containers or contaminated puddles and thus poison themselves.

Symptoms of phenols are more easily recognized and are of greater concern than are the other types of antiseptics and disinfectants. Usually calves are affected because they are most susceptible. The signs are apathy, weakness, convulsions, coma, ulcerations of the mouth and throat, and respiratory paralysis. These result in death in a few days. There may be an accumulative effect caused by calves licking or chewing on wood posts treated with phenols; however, phenols can also be absorbed through the skin and cause the same problem.

Cause. Phenols are extremely corrosive, especially to the gastrointestinal tract, and this corrosion can bring on shock or a collapse of the respiratory system.

Prevention Separate any of these products from the feed storage area or from the second floor of a barn where they might accidentally contaminate hay or feed.

Treatment. Any gastrointestinal flushing material may be useful. Stomach coatings should also be used, and any external phenols should be removed from the skin with soap and water.

Barbiturates and Sedatives. Barbiturates and sedatives are used by veterinarians as anesthetics. Chloral hydrate was used commonly in earlier times but has been replaced by more advanced preparations. Most tranquilizers on the market today contain chloropromazine or similar compounds that are safer than chloral hydrate, but there is always the possibility that respiratory problems can occur. The recommended dosage should be adhered to with extreme caution and administered by a veterinarian.

Cantharide Poisoning. Cantharides are substances compounded from the Spanish blister beetle; they are found during certain times of the year along the Gulf Coast of the United States. Alfalfa hay especially attracts the blister beetles, and if they are in large numbers, as happens during certain times of the year, they may be baled along with the hay. If eaten by cattle, these beetles release a potent irritant, which is absorbed through the gastrointestinal tract and produces a tremendous inflammation of the kidneys.

Calves are more often affected by cantharides because older cattle usually get to the hay first and eat the longer stems, shaking out the beetles in the process. Younger calves clean up the finer material and thus eat the bulk of the beetles as well. Shortly after eating the substance, the animal's whole intestinal tract becomes irritated and the kidneys are greatly inflamed. Blisters may be seen over the mouth, lips, and internal areas that are visible to the eye.

Gastrointestinal coatings should be given and a lotion used for external blisters or lesions.

Strychnine Poisoning. Cattle are somewhat resistant to strychnine poisoning because it is partly destroyed by the rumen. However, accidental poisonings do occur, and cattle are certainly not immune. The most common occurrences are caused by cattle consuming mole baits, or certain plants that are natural producers of strychnine.

The signs of strychnine poisoning are nervousness, restlessness, twitching of muscles, a stiff neck, and convulsions that may be brought on by any excitement or noise. Death is caused by respiratory paralysis.

Treatment of strychnine poisoning is with tranquilizers and anesthetics to control the convulsions until the poison can be excreted.

Pesticides, Insecticides, and Rodenticides

Acariacides. Acariacide compounds are used in the control of mites and lice. There are two groups of these compounds. One is the agricultural acariacides; these are used for the control of mites on trees and crops. The other group is used mainly by veterinarians for animals. A couple of common acariacides are lindane (for animals) and dieldrin (for plants).

Accidental ingestion of these products or inhalation of insecticide due to prolonged exposure to drift will bring on depression, a discharge of tears, diarrhea along with obvious intestinal irritation (bloody discharge), and deep, rapid respiration.

An animal that is suspected of being poisoned with these products should be treated as you would one that has diarrhea. The use of intestinal protectants or coatings is recommended.

Fungicides. Seed to be planted is generally treated with a fungicide. Although cattle frequently consume small amounts of fungicides along with treated seed, it is usually not a toxic problem to cattle; but it is mentioned here because it could be poisonous to humans under unusual circumstances. One of the most tragic cases of poisoning in this way came about in Texas when a migrant farm family got free grain from an outdated storage area that had been treated with a fungicide. They fed this treated seed to hogs, slaughtered the hogs after the normal period of time, and ate the meat. Several members of the family died, and the rest of them were disabled with varying degrees of blindness or muscular disorders. Even though the hogs had lived with a toxic level of fungicide in their system, it had been passed on to the human consumer in the final chain of events. For this reason, treated seed should never be used as an animal feed.

Herbicides. Herbicides are generally called *weed killers* and are not a problem when used properly. However, these compounds could become a problem if cattle are not removed from the pasture when herbicides are being sprayed or if they are turned in to a field within a few hours after spraying has taken place.

Insecticides.

1. Chlorinated hydrocarbons. DDT (now off the market), lindane (benzene hexachloride), dieldrin, toxaphene, methoxychlor, and heptachlor are among the more common compounds in this group.

Occasionally these hydrocarbons do present a toxic hazard. The first signs of poisoning are muscular tremors. Grinding of the teeth comes next, followed by or along with labored respiration, frequent urination, increased excitability, tendency to walk backward, irritability, and an attempt to "climb the walls" for no apparent reason. Muscular paralysis and convulsions eventually lead to death.

The cause of this poisoning is most often a downed fence, which allows cattle to get into a freshly sprayed field or crop and absorb material through the skin. The chlorinated hydrocarbons are toxic for only 4 to 5 hours after spraying, but caution should be taken to keep cattle out of treated areas for at least half a day. Some products on the market are to be used directly on the animals. These are safe if they are used at the recommended dosage but don't overdose. Spraying is usually considered superior to dipping when used with animals because you don't have the hazard of other portals of entry such as inhaling, swallowing, and so forth.

In poison cases the toxic material is eventually concentrated in the body fat (and in the butterfat in the cow's milk). There have been cases where animals have been poisoned many months after the initial exposure occurred due to a reduction in diet. This brings on a mobilization of the fat reserves, thus releasing poison into the system again.

Treatment consists of washing the animals as quickly as possible after it is known they have been contaminated, in order to remove the source. Then, if signs do appear, sedatives should be given until the signs diminish.

2. Pyrethrums. Pyrethrums are usually safe even to young animals. They are one of the least toxic insecticide materials used on domestic animals.

3. Organophosphate insecticides. This is the most poisonous group of materials normally encountered in animal husbandry. These substances are in common use, which brings about a greater chance of poisoning. Organophosphates are used to treat bots (intestinal larvae stage of botflies), soil nematodes, etc. The compounds are now widely used and they vary in their hazard rating. For practical discussion purposes all of these are considered dangerous. Some of the more common names of these products that you might encounter are malathion, parathion, and chlorothion. The dangerous thing about these materials is that they are absorbed as readily through the skin as when given orally, and they are equally dangerous to humans. The action of the poison is on various areas of the nervous system.

Within a few minutes of exposure either by accidental spill, spray, etc., there is salivation, smooth muscle contraction (contractions of the intestine), diarrhea, and muscular stiffness. Signs vary with the level of the material ingested. The range of observations may vary from mild salivation to blind staggers and death by respiratory distress. Death can come as early as 5 minutes after exposure, but nearly always within 24 hours. These compounds are highly lethal and should be used with a high regard for the potential hazard.

These chemical preparations are often used in aerial spraying as crop insecticides. Therefore, poisoning is not to be expected except in cases where wind conditions may cause drift. They are also used widely as pour-on and sprays or dyes to control cattle pests such as mites, grubs, or flies.

Atropine is often used as a treatment. It is given at the rate of $\frac{1}{2}$ mg per pound of body weight: one-third intravenously and two-thirds subcutaneously. The dosage is repeated until effective, as necessary. If the material was eaten, activated charcoal in water should be given by stomach tube. If external exposure occurs, wash the material off with water and detergents.

Molluscocide (Slug Bait). The most common slug bait is metaldehyde. It is widely used in gardens, so the exposure to domestic animals is quite possible. Although dogs and cats are the more normal consumers of this bait, it is also a potential threat to cattle. Signs are incoordination, rapid breathing, loss of consciousness, and possibly death due to respiratory failure.

Copper sulfate is also used to control slugs, and cattle may also be poisoned with this compound. Treatment for either case of poisoning is usually pumping of stomach contents, which should only be attempted by a veterinarian.

Warfarin (Rat Bait). The active ingredient, dicoumarol, is found in nature in spoiled sweet clover and white clover. It is also manufactured synthetically. There is a substance in some clovers called *coumarin*, which may be converted to dicoumarol due to weather damage and a moldy condition; a factor develops within 24 to 48 hours after weather damage to produce the dicoumarol. Whether it is rat bait or sweet-clover poisoning, the effect is the same. An impairment of the blood-clotting mechanism occurs, which creates small hemorrhages throughout the body. These result from normal bumps and bruises, but because of the lack of normal blood clotting, the internal bleeding takes palce.

Vitamin K is one of the factors that normally is involved in blood clotting. Therefore, in the case of dicoumarol poisoning, increased levels of Vitamin K can be effective in preventing the internal bleeding. Young calves may occasionally need blood transfusions, but this is rare.

Chlorinated Naphthalenes ("X Disease"). The veterinary term for the condition caused by chlorinated naphthalenes is *hyperkeratosis*, which means an increased thickening and crusting of the skin. This condition first occurred on a large scale in 1941 and cost as much as $20 million in death and lowered production losses of livestock per year. At first there was no hint of what could be causing the problem, and researchers required considerable time to track down the cause. Since it appeared to be a new disease and since the cause was unknown, they referred to it as the *X Disease*. Later, researchers found the problem was due to ingestion of chlorinated naphthalene derivatives, which were used in petroleum products at that time. Most of these derivatives have now been taken off the market, but some wood preservatives still contain these substances. Thus, hot weather occasionally can precipitate a problem due to the heat's increasing the viscosity of the preservative, even in old wood, which cattle may then lick.

Cattle that have been exposed to this problem will appear listless, depressed, have a variable appetite, watery nose and eyes, and salivate. They show intermittent diarrhea, red swollen areas on the mouth and muzzle, frequent urination, and weight losses; and in the later stages the condition appears from which the name *hyperkeratosis* is derived; that is, the skin loses elasticity, hardens, wrinkles, develops loose folds, and cracks open. The neck and withers are most affected, but the whole body may be involved. A high death rate is not unusual, although many may recover completely.

There is no treatment; so prevention is the best method of control.

Plant Poisons

Oak Bud Poisoning. During drought or overgrazing of pastures, cattle may be forced to eat young oak leaves or acorns in areas where they grow. The shin oak is especially noted for its potential for poisoning. Under normal conditions, small quantities are of no concern, but when a major part of the diet comes from the oak leaves or acorns, it causes polyuria (frequent urination). There is a swelling along the middle of the belly, abdominal pain, severe gastrointestinal upset, and inflammation of the kidneys. Bloody mucus on the excrement may also be observed.

Treatment involves removing the source of the irritation by taking cattle out of the area or by providing supplemental feeding. Intestinal coatings should also be used to soothe the tract and to promote healing.

Bracken. Bracken is a plant that is found worldwide. All portions of the plant are poisonous, whether it is growing or dried. The agents that cause the poisoning are numerous types of compounds, but an aplastic anemia factor and a product that causes blood in the urine are the chief culprits.

Bracken poisoning is very hard to diagnose, and the signs vary with the age of the animal. The affected adult will show signs of depression, no appetite, bleeding from the nose or urinary tract, passage of bloody excrement, small hemorrhagic areas around the mouth or other body openings, and a marked elevation in temperature just before death. Death is caused by extensive ulcers in the gastrointestinal tract.

Young animals evidence similar signs but do not have external bleeding and ulcers. There is a swelling of the throat area that produces difficult breathing or a "roaring" sound, which is the main diagnostic sign in calves. The temperature is elevated, and death is caused by anemia rather than ulcers as in adults. The development of red blood cells in the bone marrow is suppressed; so an autopsy may show little.

Treatment has been uniformly unsuccessful. Perhaps the only key to control is learning to identify the plant and controlling with herbicides or other methods.

Ergot. Ergot is a type of fungus that grows on flowers, cereal grains, and some grasses, especially smut grass. It produces a substance that affects the central nervous system.

Animals usually walk in a wobbly stupor. Other signs include weak convulsions, depression, diarrhea, and lameness and stiffness, especially of the lower parts of the legs. The extremities such as the ears, nose, and tail lose warmth and pain sensitivity. Ergot causes a blockage in the small blood vessels (capillaries) that supply the extremities with blood. This blockage creates dry gangrene. Therefore, parts of the animal actually die and slough off, often resulting in the loss of the tail or part of the ears.

There is no treatment. Rest and removal of the source are the only recourse. Most grasses and flowers have the fungus only on the seed head, where it has a tendency to grow exclusively. Removing the seed heads of these flowers and grasses by periodic shredding has been a very effective preventive.

Legume and Fescue Poisoning. Sweet-clovers and white-clover problems are covered in the discussion on warfarin. For other related problems see the discussion of bloat.

A condition similar to ergot poisoning is caused by a toxic substance in fescue grass. Lameness in one or both hind feet characterizes this poisoning, known as *fescue foot*. The tail and ears may also be affected.

Nightshade. There is a wide distribution of black nightshade in weeds in pastures from Missouri to Texas, and from California southward into Mexico. It is not a problem when other forage or feed is plentiful; but when cattle are forced to forage on it, due to drought conditions, they will eat it.

Signs. There is difficult breathing with a characteristic expiratory grunt, salivation, nasal discharge, jaundice, weakness, a trembling of muscles in the hind legs, an increased heart rate, and occasionally bloat. The temperature is near normal or slightly elevated.

Cause. The cause is actually an alkaloid found in the leaves and fruit of the nightshade weed. Tomato and potato plants are in the nightshade family, and their leaves and fruit may also be toxic to cattle.

Treatment. Management is the only key. Hungry animals should be kept out of nightshade pastures, and if supplementally fed, they should not be fed on the ground where some of this material might be picked up. Animals showing signs should be placed in the shade to rest. If they survive the first 24 hours, they will usually recover.

Loco Weed.   Loco weed is found in the central and the western states of the United States. Although horses are most susceptible, cattle, sheep, and goats may also develop problems. The plant is toxic only in the early growth stages; these stages vary across the country depending on the amount of rainfall received. Thus, a fresh rain and new growth may occur even in a winter season in areas where temperatures are rather warm such as the Southwest.

The acute form occurs when large quantities of loco weed are eaten at one time. The chronic form is caused from a small intake over a longer period of time.

In cattle, consumption of about 90% of their body weight is needed before signs develop. Approximately 250% of their body weight normally must be consumed over a 3 to 4 month period before death occurs.

Signs.   A nervous, slow-staggering gait, rough haircoat, weight loss, muscular incoordination, and a characteristic blank stare are signs of loco-weed poisoning. Cattle at rest will show few signs but if excited, they may act *loco*, the Spanish word for "crazy."

Treatment.   Cattle return to normal if fed forage free of loco weed. Once cattle start eating the loco weed, it is hard to stop them. They seem to acquire a taste for it, and most will eventually die from it if turned back out to pasture. Cattle recently brought into the area are more likely to become addicted than those raised around it. At the first signs, affected cattle should be pulled out of the pasture, put on regular forage or feed, and shipped out as soon as they appear normal.

Loco weed may be controlled by spraying the pasture with 1 lb of 2-4-D per acre. The recommended time for spraying is between October and April, depending on the location.

Oleander.   The oleander shrub grows 15 to 20 ft high and is used quite commonly throughout the South as a yard decoration. There are times when cuttings are thrown into pastures or cattle are able to reach over a fence and eat them, bringing about the poisoning. The oleander is toxic throughout the entire plant, a little known fact considering its wide usage as an attractive landscape item. However, there have been reports of humans being poisoned with the oleander simply by using a twig as a meat skewer.

Signs.   Abdominal pain, vomiting, diarrhea, a rapid heartbeat due to constriction of the blood vessels, trembling, coma, and death are the signs.

Cause.   Cardiac glycosides—toxic substances found in heaviest concentration in the seeds but distributed throughout the plant—are the cause of toxicity. They actually bring on a heart attack.

Treatment.   Keep the animal warm, administer atropine, and drench with any substance that will induce vomiting.

Mesquite.   The mesquite tree produces a bean in the spring of the year throughout many parts of the desert Southwest. Some animals develop a peculiar affliction upon consuming these beans. Although normally the beans do not cause any harmful effect, there is individual susceptibility in cattle to impaction in the rumen by the undigested hulls of the beans. The affected animal simply ceases to have a functioning rumen due to this impaction, and for some reason the bean hulls tend to remain there (in the rumen) for the life of the animal. The animal can then literally starve to death because of its inability to digest other forages.

The affected cattle can be put in a feed lot and fed a high concentrate and recover very quickly; but once returned to the pasture, the condition recurs. The only sensible solution is to take such affected cattle from mesquite pastures, fatten them on grain, and ship them to slaughter.

In most cases, the mesquite bean does little damage and cattle are not affected by it.

Castor Bean

Signs. Nausea, violent digestive upsets, bloody excrement, and muscular tremors are the basic signs.

Cause. The cause is a toxic chemical, ricin, found throughout the plant but very heavily concentrated in the seed.

Treatment. There is no known treatment. An animal often will survive castor bean poisoning and have a prolonged seige of the condition. In this case, intestinal coatings are recommended.

Yew. Yew is a type of ornamental evergreen shrub that is planted around public buildings, driveways, and foundations of homes. It is popular especially in Kentucky and in the surrounding states. Also known as *ground hemlock*, *English yew*, and *Japanese yew*, it is a stiff needlelike bright green plant that produces red seeds.

Signs. The yew is extremely toxic and its effect requires a very short period of time. An animal is usually found dead without signs of struggle. Occasionally pieces of the yew will be found intact in the animal's mouth. Less severely affected animals show signs of trembling, difficult breathing, and collapse. After the onset of these signs, the duration of the illness is usually short with death the end result.

Cause. The cause of death from yew is a toxic substance that acts upon the heart, creating heart failure. It is also toxic to man and all classes of livestock. For horses and sheep, the poisonous amount is 4 to 8 oz; for cattle, it is 1 lb; for the pig it is 3 oz.

Prevention. The way to prevent the disorder is to keep domestic animals from direct contact with the plant.

Treatment. Although atropine has been beneficial in a few rare cases, no treatment has been effective.

Mycotoxins (Moldy Feed). The word *mycotoxin* comes from the Greek *mykes* meaning "fungus" and the Latin *toxicun* meaning "poison." Fungi are capable of both good and bad deeds in agriculture. Various fungi growing on cereal grains, foodstuffs, and mixed animal feeds are capable of producing toxic effects on animals that can result in death. This toxic characteristic can be used for some good purposes also. For instance, penicillin is a mycotoxin that is responsible for eradication of certain susceptible types of bacteria.

Although some mycotoxins like the ones derived from penicillin are harmless to man and animals, others can create serious difficulties. For example, rye, infested with fungus, was ground into bread and consumed by populations during feudal days, bringing about a nervous derangement in man known as "St. Anthony's Fire" or "Holy Fire," which swept through Europe and poisoned tremendous numbers of people.

Because of our advanced harvesting and storage techniques, the problem of mycotoxins is minimal, but it occasionally occurs in animals that are fed feed that has been improperly harvested or stored. If a feed becomes moldy, the chances are quite good that some slight to moderate poisoning can occur. Animal production can be severely limited, or in cases where large amounts are consumed, the animals can die.

Signs.   Reduced growth rate, stunting, poor performance, increased salivation, internal bleeding, kidney and liver damage, depression, poor appetite, weakness, staggering, nervous signs, intestinal disorders, and possibly death are signs of this mycotoxin poisoning. Young animals are more severely affected than older animals. Moldy feeds have also been reported to stimulate estrogen production, particularly in swine, causing prolapses of the vulva and abortions.

Cause.   Many toxic substances are produced by molds, but the aflatoxins receive the most attention because they are capable of producing cancer in animals, suppressing growth, and damaging the liver. Death occurs from internal bleeding and kidney and liver damage.

Prevention.   Although moldy feed is rarely toxic, caution should be exercised in its use. Damaged corn and grains are probably more susceptible to molds than other types of feeds. Under ideal growing conditions (frequent rainfall and high temperature), a mold growth can become toxic within a week. Cracked grains or screenings are most apt to have high mycotoxin content.

Stored grain should contain less than 13% moisture to keep fungi from developing to toxic levels. If there is any question about grain's being safe to feed livestock, diagnostic laboratories are available to assist veterinarians in evaluating any suspected feeds.

In addition to lowering and maintaining moisture content to less than 13%, it has been proposed that 1% proprionic acid would prevent mold from occurring, thus insuring good feed quality. The U.S. Food and Drug Administration has established a maximum allowance level of 20 parts per billion (ppb) of alfatoxin for a safe level of feed to be shipped interstate. This has been done to protect humans from eating meats from animals that have consumed mycotoxins, as these could be passed on to the human population.

167
NUTRITIONAL
DEFICIENCIES
AND
METABOLIC
DISEASES

Although a small amount of mold in feed may not be of concern, any obviously moldy feed should be destroyed. The following suggestions will help to avoid losses in livestock and will aid in utilization of feeds that have some mold present.

1. Feeds containing aflatoxin levels greater than 20 ppb cannot be shipped interstate; however, this is still a low level and is not toxic to animals. Research has shown that feed containing up to 100 ppb aflatoxins can be fed to nonlactating animals without causing toxicity. Anything over 200 ppb is more hazardous and should not be fed.

2. If moldy feed does cause problems, it still may be utilized by diluting it with good quality feed and watching closely for signs of toxicity. A general recommendation is three parts good feed to one part moldy feed.

3. If signs of prolapse or abortion occur, the feed should be withheld from animals of any age.

4. If possible, do not feed moldy feeds to younger stock as they are the most susceptible to the toxins.

Treatment. At the first sign of any problems feed should be withdrawn and good quality feed given, while the suspected feed is being checked by a veterinarian with the help of a diagnostic laboratory.

NUTRITIONAL DEFICIENCIES AND METABOLIC DISEASES

Milk Fever (Eclampsia)

Milk fever occurs most commonly at calving time in the adult female, although it is unlikely to occur until a second calf is born. It is more likely to occur in high milk-producers, both beef and dairy cows; and once a cow develops the condition, it is not unusual for it to occur at every calving thereafter.

Signs. Just after calving, there is a general muscular weakness; excitement may create head and limb tremors, and this is followed by a tendency to appear drowsy or even to lose consciousness. The affected cow doesn't want to move, has no appetite, will shake her head, grind her teeth, and eventually go down in a "curled" position similar to a sleeping dog. In spite of the name given to the disease, the body temperature is normal and in the advanced stages may even be subnormal.

An old method of diagnosis has been to straighten the head of the cow from the curled position and if her head immediately goes back as if on a spring, it is probably milk fever. The eyes are dry and staring, with pupils dilated. The pulse is weak, although the heart rate is increased. In more advanced stages the cow may lie flat on her side and bloat may develop. If the animal is not treated at this stage, death can occur within 6 to 12 hours or less. Treated animals have a good chance of recovering.

Cause. A low level of calcium in the blood brings on the condition, although the problem is also related to a deficiency of vitamin D and phosphorus. There may be some cases where treatment with substances other than calcium is necessary to bring about a response.

Prevention. There is an old farm tale that milking before calving will prevent milk fever. This is definitely not true and should not be followed.

Once cattle develop milk fever, they often become repeaters, accumulating a history of attacks. These known suspects can be given a vitamin D injection within 2 to 5 days before calving to create favorable response in most cases. Two hundred million units per day of vitamin D_2 are recommended for 5 days if given orally. If administered in an injectable form, vitamin D_3 is recommended as a single dose of 10,000,000 units 2 to 8 days prior to calving, given intramuscularly.

Treatment. The animal should be injected with a 20% solution of calcium borogluconate, given intravenously at a dosage of 400 to 800 cc. The solution should be given very slowly because if given too rapidly, it could cause a heart block and sudden death. It is important to give an accurate dose. Too little can cause an incomplete response and a return of the condition.

If the cow is found in the early stages of milk fever and is still standing and only showing muscular tremors, it can be given the injection subcutaneously or intraperitoneally.

Another treatment that may be used is a solution of glucose, magnesium sulfate, and steroids.

Avoid feeding a high calcium ration, even though this may seem to be the thing to do. Oral calcium can shock the system in its weakened condition.

Grass Tetany ("Grass Staggers")

Grass tetany occurs in lactating cows and is characterized by low levels of magnesium (and often low levels of calcium) in the blood. The name *grass staggers* is derived from the fact that this disorder most often occurs in the spring when cattle graze on lush, fast-growing grass pasture, and the cattle invariably assume a staggering gait at some point in their affliction.

Signs. Clinical signs include muscular spasms, convulsions, and death due to respiratory failure. An animal that has been grazing peacefully will suddenly cease grazing, begin twitching in the muscles of the legs and ears, and appear very uncomfortable. It will take on a characteristic alertness, and any minor disturbance may precipitate frenzied galloping, bellowing, even attack.

Cause. The body does not have a very large natural storehouse for magnesium. Reserves are depleted very quickly; therefore there must be magnesium in the daily rations in an absorbable form. Under normal circumstances there is enough magnesium in the daily ration; but under unusual circumstances, such as in highly fertilized, fast-growing spring grass pasturage, the potassium levels in the grass rise dramatically, and the potassium then inhibits the absorption of magnesium by the cow. It is thought that this is the reason for magnesium deficiency, and since magnesium has an important role in muscle functions, a deficiency brings on muscular incoordination, "staggers", and convulsions. The obvious remedy for a deficiency of this sort is to either reduce the level of potassium or increase the level of magnesium. On a practical basis the level of magnesium can be increased by feeding 1 to 2 oz of magnesium oxide per cow each day. The supplementary magnesium can be fed in a small daily feed of grain and molasses or in other palatable forms such as mineral mixes.

169
NUTRITIONAL
DEFICIENCIES
AND
METABOLIC
DISEASES

Downer Cow Syndrome

Signs. The "downer" cow syndrome is brought about by a variety of problems, all resulting in a down cow that is unable or unwilling to rise. The cow will have normal signs. She will eat and drink, and have normal temperature and normal pulse, but just be too weak to rise.

Cause. The name *downer cow* is probably a misnomer because a variety of conditions that cause a cow to be unable to rise have been grouped together under this one category. The cow is "downed" most often just before or just after calving because of damage to the nerves that are located just inside the pelvis. This damage is brought about by passage of the fetus through the pelvic canal, causing pressure on the nerves. Many times in a difficult or lengthy birth, this pressure is sufficient to cause the damage. In other cases just the presence of the fetus for a long time in this position can cause damage because of the continued pressure.

The condition can also be caused by numerous mineral deficiencies or metabolic disorders, and serious infections can give rise to the syndrome. This is actually a catchall term. Not even the exact cause of the disorder is known, but it is different from other "down" conditions such as milk fever because there is no response to injections of calcium gluconate. The affected cow just appears to give up, and many "old timers" speculate that it is a mental situation as much as physical. At least, it does appear that way because of a lack of abnormal signs other than the inability of the cow to put weight on its hind legs.

Prevention. The sooner a cow is observed with the downer cow syndrome and the sooner she can be replaced on her feet, the more likely she is to recover. Good observation and swift attention are the best preventives.

Treatment. There has been very little success with any treatment even though magnesium, calcium, steroids, and stimulants of every type have been tried.

A sling is normally used to hoist the "downed" cow to its feet once or twice a day. If this cannot be done, the cow should at least be turned from side to side and should be well bedded to prevent urine scalds and other bedsores from occurring. The normal recommendation is to provide feed, water, shade, and comfort, and to try to lift the cow once or twice a day in a sling to stand some weight on the hind legs for 5 or 10 minutes and hope that she will eventually recover.

Another common cause of the downer cow syndrome is a fracture of the bones of the legs or pelvis. Downer cows should be carefully examined for fractures by a veterinarian to eliminate this as a cause of the cow's inability to rise.

Ketosis (Acetonemia)

Signs. The name *ketosis* comes from the fact that there is a characteristic odor of ketones on the breath and sometimes in the milk of cattle, along with other signs. This ketone odor is difficult to describe, but once experienced, it will never be forgotten. Acetone is one of the ketones that is commonly used in fingernail polish remover. Therefore, think of the odor of fingernail polish remover on the breath of a cow with ketosis. It has been described by some as a sick, sweet odor; and when this odor is detected on the breath of cattle, ketosis can fairly safely be assumed to be the problem although a definite diagnosis must come from a veterinarian because there are several other conditions that can create the same signs.

There are two forms of ketosis. The first is called the *wasting form*. Clinical signs include a decrease in appetite and milk production over a period of 2 to 4 days; an extremely fast loss in body weight; dry, firm feces and often severe constipation; temperature, pulse, and respiration are normal. These animals may die. Milk production will drop severely if they do not die, and it may take as long as 30 days to recover. Even then, cows will not regain their former production levels until the next lactation. This is a disease that is much more common to dairy than to beef cattle. All domestic animals are subject to having ketosis, however.

The second form of ketosis is called the *nervous form*. Clinical signs include mild staggering, partial blindness, delirium, walking in circles, crossing of the legs, leaning on stanchions, depraved appetite, and chewing and salivation. These signs may be intermittent, occurring every 1 to 2 hours, or they may occur every 10 to 12 hours.

This is one disorder that will definitely require the use of a veterinarian who has had experience with the condition. It is a very complicated metabolic disorder. Biochemically, ketones are eliminated in the urine, and there is low blood sugar (hypoglycemia) and a low level of glycogen in the liver. Carbohydrates and fats are broken down in the rumen to produce propionic acid and acetic acid in a ratio of four to one. When this ratio is disturbed, the system produces ketone bodies that disrupt the normal pathways, bringing on an exhaustion of the glucose stored in the liver. Since cattle have very small storages of glucose, the condition can quickly become serious.

171
NUTRITIONAL
DEFICIENCIES
AND
METABOLIC
DISEASES

Cause. The cause is a disruption in the metabolism of carbohydrates and fatty acids to produce ketones. This condition is associated with dairy cattle on a high level of feed. It is uncommon in beef cattle or any cattle on grass pastures. In general, the cause is a higher demand made on body production, such as milk production, than can be met through the normal digestive and metabolic processes.

Prevention. The best precaution is to have animals neither too fat nor too thin before calving because ketosis often occurs just prior to or just after birth. Keeping an adequate mineral mix available is definitely recommended, and problem herds that have a history of this condition may be fed sodium proprionate at the rate of 100 grams per day for 6 weeks. Also, a reduction of the high level of feeding, particularly ensilage, just prior to calving, may be of some help as a preventive.

Treatment. A veterinarian should be consulted because of the complexity of the disorder. Generally, glucose replacement therapy at the rate of 500 to 1000 cc of 50% dextrose is administered along with steroid therapy. There are many steroids on the market, and administration will vary according to type used and the manufacturer's direction. This treatment will need to be repeated periodically.

Rickets

In general, rickets is a condition of young, growing animals that causes a defective calcification of the skeleton, usually resulting in distorted or malformed bones. It is very unusual to find rickets in recent years because so many livestock owners now recognize the importance of proper calcium and phosphorus supplementation. However, clinical signs are covered here in the interest of historical classic signs of a mineral or vitamin deficiency.

Signs. Clinical signs include stiff gait, enlarged legs (especially the forelegs), lameness, abnormal curvature of the bone, easily fractured bones, and maybe a collapse of the pelvis. Teeth are also affected by rickets, and enlarged jawbones and a protrusion of the tongue are sometimes seen.

Cause. The cause is a deficiency of calcium, phosphorus, or vitamin D. All three of these essential nutrients are necessary for proper bone development. Calcium and phosphorus are minerals used in making up the major portion of bone structure, and vitamin D is necessary in order for these two minerals to be properly absorbed and laid down in the form of bone.

Prevention. A mineral mix containing calcium and phosphorus should be provided and put out free-choice. There are numerous commercial mixtures available, or you may mix your own using one-third salt, one-third ground limestone or ground oyster shell, and one-third monosodium phosphate.

Treatment. If the disease is caught early—before the bones are distorted—recovery is rapid when calcium and phosphorus are simply restored to the diet. If the animal has been housed and rickets have developed, it is possible that calcium and phosphorus were adequate in the diet, but vitamin D, which comes from sunshine, was absent and therefore precipitated the disease. A dose of injectable vitamin D in this case will produce marked improvement within a few days. Animals that could not stand or could not straighten their legs completely are standing straight and moving with noticeable ease within 7 to 10 days or less. However, if treatment is not started until after there has been obvious deformation of the bones, there usually is permanent damage that will not respond to treatment no matter what is done.

Founder (laminitis)

Signs. The condition of founder is most common in cattle and horses, although it can affect most domestic farm animals. The clinical sign is an inflammation of the area between the bony part of the foot and the hoof wall. In cattle the disorder generally occurs in a chronic form in which the hoof wall separates from the bony tissue and the toes grow long and turn up without touching the ground. The toes often cross over and step on each other when the animal walks. In the acute form the signs include a condition of lameness, stiffness in the joints, and a painful straight-legged gait.

Cause. Founder is listed here under nutritional deficiencies, but actually it is more likely an allergic reaction to grain components due to overfeeding of grain or an animal accidentally getting into feed and gorging itself when it is not used to high-concentrate feeds. Signs usually begin to appear within 24 hours after the animal has gorged itself.

Prevention. If an increased level of grain is needed for milk production or fattening, the increase should be gradual. A reasonable "warm-up" period of gradually increasing the feed to new levels within 2 to 4 weeks will generally prevent an occurrence of founder. Storeroom doors should be kept secured so that the possibility of a break-in by cattle is avoided. The condition is most often found when cattle accidentally stumble onto an unexpected feast and gorge themselves.

Treatment. In the chronic form the elongated toes should be trimmed back to normal using hoof shears, so that the animal can get around with as little pain as possible. Disposal of the animal through sale or slaughter should be as soon as practical because the condition generally recurs and is difficult to completely cure.

If the acute form is in evidence, treatment with antihistamine and steroid therapy is recommended. This will provide a good chance of recovery.

PARASITES

Internal Parasites

Lungworms. Lungworms are parasites that cause lungworm disease and also a condition known as *verminous pneumonia*.

Signs. The signs vary greatly with the individual animal. Generally the disease is seen only in the severe stages, usually with young animals. If the infestation is mild, there may only be a hacking, noticeable cough. In heavy infestations, there is a loss of appetite, diarrhea, and very stunted growth. A secondary bacterial infection may also occur in severe cases, causing verminous pneumonia and death.

Cause. The cause is Dictyocaulus, a parasite that lives in the host, commonly referred to as the *lungworm.* The disorder may cause death by pneumonia, but generally it is only an irritating condition. The adult lungworm lives in the upper part of the lung where the trachea (windpipe) joins the lungs. The parasite lays eggs there. These eggs may be coughed up and swallowed, and the larvae stage then develops in the digestive tract; the larvae pass on out to the pasture and are picked up by other grazing cattle. If the larvae are not coughed up, the eggs develop where they are, in the lung, to continue the infestation.

Treatment. If pneumonia is present, it must be treated separately, in addition to getting rid of the lungworms. Levamisole is a good deworming agent. It is available in an injectable form or in an oral powder or tablet form. Pneumonia, if present, should be treated with antibiotics and steroids at the discretion of a veterinarian (see section on pneumonia).

In areas where lungworms are a continuing problem, the whole herd is generally treated in the spring and fall, varying the type of dewormer used so that the parasites will not become immune to the deworming agent. (See Herd Health for specific recommendations of products and amounts.)

Hookworms

Signs. Hookworms generally are more of a threat to young calves ranging from 4 to 12 months of age than they are to older cattle. The older cattle tend to develop an immunity to hookworm and are able to survive even though the infestation may be severe. Young calves most often show clinical signs of infestation during the winter months when nutrition is generally at a low level; so this time there may not be adequate levels of high-energy feed supplied to both animal and parasite. Clinical symptoms are mild abdominal pain, bouts with diarrhea, unthriftiness, a characteristic "bottle-jaw" anemia, and weakness. On occasions the infestation is severe enough that calves go down, and death occurs within 2 to 3 days.

Cause. The Bunostomum species of worm attaches itself to the gut by a hooklike connection and sucks blood, creating internal hemorrhaging. There is also a loss of nutrients to the parasite. The hookworms are very small; so they probably would not be seen with the naked eye. The eggs are even smaller and can only be seen under a microscope. The eggs are passed in the feces and may be detected by microscopic examination by a veterinarian. These eggs develop into larvae in one week, and then go through several stages before reinfesting the animal. Reinfestation may be by skin penetration where the larvae enter the bloodstream, and then go to the heart, or to the lungs where they are coughed up and swallowed, thus entering the small intestine for the completion of the cycle. Or the larvae may be simply picked up by grazing animals and go directly to the small intestine.

Prevention. Quite often calves are not wormed until after they have been weaned. A good preventive is to worm at about 4 months of age with a mild wormer. This is particularly important when young calves are going into the winter where poorer nutrition will cause additional stress if they do become infested.

Treatment. Specific products and recommendations for intestinal parasites in general are discussed at the end of this section.

Intestinal Worms. Intestinal worms come in a wide variety of species; they attack the gastrointestinal tract from the abomasum down to and throughout the small intestine. Most types are closely related, and if you have one type of intestinal worm, you usually have another. Therefore, to simplify the discussion, intestinal worms will be treated as a group.

These parasites mainly attack young animals, and older animals with poor nutrition; they may rob their victims of as much as 50% of their nutritional intake. Many cattle appear to do quite well in spite of having relatively high infestations, but young calves are not able to cope as well and usually are "poor doers" right from the start.

Signs. Weight loss, reduced growth, unthriftiness, dull haircoat, and persistent diarrhea are all signs of intestinal worms. In severe cases, a deworming agent may be used, and even though the worm is removed by it, there is still sufficient damage to the intestinal tract, so that the diarrhea continues and recovery may be very slow. For this reason it is most important to control intestinal parasites rather than treat the animal after there is an obvious problem. Some cattle may eat right up to the day of their death in cases where heavy infestation exacts the final toll.

Cause. Several closely related intestinal worms, the most common of which are *Cooperia*, *Ostertagia*, *Trichostrongyl*, and *Nematodirus* are the cause.

Prevention. Cattle frequently contract a condition of intestinal worms on heavily-grazed pastures where they are forced to pick up the larval stage by grazing around manure-contaminated forage. If the stocking rate cannot be lowered, a common preventive is to drag the pasture with a heavy object, such as a railroad iron, to spread the manure out, allowing direct access by sunlight. This will kill the developing worms if enough exposure is allowed. It is also recommended that young cattle be wormed at least 4 times per year, and older cattle should be wormed at least twice a year.

Treatment. Thiabendazole (TBZ, Omnizol) in paste, liquid, or bolus form given 3 to 4 times per year is recommended. Levamisol, Rulene, phenothiazine, and other dewormers will work well if used regularly.

Coccidiosis. Coccidiosis causes little death loss, but it is a very common problem in young animals. Older cattle generally develop an immunity to it and are not impaired by the condition unless they have not been exposed to it in their lifetime, in which case they react in the same way as a newly infected young animal.

Signs. Clinical signs include diarrhea, anemia, and weight loss. The most common sign is bloody or brown-colored manure. This condition generally occurs in housed cattle that are in close confinement during the winter months. It is also commonly found in pasture conditions. The incubation period is 18 days, so it will not be seen in calves younger than about 3 weeks.

Cause. The cause is a microscopic protozoan. The parasite is transmitted by spores called *oocysts*, which get their name from the fact that the organisms spend their entire lifetime in the mucosa (lining) of the bowel, producing a cyst (small blister) that ruptures. This in turn releases a spore that may contaminate feed, water, and even the haircoat of nearby cattle. It is easy to see how food, drink, or licking of the haircoat by close-quartered cattle could cause a widespread outbreak. The ruptured cyst in the intestine also produces some blood loss, which brings on the anemia.

Prevention. Good hygiene, no crowding, and feed troughs that are high enough to prevent accidental contamination with manure will help prevent the disease. Feeding amprolium is also a good preventive.

Treatment. The aim is to destroy the protozoa and treat the ulceration of the intestine caused by the cysts. Sulfa drugs, given orally, are good for this. The disease is mainly self-limiting because if an animal lives through it, he usually will recover on his own. Coatings and astringents may be used if there is an animal that is very weak.

Tapeworms

Signs. Tapeworms are generally a problem in younger calves. The chief signs are unthriftiness, poor haircoat, mild digestive upset, and constipation. This is not an obvious condition, especially if nutrition has been adequate, because the animal is able to sustain his own body functions as well as those of the parasite as long as sufficient feed is available. It is a most common problem in calves, but does not always result in clinical illness.

Cause. The condition is spread from one animal to another through the life cycle evolution of the tapeworm. Eggs from the tapeworm, which contain a living embryo, are passed in the feces; the embryo then develops -within an intermediate host, usually a mite. Cattle pick up the mite by licking their haircoat or the haircoat of other cattle; they ingest the intermediate form, and so develop a tapeworm.

Treatment. The product Yomesan is the most common dewormer recommended today; it does an effective job in ridding the animal of tapeworms.

Flukes. Flukes are a most common problem along the Gulf Coast areas of the United States and Central and South America. Flukes are also prevalent in Africa and any other part of the world where there are low-lying, wet areas. There are two main forms of flukes—the cattle fluke and the deer fluke. The latter is extremely difficult if not impossible to control because of the wild nature of the deer population and the inability of most drugs to kill the parasite.

Signs. The acute form of cattle fluke disease will be indicated by the clinical signs of a lack of appetite, edema (an accumulation of fluid, especially "bottle jaw"), pallor (a lack of natural color), pain when pressure is exerted over the area of the liver, and death within 48 hours. The cause of death is a swollen liver that restricts the blood flow through it, and if afflicted subjects are stressed too much, death can occur quite quickly.

The chronic form is the more common problem and can cause great economic loss. The signs are "bottle jaw," unthriftiness, and diarrhea. The main worry with flukes is that they weaken the animal to other diseases—diseases that can kill. Redwater is one of the common diseases that results from the weakened condition caused by flukes.

Cause. The term *liver fluke* is most often used, and it indicates where the parasite normally resides. The fluke grows in the bile ducts of the liver, producing eggs; these eggs later migrate into the intestines, are passed out in the feces, and are picked up by an intermediate host, the common snail. The parasite lives in the snail until it develops into the next stage; it then leaves the snail and crawls up on grass; the grass is eaten by cattle, thus causing a reinfestation and completion of the life cycle.

Prevention. Controlling snails, keeping cattle out of standing water, and/or draining low-lying areas to reduce the habitat of the snail are the most common ways of reducing the possibility of infestations. Snail baits have also been used, but there are some situations that are not economically feasible to change, and treatment is still the cheapest way out.

Treatment. There is no drug that is effective in complete eradication of flukes because you must kill the migrating stage found in the snail as well as the fluke found in the bile duct. Hexachloroethane is most often used as a drench. It is relatively nontoxic, but it is only effective against the early, immature stages of the fluke, before it becomes entrenched in the liver. Treatment must be started before the flukes have had a chance to build up levels of mature infestations. Three treatments per year are recommended in low-lying, wet areas to control the condition. There are many cattlemen who have been able to maintain herds in these wet areas only because they faithfully treat for flukes in the winter, spring, and fall of each year.

Parasite Control in General. There are several factors to consider in an overall program of parasite control. First, the nutritional status of the herd is of the utmost importance. If the herd is well-fed with no nutritional deficiencies, parasites will seldom be a health problem because enough feed is being consumed for both animal and parasite. Treatment here would be much less stressful and much more effective since the nutritional status is sound.

Another important factor in parasite control is pasture management. Dragging the pastures with a heavy iron will not only kill the eggs of many parasites by exposing them to the sunlight, but grass will grow evenly over the pasture, increasing the stocking rate, and the pasture will be fertilized with the manure at the same time.

Dewormers. There are many dewormers on the market, but perhaps a few have been accepted more readily because of their effectiveness. These are:

1. Levamisole (Tramisol)—This drug is a good all-purpose dewormer that is effective on lungworms, hookworms, and intestinal worms. Although it will not control flukes or coccidia, it is a popular product that is available both in an injectable form and as an oral drench. However, it is not recommended for use on very weak animals.

2. Thiabendazole (Thiomnizol TBZ)—This drug is a dewormer that is very effective against intestinal worms of all types. It is *not* effective on tapeworms, flukes, lungworms, or coccidia. However, the intestinal worms (parasites) that cause the greatest economic loss are easily controlled by TBZ. It has a mild reaction on the animal; the medication can be given with little concern, even if a mistake is made and an overdose is given. In very high infestations of intestinal parasites, an even higher than recommended dose of TBZ should be considered. Dosages two or even three times higher than the label recommends can be given without worry. It is available in a liquid drench, bolus, and oral paste form.

Because of its mild properties, it is highly recommended for calves and any animal that is weak.

3. Phenothiazine—Phenothiazine is the old green standby that has been used for many years. It is a toxic substance that must be used in a controlled dose, however, and should not be used on animals that are already sick with parasites as this could cause enough additional stress to kill the patient. There are several different forms of phenothiazine that vary with the particle size. Look closely at the forms available because the cheapest priced product may not give the most economical returns nor be the most effective.

4. Hexachloroethane—This drug is used for the control of the immature stages of liver flukes. It is a good, relatively safe drug.

5. Crufomate (Ruelene)—This drug does an excellent job but is toxic and should be used with extreme caution on any animals that are sick.

There are many other products on the market that can be used as deworming agents, but we have listed here only the ones most commonly adaptable to the average cattleman's needs and capabilities. These should give you the best program. A veterinarian may want to supplement this program with more effective dewormers that can control a specific parasite in a specific situation or part of the country. A more complete outline of what to use and in what dosages is given in Table 6-3.

Table 6-3. Internal Parasite Recommendations

CONTROL OF COMMON CATTLE WORM

Chemical (Example brand)	Stomach worms	Nodular worms	Cooper's worms	Thread-necked Strongyle	Hookworms	Lungworms
Thiabendazole (Thiomnizole, TBZ)	+	+	+	+		
Levamisole (Tramisol)	+	+	+	+	+	+
Coumaphos[a] (Baymix)	+		+	+		
Haloxon (Loxon)	+		+			
Crufomate (Ruelene)	+	+[b]	+	+[b]		
Phenothiazine	+	+				

WORM MEDICATION

Chemical	Brand Example	Bolus	Drench	Feed[c]	Paste	Injectable	Water
Dichlorvos	Atgard			●			
Hygromycin B	Hygromix			●			
Levamisole	Tramisol	●	●	●		●	●
Piperazine				●			●
Pyrantel	Banminth			●			
Thiabendazole	TBZ	●	●	●	●		
Coumaphos	Baymix			●			
Haloxon	Loxon	●	●				
Crufomate	Ruelene		●				
Phenothiazine		●	●	●			

178

Parasite	Cause	Prevention	Treatment	Withholding Period
Gastrointestinal (all types) and Lungworms.	Anemia, unthriftiness, slow weight gain, feed utilization and weight gains affected. Internal parasitism is frequently not clinically detected.	Phenothiazine—0.15 g/100 lb average body weight/day. (Average daily dose =2 g in salt.) Rotate pastures. Feed in bunks, feed adequately for maximum results.	Phenothiazine—20 g/100 lb body weight/day. Maximum 70 g. Rotate pastures. Feed in bunks. Feed adequately. Thiabendazole—3–5 g/100 lb body weight. Levamisole hydrochloride—0.08 –0.8% (0.36–3.6 g/lb) 0.09 g/100 lb body weight per day for 6 days. Haloxon—7 days.	Phenothiazine—Do not feed to animals during last four weeks of pregnancy. Don't feed to lactating animals. Thiabendazole—Don't use milk for human consumption for 96 hours after last treatment. Levamisole hydrochloride 48 hr. Injectable Levamisole—7 days.
Cysticerosis (Beef Measles): Invasion of muscles by beef tapeworm of man (*Taenia saginata*)	No symptoms found on post-mortem.	Strict human sanitation around feedlots.	None	
Echinococcosis: Cysts caused by dog tapeworm: a public health hazard.	No symptoms found on post-mortem.	Keep dogs out of feed lots.	None	
Liver flukes: *Fasciola hepatica* (Common liver fluke)	Unthriftiness, weakness, emaciation.	Destroy the intermediate host by keeping cattle away from areas frequented by the snail.	Hexachloroethane 10 gm/100 lb of body weight.	None

Source: John B. Herrick, *Feedstuffs*. (Minneapolis, Minn.: Miller Publishing Company, Reference Issue, Volume 49, No. 30, 1977), p. 83. Reprinted by permission.

[a]Cleared for lactating dairy cattle.

[b]Aids in controlling.

[c]Feed form may include top dress, premix, medicated block, supplements, complete feeds, range cubes, and minerals, depending on chemical.

External Parasites

Lice. Lice are very small parasites that are a problem mostly in the winter. They cause economic loss because of an invasion of the skin, creating an itching that causes cattle to look unthrifty and to scratch when they should be eating. Weight loss results simply due to the irritation. Lice are also vectors of some diseases. Lice can be controlled by a variety of products used in backrubbers, dusters, and spray-on materials.

Ticks. There are many species of ticks, and the type may need to be identified before effective control is possible as some species will be killed only by certain insecticides. Occasionally these species will build up an immunity to one product, and another product may need to be substituted. Ticks suck blood from cattle, creating anemia, and in production-type cattle (milk cows and feed-lot cattle) ticks do pose a threat to the pocketbook. The main problem is that ticks get down into the ears of the cattle causing them to go berserk because of· the mere sensation of the ticks' activity. Ticks also transmit many diseases such as anaplasmosis, tick paralysis (which affects both calves and humans), bacterial diseases, and many viral diseases.

Control is the main concern rather than complete eradication, which appears to be unlikely. There are a variety of products on the market, including dips, sprays, and powders. The form chosen will depend on whether cattle are show animals, or whether they are being milked in a parlor or out on the range. Some products may be restricted as to their use indoors. Specific recommendations depend on the particular species of tick and what will work against it. Arsenic compounds are still being used for control, but generally arsenic-based products are not recommended because of the potential danger of residues. In general, rotenone and pyrethrum can be used safely. Lindane in a .025% solution or toxaphene in a .05% solution may both be used as a dip or spray. The latter two insecticides have wide acceptance by cattlemen across the country.

A chemically impregnated ear tag has proven quite effective in killing most species of ticks. It is used extensively along the Mexican border with good results. Specific recommendations for most external parasite control are given at the end of this chapter in Table 6-4.

Dermatophytes (Fungi). Dermatophytes cause infections of the skin, the most common of which is ringworm. The name is really a misnomer because the condition is caused by a fungus. The lesion occurs in a circular shape that ranges from the size of a nickel to a 50¢ piece, or even larger. The hair falls out and a crust develops over the area. It is not a severe economic problem and is most common on show animals. It is a condition that usually can be cleared up simply by time, but show animals in particular need a quick solution to the problem. A very effective treatment is a 10% solution of Clorox (one part common Clorox and nine parts water). Bathe the affected area two to three times per week and the ringworm will be gone in 2 to 3 weeks. Iodine is also effective as a treatment.

Ants. The most pressing problem for the cattle industry in the ant category is the fire ant, which is distributed across the southern half of the United States. If a hill of these ants is disturbed, there is an immediate swarming, and the bite of these ants is very painful, much like falling into a fire. They will swarm on a young calf if it accidentally lies down next to a hill and can sting it so severely that shock and even death may result. Cows have been known to calve near an anthill and being unable to get up, have lost the calf and gone into shock from the fire ant stings. There are many instances of cattle that accidentally become exposed to fire ants, and before they can move out of the area, they have large welts over many parts of their bodies. There is a tremendous economic loss to cattlemen as well as severe irritation caused to both cattle and men in the South due to these fire ants.

In the case of severe stings and welts, systemic steroids and antibiotics are recommended. The Environmental Protection Agency has taken Mirex off the market; so there is little chemical control available that is sanctioned by the government. About the only recommendation that can be made for control is to keep the ground worked as much as possible. Perhaps dragging a heavy railroad iron, keeping the hills disturbed, will be of some assistance because fire ants will not develop in plowed fields or areas where the ground is frequently worked.

Flies and Mosquitoes. Flies are not only a concern to the animal, but they are also a menace to the cattleman because face flies are vectors (carriers) of pinkeye. Other flies carry anaplasmosis, brucellosis, and many viral and bacterial diseases. This is especially true of the biting-type of flies. Flies also cause severe irritation and itching of the skin, loss of hair, and occasionally maggots. In the Southwest the screwworm fly is always a threat because of the maggots that eat out the flesh in a wound. Although sterile male flies have been regularly released in the Southwest along the Mexican border to keep most female flies barren, there have been numerous outbreaks of screwworms reported recently, and a general fly-control program should be a part of the cattleman's management plans.

Mosquitoes are also responsible for weight loss, irritation, and discomfort; they too can serve as carriers of disease, either directly or as an intermediate host.

Grubs (Ox Warbles). In the spring the heel fly lays its eggs in the hair of the legs and bellies of cattle. The eggs hatch in 3 to 5 days, and the small larvae penetrate the skin, migrating toward the throat area where they remain until late winter. Further migration is then to the animal's back, just under the skin. The grubs make a small puncture or "air hole" in the hide; eventually they mature and "pop out" onto the ground to form pupae, which emerge as flies to start the cycle over again.

The common grub migrates to the area around the esophagus, while the northern grub migrates toward the spinal canal. Bloat can occur from grubs around the esophagus. "Downer" cattle can occur when the spinal canal is the location of the grub.

There is considerable discomfort to cattle, not to mention economic loss due to weight loss, lowered milk production, and destruction of the prime portion of the hide. Although there is no pain to the animal when the heel flies lay their eggs, cattle are terrified, perhaps by instinct, and run around wildly, creating numerous possibilities for injury.

Treatment with a pour-on grubicide is very effective. Products containing Coumaphas (Co-Ral), Triclorofon (Neguvon), or Ruelene are available and are recommended in areas where grubs are a known menace. A grubicide is absorbed through the skin and is transported in the bloodstream (systemic) to kill the grubs in the tissues. It should be applied annually after the first killing frost, not less than 14 days before calving and not more than 21 days prior to slaughter. Do not apply to lactating cows.

Mites. *Sarcoptic mange* is a condition caused by mites. Although it is not widespread in cattle, it does occur with enough frequency to alert you to the potential threat to animal comfort and to its possible spreading to the herd.

The tiny mite burrows in the skin, forming a tunnel or burrow where eggs are laid. This causes skin irritation, inflammation, and hair loss due to rubbing. The mite eggs mature in about 17 days. The mite can live only a few days off the host, but spreads readily by contact.

Treatment at the first sign of hair loss, especially about the neck, shoulders, and tail, is very effective. Toxaphene or any approved external insecticide for spraying or dipping will readily control an outbreak.

External Parasites in General. Controlling flies around livestock is the key to controlling most other external parasites. Since fly larvae develop in manure and moist areas, removing manure build-up and providing good drainage are the first steps in controlling flies and thus most external and a few internal parasites around the farm.

Sprays, rubbing devices, and dust are common methods of applying insecticides. Sprays can be applied directly to the animals or they may be applied by foggers and mist sprayers while animals are in groups. Dusts can be distributed by hand or applied through dust bags or blowers.

Backrubbers and dust bags require little labor and provide effective control, although they miss flies that congregate on the under side of the animal. Locate dusters where animals are forced to use them daily. For example, if water supplies are fenced off, use a backrubber or duster so that cattle have to walk through it to get to water. Other key areas for duster bags are any shady areas where cattle tend to loaf.

Vapor strips are effective indoors or in enclosed areas. For longer term control, residual sprays should be applied to building surfaces. In addition, outside areas where flies congregate around windows, doors, along fences, and under feed bunks should also be sprayed. Fly baits will continue to kill flies for a period of time but must be placed out of reach of animals.

Feeding systemic insecticides in loose or block form helps by killing fly larvae in the manure. Where large areas must be covered, aerial application of ultra-low volume insecticides is being used with increased frequency.

Table 6-4. Recommendations for External Parasite Control
(Beef Cow)

Diseases/Cause	Prevention	Treatment	Withdrawal Period
Lice: *Several ssp.*	Backrubber, spray. Spraying is the best method of louse control. In addition to killing lice, enough insecticide remains in the hair and coat to kill lice that hatch from eggs several days after application. Backrubbers suppress louse populations but do not effectively eradicate.	Ciodrin (S) Co-Ral (S-P.O.) Delnav (S) Lindane (S) Malathion (S) Neguvon (P.O.) Korlan (P.O.) Toxaphene (S) Warbex (P.O.) Trichlorfon Rabon Ciovap Ravap Lysoff P.O.	0 day 0 day 0 day 30 days 0 day 14 days 0 day 28 days 35 days 14 days 0 day 0 day 0 day 35 days
Grubs: *Two species*	Treat for grubs from Aug. 1 to Dec. 1 to avoid side reactions. Learn the life cycle to understand this recommended treatment period. Grubby animals are not only expensive to the producer, but are not good for the image of the industry. Grub control also provides louse control.	CoRal (S, P.O.) Ruelene (S, P.O.) Warbex (P.O.) Neguvon (S) Tiguvon (P.O.) Feed additives– Ronnel or Famphur Spotten Gx-118 Gx-130 Trichlorfon	0 day—Do not use on calves under 3 mo. of age. 7 days 35 days 7 days—Do not use on calves under 3 mo. of age. 35 days– Withdrawal depends on formulation. Check carefully. 45 days 21 days 21 days 14 days

Table 6-4. (*Continued*)

DISEASES/CAUSES	SIGNS	PREVENTION	TREATMENT	WITHHOLDING PERIOD
Flies: *Several ssp.*	Fly control in pastures is difficult. It requires the use of feed additives, backrubbers, dust bags, oilers, & sprays. Low-level feed additive—Ronnel, Phenothiazine Rabon Altosid—14 days.	Dust bags: Ciodrin Co-Ral Malathion Methoxychlor Rabon Backrubbers: Clovap Co-Ral Delnav Korlan Melathion Toxaphene Ravap	Sprays: Ciodrin Co-Ral Delnav Korlan Toxaphene Malathion Rabon Ravap	7 days 0 day 0 day 7 days 28 days 0 day 0 day 0 day
Mange: *Several ssp. mites.*	Spray or dip. Mange is a reportable disease and animals are quarantined on premises.	Toxaphene Lindane Co-Ral		28 days 30 days 15 days

Notes: S = spray.
P.O. = pour on.

Surface Treatment for Fly Control in Livestock Areas[a]

INSECTICIDE (TRADE NAME)	FORMULATION		REMARKS
Pyrethrins + Synergist Dichlorvos (Vapona) Naled (Dibrom)	0.1% 0.5% 0.3%	space sprays	Space spray with fogger or as mist. Remove animals.
Crotoxyphos (Ciodrin) Dimethoate (Cygon, De-Fend) Ronnel (Korlan) Rabon (Gardona) Fenthion (Baytex) Malathion	1.0% 1.0% 1.0% 1.0% 1.0% 1.0%	residual sprays	Remove animals. Apply to cover surface of walls and ceiling. Avoid runoff.
Malathion Naled (Dibrom) Dichlorvos (Vapona) Trichlorfon (Dipterex)	1.0% 0.5% 0.5% 1.0%	baits	Largely ineffective for adult flies in areas with manure and bedding. Kills larvae in manure.
	VAPOR STRIPS		
Dichlorvos (Vapona) Dimethilan (Snip)	1 strip per 100 sq ft of ceiling space		Place out of reach, not over feed, water or milk utensils.

[a]Only specific chemicals permitted in milk rooms. Consult milk inspector concerning local restrictions.

Table 6-4. (*Continued*)

Direct Fly Control on Animals

INSECTICIDE (TRADE NAME)	FORMULATION	WITHDRAWAL BEFORE SLAUGHTER (DAYS)
Coumaphos (Co-Ral)	0.25% spray 1.0% oil in backrubber 1.0% dust or as dust bag	0
Crotoxyphos (Ciodrin)	1.0% spray 1.0% oil in backrubber 3.0% dust	0
Crufomate (Ruelene)	9.4% oil, pour on 0.375% spray 6.2% emulsion, pour on	28
Fenthion (Tiguvon, Baytex)	1.0% oil in backrubber	0
Malathion	0.5% spray 2.0% oil in backrubber	0
Ronnel (Korlan)	0.5% spray 1.0% oil in backrubber	7 0
Trichlorfon (Neguvon)	1.0% spray	14
Toxaphene	0.5% spray 5.0% oil in backrubber	28
Methoxychlor	0.5% spray 5.0% to 6.0% oil in backrubber	0

Face Flies

INSECTICIDE (TRADE NAME)	FORMULATION	WITHDRAWAL BEFORE SLAUGHTER (DAYS)
Coumaphos (Co-Ral)	1.0% oil in face rubber	0
Crotoxyphos (Ciodrin)	1.0% oil spray daily. Not over 2 oz/head. 2.0% oil in face rubber	0
Crotoxyphos, Dichlorvos (Ciovap) Dichlorvos (DDVP, Vapona) Pyrethrins + Synergist[b]	1.25% in oil ⎱ Light mist 1.0% in oil ⎰ daily. Not 0.075% in oil ⎰ over 2 oz/head.	0
Ronnel (Korlan)	1.0% in face rubber	0
Toxaphene	5.0% in oil on face rubber	28

Source: John B. Herrick, *Feedstuffs*. (Minneapolis, Minn.: Miller Publishing Company, 1977). Reprinted by permission.

[b] For stable and horse fly control, use 0.5% oil, spray mist. Apply 2 oz/head 3 times per week.

Table 6-5. Fly Control Under Close Confinement

FEED-LOT FLY CONTROL

Flies:	Sanitation, prevention of breeding areas; use residual sprays and mists before fly population builds up. Start program early in season.	Baytex[a]		0 day
Stable fly		Cygon[a]		0 day
House fly				0 day
		Korlan[a]	Residual sprays	0 day
		Rabon[a]		0 day
		Ravop[a]		0 day Does not go on animals
		Diazinon[a]		

DAIRY CATTLE INSECT CONTROL

Flies:	Adequate fly control on lactating cows usually means good louse control.	Ciodrin[a]—spray or dust Vapona or Pyrethrins Residual wall sprays: 1% Baytex, 1% Ravap, 1% Cygon, 1% Korlan or 1% Rabon.	0 day	Mist Blowers: 0.570 Vapona—0 day 1.070 DiBrom—0 day

Source: John B. Herrick, *Feedstuffs*. (Minneapolis, Minn.: Miller Publishing Company, 1977). Reprinted by permission.

[a]Always read and follow manufacturers' directions.

186

As with any chemical, but especially so in the case of insecticides, observe the general precautions of reading the entire label before using, follow regulations and withdrawal periods, avoid contact with skin or clothing, avoid contamination of feed or water, and restrict eating and smoking while handling insecticides. Dairymen should pay particular attention to restrictions on the use of pesticides in milk rooms. Consult the milk inspector about local restrictions.

Table 6-4 lists numerous examples of chemicals available for use in controlling flies. Although not all insecticides are covered, you will find the material here to be extremely valuable and of a general nature, whether you plan to spray, dust, or use an oil-type product.

The examples given in Table 6-5 may be very useful in confined situations such as feed lots and dairies, along with a regular program for dusting or spraying.

7

Reproduction in Cattle

An understanding of the anatomy of the male and the female is fundamental to understanding the reproductive process. Although the reproductive system of cattle is basically the same as that of any other mammal, it is always a good idea to cover the specifics. Using a young male and a young female, the physiological changes that occur from the earliest age of mating through adulthood will be discussed here.

Although physiologists, veterinarians, and other scientifically minded individuals prefer to use more complicated terminology, it is the intent of this discussion to make the reproductive system easy to understand by using as many layman's terms as possible.

THE MALE

Since the male is the foundation of most herds, the anatomy of the bull will be covered first. The male reproductive system shown in Figure 7-1 indicates the location of the various organs pertaining to the male.

As can be seen from the illustration, the reproductive system of the bull has many parts. However, we can divide the reproductive system into three main sections: (1) the testes, (2) the accessory or secondary sex glands, and (3) the penis. Each of these sections has a specific function in relation to animal reproduction.

The Testes or Testicles

The testes, or testicles, are the location of the factory for the production of sperm. The testes are located inside the scrotum (or bag). In bulls, the testes descend into the scrotum from inside the body cavity shortly before birth. Nature has seen to it that this scrotum serves to provide the correct

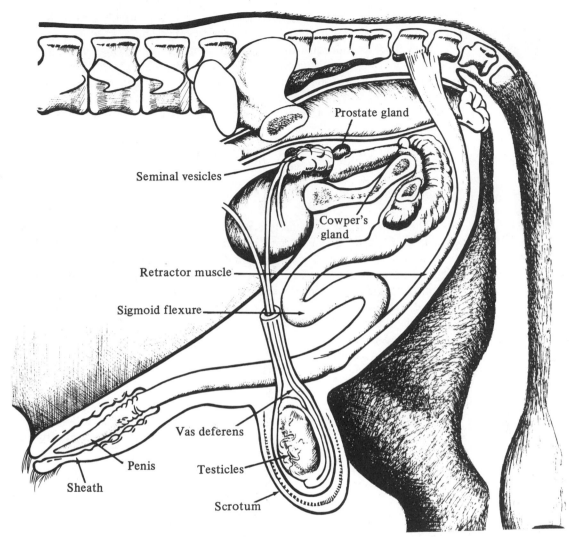

Figure 7-1. The male reproductive tract. (From Blakely and Bade, *The Science of Animal Husbandry*. Reston, Va.: Reston Publishing Company, Inc., 1976)

temperature for sperm development. (At the normal temperature inside the body cavity, heat produced for other body functions would destroy any sperm, rendering a bull infertile.) Viable sperm production is possible only within a very narrow temperature range. Therefore, the scrotum lowers the testes from the body when the environment is warm and contracts on colder days in order to provide the correct temperature.

Sometimes both of the testes do not descend from the body cavity. This condition is known as *cryptorchidism*—meaning one or both of the testes are still inside the body cavity and are not producing viable sperm. In the event both testes remain inside the body cavity, the animal would usually be sterile.

If an animal is cryptorchid on one side only, he will probably still be fertile, but the chances of full fertility are somewhat diminished.

Sperm are produced in the testicle and migrate up through a small tube called the *vas deferens* to the secondary sex glands, where fluids are secreted to increase the volume of semen (fluid). It is important to understand that the fluid produced in the natural act of mating by the male is not all sperm. In fact, the sperm cells make up only a very small percentage of the total volume of semen. The fluid serves as a transport medium to enable the sperm, which look like very small tadpoles under a microscope, to have the needed mobility in the reproductive tract to unite with the egg of the female.

Secondary Sex Glands

The secondary sex glands referred to in the diagram as *seminal vesicles*, *prostate gland*, and *Cowper's glands* are the organs that are stimulated by an electrical probe when artificial inseminators collect semen from a bull. The electrical impulse serves to artificially induce ejaculation, a condition similar to mating stimulation of nerve endings, which causes a forceable release of the fluid and accompanying sperm that have been stored. The "triggering mechanism" under natural conditions is the male hormone (testosterone), also produced by the testicle, which causes sexual excitation in bulls through normal sensory channels.

The Penis

It is important to understand the function of the penis in cattle because of two characteristics that could create problems for the average stockman. First of all, the penis has an "*S*-shaped curve" (sigmoid flexure, shown in Figure 7-1), which is held in place by a special muscle called the *retractor penis muscle*. At sexual rest, the natural muscle tone of the retractor keeps the organ in place. However, if there is some natural defect or if this muscle should become injured, the male organ would be allowed to protrude through the sheath, creating the possibility of infection or injury.

When everything is functioning normally, sexual excitation causes blood to be pumped into the chambers of the organ, causing an erection or straightening of the *S*-curve, which allows normal mating. After mating, the *S*-curve contracts, due to the action of the retractor muscle, into the protective sheath.

The second characteristic that could cause a problem is that the sheath, which is the housing mechanism for the penis, can itself be damaged, especially if it is a pendulous sheath. This could create a problem, such as a lack of desire to breed even though normal semen is being produced. Numerous cases of bulls with thorns or abrasions in the sheath are seen every year by veterinarians, especially in rocky or brushy country. Selection for a tight-sheathed bull, therefore, is something to keep in mind when selecting bulls.

Thus, it is important to understand the basic anatomy of a bull and the points to look for in order to avoid problems of infertility. In other words, a bull may be fertile but may have certain anatomical defects that prevent him from mating. Or a bull may be perfect anatomically but simply not be producing live sperm. These cases will be discussed in subsequent sections on artificial insemination and bull-testing procedures.

THE FEMALE

Even though most breeding programs emphasize the importance of the bull, the female reproductive system is more important; it is less viable but much more complicated. Therefore, it is necessary to try to visualize the anatomy of the cow and to understand the functions of the various reproductive parts of the female.

Figure 7-2 shows an artist's conception of the cow's reproductive system. Figures 7-3 and 7-4 show the actual reproductive tract and a dissected view of one side to compare with the artist's conception. The major points of interest are the ovary, the uterus, and the cervix. The other portions of the reproductive system serve to act as landmarks.

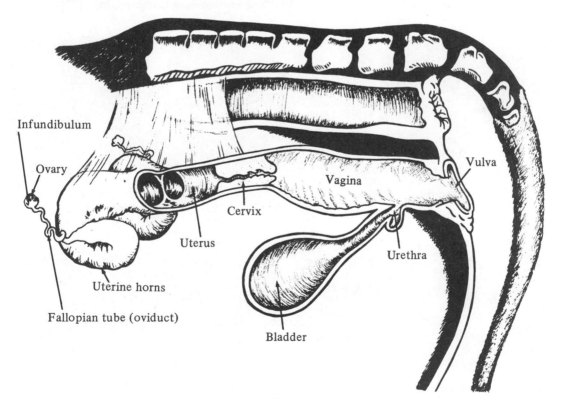

Figure 7-2. The female reproductive system. (From Blakely and Bade, *The Science of Animal Husbandry*. Reston, Va.: Reston Publishing Company, Inc., 1976)

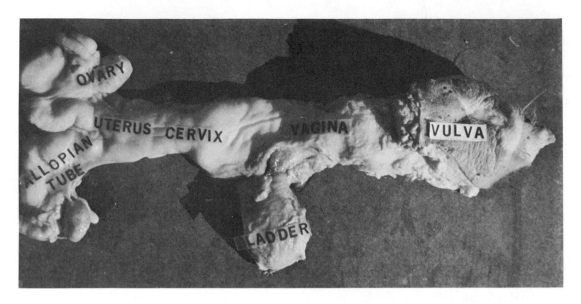

Figure 7-3. The female reproductive tract; ovaries and Fallopian tubes come in pairs. (From Blakely and Bade, *The Science of Animal Husbandry*. Reston, Va.: Reston Publishing Company, Inc., 1976)

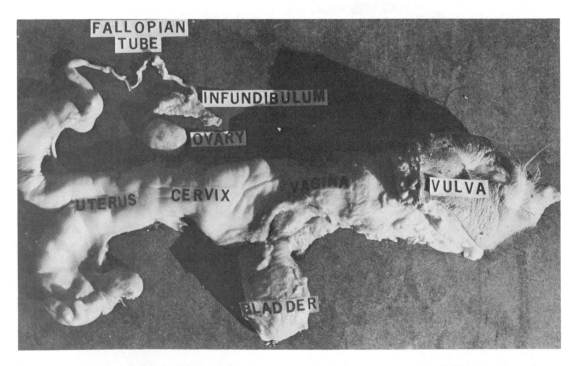

Figure 7-4. The female reproductive tract, illustrating the dissected ovary and Fallopian tubes. (From Blakely and Bade, *The Science of Animal Husbandry*. Reston, Va.: Reston Publishing Company, Inc., 1976)

192

The ovaries correspond to the testes in the male. The male testicle produces the sperm; the female ovary produces the egg. The uniting of the sperm and the egg creates the beginning of a new life.

Each of the two ovaries is about the size of a 50¢ coin or smaller. Each ovary has a number of small follicles that erupt on a regular schedule to produce an ovum or egg. Although a male may provide millions of sperm at each mating, a cow will shed relatively few eggs—perhaps 20 to 30—during her entire lifetime. It is interesting to note that researchers have estimated that during the life span of a cow, the two ovaries may contain as many as 75,000 potential eggs. If these eggs could actually be released, for instance, to produce twins or triplets through the use of certain drugs, then cattle production could be greatly increased. There are, however, numerous other problems that prevent this from being a desirable situation, such as whether a cow could produce enough milk to raise these extra calves.

The ovary produces a hormone that stimulates egg production in the female. It is called *estrogen*. Production of estrogen is activated by the pituitary gland in the brain to create mating desire at a regular heat interval of about 21 days. Another hormone called *FSH* (follicle stimulating hormone), causes a blisterlike follicle on the surface of the ovary (see Figure 7-5). This follicle is stimulated to rupture by a third hormone called *LH* (lutenizing hormone). The egg is shed and falls into a funnellike mechanism called the *infundibulum*. The egg then moves down the Fallopian tube (oviduct) into the uterus (womb). We know that, normally, somewhere in the upper part of the Fallopian tube the egg unites with the sperm, which starts the miracle of life. The united sperm and egg then take up residence in the

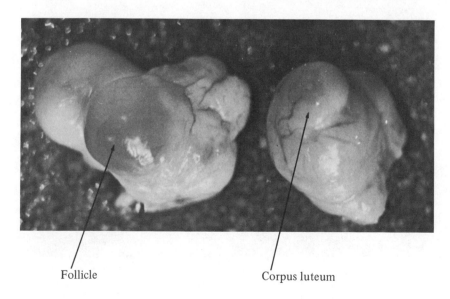

Follicle   Corpus luteum

Figure 7-5. The ovarian follicle and corpus luteum. (From Blakely and Bade, *The Science of Animal Husbandry*. Reston, Va.: Reston Publishing Company, Inc., 1976)

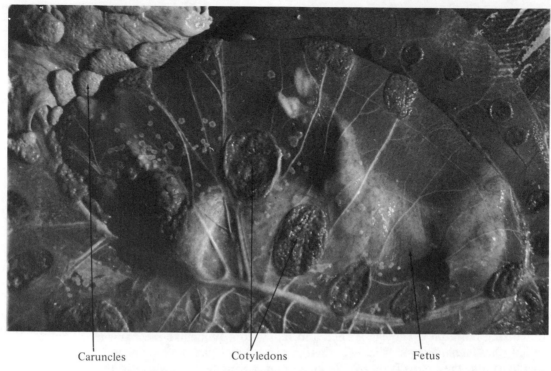

Caruncles   Cotyledons   Fetus

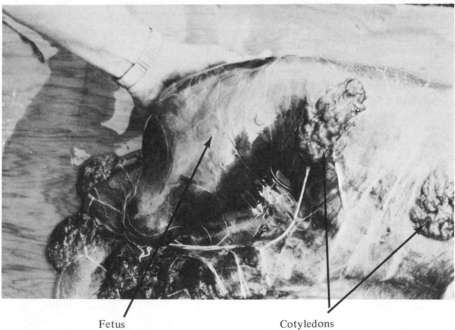

Fetus   Cotyledons

Figure 7-6. A detached placenta, illustrating cotyledons. Note the fetus floating in amniotic fluid. (From Blakely and Bade, *The Science of Animal Husbandry*. Reston, Va.: Reston Publishing Company, Inc., 1976)

uterus, and a plug of mucus seals the cervix so that no bacteria or foreign material can get to the developing fetus.

Remember the place on the ovary where the egg erupted? This scarlike area, called the *corpus luteum*, through a miracle of nature produces yet a fourth hormone called *progesterone*, which is responsible for suppressing further heat periods in the cow and for maintaining the pregnancy until birth (see Figure 7-5).

The united sperm and egg receive nourishment from secretions produced by the uterine glands and blood plasma (uterine milk). A membrane or sack (placenta) begins to develop, enclosing the newly fertilized egg, and attachments to the uterus are made at points scattered over this sack. The sack fills with amnionic fluid in which the fetus floats, and it protects the fetus somewhat like a shock absorber protects the family car from rough jolts. Within a few days the uterine milk ceases to feed the fetus because of the development of attachment points on the sack that connect with other points scattered over the uterus. These attachment points are technically called *cotyledons* on the placenta and *caruncles* on the uterus (see Figure 7-6). Cattlemen have lumped them together under the term *buttons* because they "snap up" to the cow's blood supply for nourishment of the fetus. When birth occurs, these buttons "unsnap," and the placenta (the term *afterbirth* is more commonly used) should be shed within 2 to 6 hours.

Even if the afterbirth is still hanging from the vulva 24 hours after calving, no effort should be made to remove it because serious infections and injury to the wall of the uterus can occur. (Sometimes, a gentle, steady pull will "unsnap" the buttons, but in inexperienced hands disastrous results may occur.) The use of injectable hormones such as ECP or stilbestrol is a safer method and results in more complete removal of the placenta. In either case, a bolus, commercially available, should be placed in the uterus to keep down infection. (Boluses containing starch or other insoluble material should not be used in the uterus.)

If the afterbirth is expelled, normally it is quite common for the cow to eat it as part of the ritual of cleaning up, just like licking the calf. Some cows may not eat the afterbirth. Except in special cases (see section on Brucellosis) this should not be of concern. There is an old farmer's tale that cattle have to eat the afterbirth to have normal milk production, but this is not true. Under normal pasture conditions, with no disease outbreaks, the only concern is whether or not the afterbirth is expelled.

MATING

We have covered everything from conception to birth for beef cattle. Now, perhaps, it would be best to back up a little and concern ourselves with the time of mating, how to recognize it, and at what age it occurs. The subjects of age of sexual maturity (puberty), heat (estrus), and breeding are not as widely understood as might be expected.

Puberty in the male generally comes much earlier than in the female and is marked by the production of viable sperm. A desire for mating may come somewhat earlier and is evidenced by young bulls riding heifers or cows. This activity is brought on by the male hormone, testosterone, produced as previously discussed by the testes. A similar desire for mating also takes place in the female, but it may come at a slightly later age. The determination of puberty in the female is exhibited by the first heat period (estrus). The period of estrus is activated by the female hormone (estrogen) produced by the ovaries. The heifer will accept the bull only during the period in which she is in heat. This usually lasts about 18 hours, although it will vary by several hours depending on individuals. If the female does not conceive, she will cycle and be in heat again 21 days later. This cycling is referred to as the *estrous cycle* or *heat cycle*.

The age at which heifers first come into heat will vary considerably with different breeds, but generally ranges from 8 to 18 months with an average of 12 months. Although age has some influence on when a heifer reaches maturity, the best time to breed is more a function of weight. The average weight for breeding, regardless of age, is about 600 lb. Weights may be slightly heavier for some of the larger breeds, making the general range from 500 to 800 lb. If the heifer conceives, she will not return to estrus and should have a calf approximately 283 days after conception. This is referred to as the *gestation period*.

The visual signs of approaching heat are a swelling and redness of the external sexual organs on the female and a restlessness or nervousness that is apparent to the trained observer. The most obvious sign is mounting and in turn being mounted. Most cattlemen have observed this activity taking place in the pasture or around the lots, but it is surprising how few understand the key to determining *which* heifer is in heat. Is it the one that is mounting or the one that is being mounted? The key to detecting the one that is in heat is to observe the one that will stand for a relatively long period of time (5 to 10 seconds) and allow another heifer to mount her. Although all heifers sense the sexual excitation and will mount even though they themselves may not be experiencing heat, it is important to remember that the one that is experiencing the actual heat period is the one that will stand still the longest. This is often referred to as *standing heat*.

Breeding of the female occurs only during this heat period. The bull is capable of breeding at any time. If hand mating is being conducted, that is, bringing a heifer to a specific bull, it is important to know the optimum time to breed for the highest conception rate. In cows, ovulation of the egg from the ovary is delayed until 12 hours after the end of estrus. Therefore, it is very important to breed the heifer toward the end of her estrus period so that the sperm produced by the bull has the best chance of mating with the egg, allowing conception to occur.

The average life of the egg is only 6 to 12 hours, and the average life of the sperm is approximately 30 hours. If only one breeding is expected to do the job, it is important to do it at the appropriate time. Figure 7-7 illustrates the breeding sequence of events, so that the optimum time for mating may be clearly understood. Notice that there is a preheat playtime among heifers of 6 to 10 hours. They will begin to show some swelling of the vulva and become

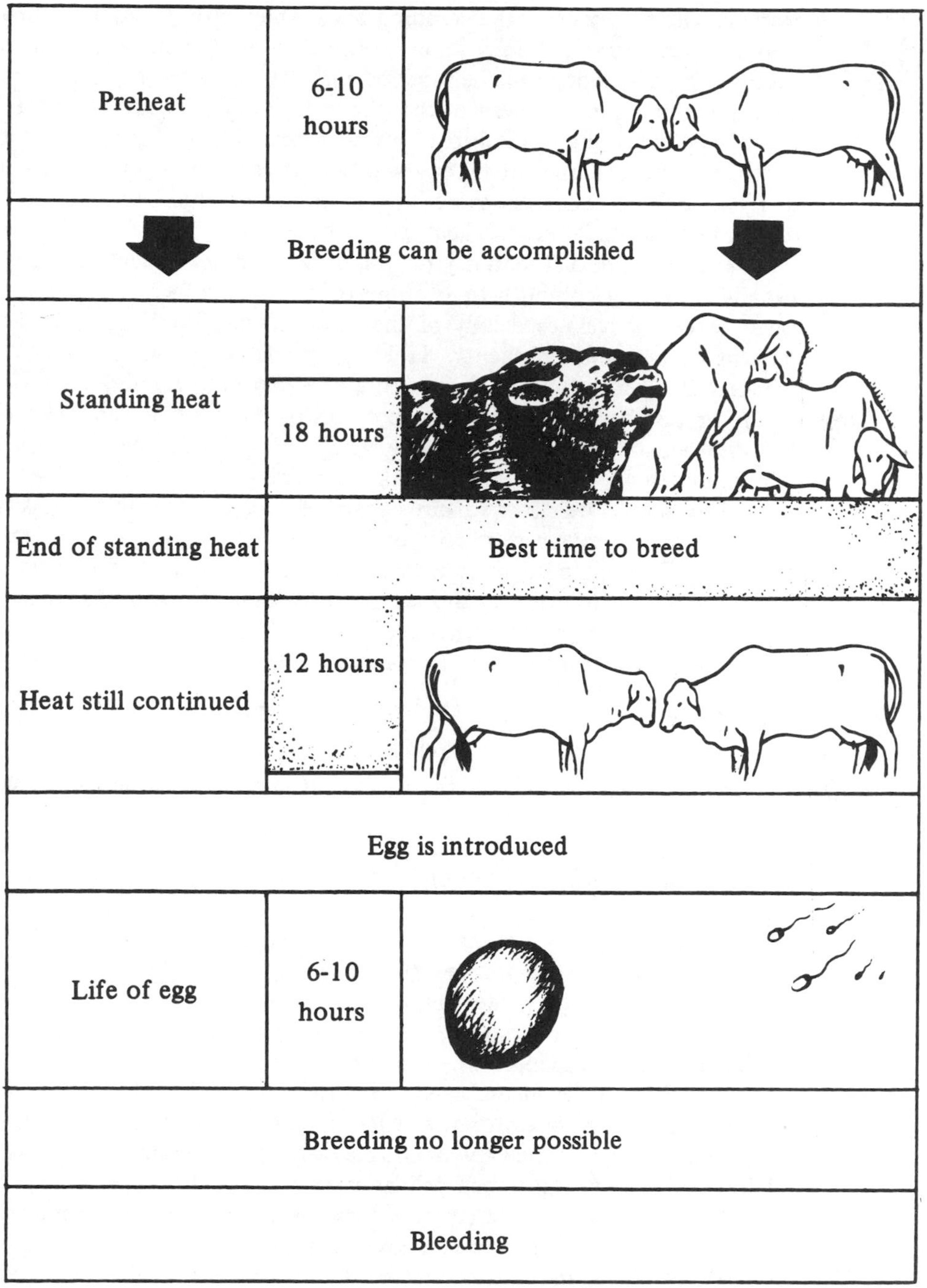

Preheat	6-10 hours	
Breeding can be accomplished		
Standing heat	18 hours	
End of standing heat	Best time to breed	
Heat still continued	12 hours	
Egg is introduced		
Life of egg	6-10 hours	
Breeding no longer possible		
Bleeding		

Figure 7-7. The sequence of events in breeding. (From Blakely and Bade, *The Science of Animal Husbandry*. Reston, Va.: Reston Publishing Company, Inc., 1976)

restless. The next stage is the standing heat, which lasts about 18 hours. It is best to breed either naturally or by artificial insemination at the end of the standing heat. Although the heat period may be continued for approximately 12 hours, the egg is not released from the ovary until after the heifer has gone "out." The life of the egg is 6 to 12 hours. After that, conception is no longer possible, and the desire for mating will not recur for another 21 days. If the heifer does not conceive, there will often be a small amount of blood discharged about 2 days after heat has ended.

The age of sexual maturity for the male is similar to that of the female, usually occurring around 8 to 12 months. There have been several reported cases of bull calves, especially of the smaller type, breeding as early as 6 months of age and producing viable sperm. However, it is rarely recommended that young bulls be used before one year of age and if then, only on a very limited basis with a maximum of 10 to 15 cows being served during a breeding season. Normally, a mature bull is used full-time for a herd of approximately 25 cows. A mature bull has passed the two-year-old stage and preferably should be closer to three years of age. The reason for this is that the bull could become sterile if used at too early an age or if used too frequently. The cause is simply a lack of sperm production, so that accessory gland fluids have to make up the semen. If the bull is used too frequently, his fertility could be impaired permanently.

The keys to a high level of production in beef cattle are:

1. Understanding the anatomy of both the male and female.

2. Recognizing the heat cycle in the female.

3. Knowing something about the time of ovulation and therefore the best time for insemination.

DYSTOCIA (Difficult Calving)

Many cattlemen attempt to correct calving problems when they have neither the instruments nor the knowledge to do so. Others may refuse to assist the cow for even the simplest problem. Neither of these is a good approach. All cattlemen should be able to recognize early signs of calving problems and to determine when to assist or when to call for aid.

The basic instruments needed to assist in calving difficulties are obstetrical chains or ropes for use when traction is needed to pull the calf. Obstetrical handles attach to chains, making traction easier. Mechanical calf pullers are also used in forced deliveries.

Chains are not absolutely necessary because a clean, soft rope will also serve well. The rope should be discarded and not used again for that purpose, unless it is plastic and can be sterilized. If obstetrical chains are used, they may be disinfected between uses. If kept wrapped in a clean cloth, they will be ready for the next use. They should not be boiled in water because it will cause them to rust.

Since the calf and birth canal must be heavily lubricated when manipulations are necessary, it is advisable to have obstetrical soaps on hand. If none are available, a satisfactory lubricant can be made by dissolving a mild soap in warm water.

Some drugs should be kept handy, particularly 1 to 3 grams of a broad-range antibiotic, such as oxytetracycline or chlortetracycline in 200 to 500 ml of physiological saline solution. It is also recommended that furacin boluses be on hand for use as a medication within the uterus, should a retained placenta (afterbirth) occur. Tincture of iodine also should be kept for treating the navel cord of the calf following delivery.

THE CALVING PROCESS

Parturition (calving) may be divided into three stages. Stage one is when the cow tries to isolate herself and shows general restlessness and tail switching or kicks at her sides. In a pasture situation, the cow will invariably drift off by herself. The uterine contractions in this early stage occur at about 15-minute intervals. The water sac passes through the cervix and often ruptures at this stage, releasing water to the outside. In normal labor, delivery may take from 2 to 6 hours but may be as brief as 30 minutes or as long as 24 hours. Stage one usually takes longer in first-calf heifers than for cows who have calved before.

Stage two is the beginning of expulsion. At this point, uterine contractions will occur at intervals of about 2 minutes, and each contraction will last about $1\frac{1}{2}$ minutes. It is important not to excite or hurry the cow at this time, but be prepared to help. Delivery should be completed within 2 hours after the water sac first appears. If this does not happen, then intervention is justified.

Stage three is the final expulsion of the calf. The placenta is usually expelled from 30 minutes to 8 hours following birth. If it is retained for more than 12 hours, some attention to the cow may be necessary to correct this malfunction and to prevent infection.

If problems should arise, they generally show up after the water sac appears. If labor proceeds for 2 to 3 hours with no progress, or if the water sac appears and delivery is not complete within 2 hours, a vaginal examination (by hand) is in order. Speed is important for extracting a live calf. Therefore, any signs of life should be checked before a decision is made to intervene. If the calf is alive, pulling or pinching the foot will cause movement of the leg, pinching the eyes will cause movement of the head, or placing the fingers in the calf's mouth will elicit sucking or movement of the tongue. With posterior or breech presentations, inserting a finger into the rectum will cause constriction if the calf is alive.

Calving Positions

The final step in examination is to determine the position of the calf in the uterus birth canal. The various positions in which calves can be born are as follows:

Normal Presentation. The normal presentation of calves is two front feet followed by the head. The correct posture of the fetus is to have both front legs outstretched in the birth canal, with the head and neck extended between or along the legs. Any deviation from this posture should be corrected before the calf is pulled. About 95% of all births occur in this fashion. It is important to remember that calving problems are most common in first-calf heifers. Only about 3% of mature cows have any trouble, but for heifers the figure can be 50% or higher. The reason is simply that their bodies have not developed to maturity, and their pelvic openings may be too small. Mature cows usually will calve without difficulty. Therefore, the main reason for calving difficulties—when the calf is in the correct posture—is simply an oversized calf or an immature heifer.

Occasionally, the calf will be coming in the correct position, but with one leg back. This is still a headfirst presentation, but it will necessitate intervention for normal birth to occur (see Figure 7-8). Correction of flexion of one leg is generally not difficult. The calf is first pushed back into the uterus and the retained foot pulled up in the proper position with the cupped hand. The hand of the assistant is cupped over the calf's foot to avoid injuring the uterus. More difficult cases may require the attachment of obstetrical chains to help extend the leg to the proper position. The chain should be positioned around the ankle and then between the claws from back to front so that the pull is at the foot, not at the cannon bone. Reposition the chain after the leg is in the normal birth position.

Another abnormality in the correct presentation is evident when two front feet are showing past the elbows but there is no head. This is an indication of a "head back" condition (see Figure 7-8). Correcting difficult cases may require pulling the head and neck around with the hand or with a snare placed on the lower jaw. The calf is first pushed back into the uterus and the hand quickly moved to grasp the calf's muzzle. The head is pulled around in line with the birth canal. In some cases it may be necessary to apply a snare to the lower jaw for additional traction. Excessive traction on a snare should be avoided because the jaw is easily fractured. A safer practice is looping the obstetrical chain around the poll, under the ears, and through the mouth in the manner of a "war bridle." This attachment allows greater traction and permits more safety to the calf's jaw. Care should be taken to avoid cutting the birth canal with the calf's sharp incisor teeth during extraction.

Breech. A condition that normally requires both traction and lubrication is a breech (backward) birth. Delivery often proceeds without complications in a posterior presentation in cattle. Assistance may be needed if labor is prolonged and if there is the possibility of death of the calf from rupture of the navel cord, which would cut off the oxygen supply to the calf.

A serious type of malpresentation is when one or both legs are tucked up in the breech position with the calf's tail protruding from the vulva of the cow. The legs must be straightened in this case before pulling. The calf is first pushed into the uterus (see Figure 7-8f), and the hand grasps one foot at a time drawing it back to present the calf in a deliverable position. The calf is usually pushed forward and its foot is guided over the pelvic brim while an assistant pulls on the obstetrical chains to straighten the legs.

A rare condition that must be determined by feel is a calf that is presented upside down and in breech position. In this case, the feet will need to be guided through the birth canal in the same manner as other breech presentations.

If a calf is dead before birth, in many cases it is already swollen before it can be removed. This may require an embryotomy (cutting the calf into pieces for removal) and will need the use of a trained veterinarian not only to remove the calf but to prevent infection of the cow.

If a calf puller is used, traction should always be increased in a downward direction. If this does not help, release the calf puller, and push the calf back far enough to relieve hip lock. This often happens in young heifers that simply do not have a passage wide enough to allow the calf's hips to pass through the birth canal. Pulling downward at a 45° angle is the most help. By pushing the calf back and by rotating the calf as much as possible, the situation may allow a position in which delivery is possible. Rotation can be accomplished by placing a pitchfork handle or similar instrument between the front legs to act as a lever.

Occasionally a calf will have trouble breathing after delivery. In such instances it is important to quickly remove the mucus from its nose and mouth. If the calf continues to have trouble breathing, pick it up by the hind legs and swing it back and forth or around in a circle to dislodge the mucus. A gentle swinging is all that is needed. Rubbing or scratching the inside of the calf's nostrils with a straw may also cause it to sneeze, cough, or otherwise clear out the breathing passages. A form of artificial respiration may also be employed by using a short section of $\frac{3}{8}$ in. or $\frac{1}{2}$ in. garden hose in one nostril. Clamp the other nostril with your hands so that you make an airtight passage and blow into the hose, allowing the lungs to be filled with your exhaled breath. This should be repeated every 6 to 7 seconds until the calf starts breathing. The results of these simple resuscitation methods can be very dramatic.

After birth has been completed, remember to treat the calf's navel cord with tincture of iodine, and be sure to check the cow for retained placenta (afterbirth) 12 hours after delivery. Also, watch the cow or heifer, especially if it has been a very difficult birth, to make sure that she can regain her feet. Occasionally difficult births cause paralysis in the hind quarters of the cow, preventing her from standing. Sometimes this is a very temporary effect. On other occasions the cow needs assistance to regain her feet. In severe cases the cow may need assistance to regain her feet for several days or weeks. In rare instances the nerves are damaged and permanent paralysis is the result.

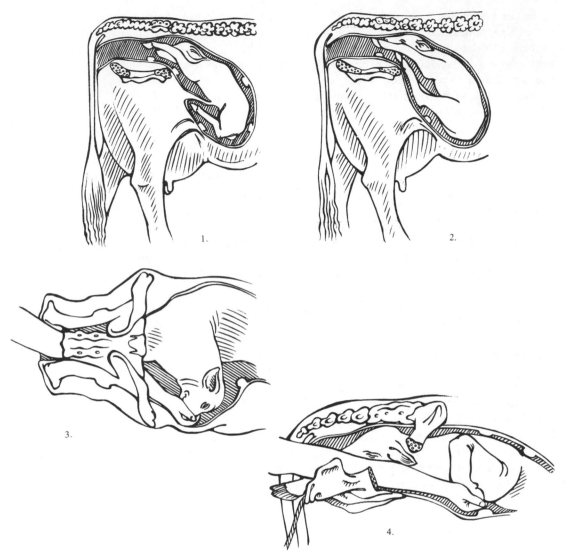

Figure 7-8. Normal and malpresentations. (1) Normal anterior presentation of the calf in the proper position for delivery. (2) A "dog-sitting posture." A very serious malpresentation. The rear legs must be retracted before normal birth can occur. Early professional assistance is needed in this case. (3) A "head back" condition that may require pulling the head and neck around with the hand. The calf is pushed back and quickly released in order to grasp the calf's muzzle. The head is then pulled around in line with the birth canal. In some cases an obstetrical chain is looped around the poll, under the ears, and through the mouth in a "war bridle" manner. This allows for greater traction to line up the head. Care should be taken not to cut the birth canal with the gaping jaws of the calf in traction. (4) Correction of a "leg back" condition. The calf is pushed forward and the retained foot grasped in the cupped hand. The foot is carried outward and then forward in an arc over the pelvic brim. More difficult cases may require the use of obstetrical chains on the foot.

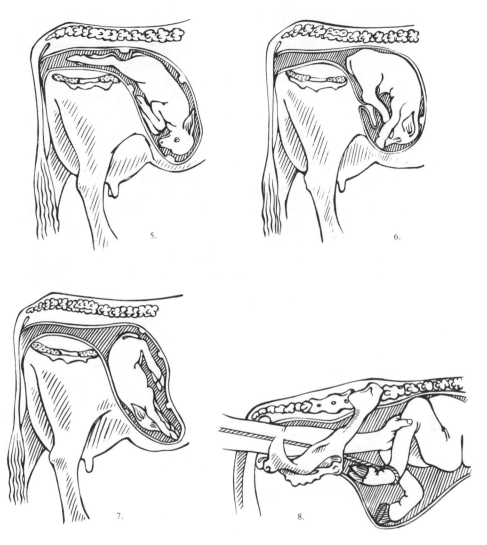

Figure 7-8. Normal and malpresentation (continued). (5) A backward presentation with rear legs extended. Birth in this presentation often occurs without incident; however, assistance may be needed if birth is delayed because of the danger of breaking the navel cord and subsequent suffocation of the calf. (6) The breech position is a serious malpresentation. It may be corrected by pushing the calf forward and pulling the rear legs into the birth canal (see number 8). (7) The upside down and backward position. A serious type of malpresentation, this is often caused by twisting of the uterus or rotation of the calf. Delivery should never be attempted in this position. Professional assistance is required. (8) Correction of a breech position. The calf is first pushed forward. Then one foot at a time is drawn back with the hand, as the hock is flexed. The foot is lifted over the pelvic brim into the birth canal. An alternate method is to place a snare around the pastern joint, close to the foot. The snare is then pulled by an assistant while the calf is pushed forward and its foot is guided over the pelvic brim.

FERTILITY TESTING OF BULLS

Bulls must be evaluated for breeding soundness in order to meet certain minimum standards both of physical condition and semen quality.

Examination of the bull should include his general condition, legs, feet, age, teeth, and eyes. In addition, the reproductive organs should be examined, and any infectious diseases, parasites, and physical defects should be ruled out. The physical act of mounting, ejaculating, and dismounting should be observed.

Semen should be collected and evaluated under a microscope by a professional, usually a veterinarian, but there may be other qualified people who can do this as well. Remember that evaluation is more than just looking for wiggles under a microscope. Movement, numbers, structure, shape, and the percentage of live sperm, etc., must all be observed with accuracy if a knowledgeable evaluation of bull fertility is to be obtained.

If a bull is to be used for heavy service, he should be given extra feed 30 to 40 days prior to breeding. A bull's feet should be cared for properly, toes kept short, and hoof walls trimmed to support weight. Control of internal and external parasites is also important.

As mentioned earlier, young bulls should serve only a limited number of cows because heavy service may cause infertility (about 15 cows for pasture mating is maximum). A two-year-old bull can serve 25 to 35 cows with hand mating, and a mature bull can serve as many as 35 to 50 cows.

Good management of the bulls after they have been fertility tested will further improve conception rates. A single mature bull in a lot with 25 to 30 cows will produce a bigger calf crop than three or four bulls turned in with 100 cows because the bulls spend a great deal of time either fighting or with only one female. When several bulls are used in the same pasture, the calf crop percentage will decrease if there are over 16 to 18 cows per bull.

Rotating bulls after 10 to 15 days of breeding has increased calf crops by as much as 18%. This practice allows bulls to rest, and it keeps fresh bulls with the cows at all times. After the second 10 to 15 day service period, all of the bulls can be turned in to serve cows that are not yet pregnant.

PALPATION

Pregnancy examination in the female can be done by the trained professional as early as 30 to 60 days after breeding and at about 90 days by those less competent at the technique. If the reproductive physiology previously discussed is understood, the technique is relatively simple and is easily learned. Basically, the examiner is feeling through the wall of the rectum and picking up landmarks of the reproductive tract to physically feel with the fingers an enlargement containing the fetus. This procedure is called *palpation* and is discussed in more detail later in Chapter 8 under herd management of beef cows.

ARTIFICIAL INSEMINATION (AI) PROGRAM

A good AI program requires planning and a commitment to do quality work. The key to an AI program is the identification of all cows in a herd by ear tags that are easy to read; this is backed up by secondary identification with a brand (freeze or hot) in case an ear tag is lost. Careful identification permits selection and observation of cows or heifers that are in heat in order to determine the best time for insemination.

Another important factor in the program is well-designed handling facilities, conveniently located so that cows can be moved into them with a minimum of disturbance.

Total energy in the ration appears to be the most important single factor in determining efficient reproduction and high conception rates. An important rule of thumb is that cows nursing calves must be fed enough to be gaining between $\frac{1}{2}$ lb and 1 lb per day prior to and during the early part of the breeding season. This requires 12 to 16 lb of TDN (total digestible nutrients) per day. Other factors known to be involved are vitamin A, protein, calcium, and phosphorus. The number one factor in any herd health program, or reproductive program, is nutrition.

An adequate interval from calving to breeding is important in maintaining high conception rates in an AI program. There is a much better chance of success if cows are not bred for 40 days after calving. It is reported that conception rates of 33% were obtained when cows were inseminated 30 days after calving compared to 62% for cows inseminated 60 days after calving.

A cow herd that is calving over a 3 to 6 month period will not lend itself to an AI program. The management level in the herd must reach a 60-day breeding season for all cows if you are to achieve a high conception rate and an efficient AI program. This is simply a management procedure to group calves as well as labor requirements to a minimum period of time.

Disease factors can also destroy an AI program. For this reason, careful sanitation and vaccination programs must be worked out. The logical course of action is the development of a complete herd health plan with your veterinarian.

Once the decision is made to breed artificially, extreme care must be taken when purchasing semen. Collecting, processing, and freezing semen requires excellent technical skills.

Given the management skills and a source of semen supply, the next step is learning to detect heat in cows. This requires considerable effort and is extremely important if success is to be assured. As discussed previously, heat is defined as a desire on the part of the cow to receive the bull and is exhibited by standing heat. In other words, a cow in heat will stand to be mounted by a bull, another cow, or a steer. Emphasis is placed on the willingness of the cow to stand. Standing heat is the only acceptable sign for determining the optimum time for insemination.

Today there is specialized equipment on the market to detect heat in cows. Originally, the method was simply the observations made by a herdsman from daybreak to about 8:30 A.M. and from 4 P.M. until dark. This results in a good rate of detection if the cow herd is not disturbed during this time. Aids for heat detection, such as heat detection pads, which mark cows when they are mounted by other cows, have proven useful. Use of "teaser" bulls have also proven successful. These are usually bulls that have been altered to render them sterile through such methods as vasectomy. Use of chin ball markers also identify cows that are in heat by leaving a mark on the back of the cow that will stand. All these methods still require individual observation at least twice a day. Recent studies have revealed that a high percentage of dairy cows are in standing heat from midnight to 6 A.M.

Once it has been determined that a cow is in heat, the highest conception rates are obtained when cows are bred during the 10-hour period at the end of the standing heat. The general rule is to observe cows that are in standing heat in the morning and breed them in the evening; and to breed cows observed in heat in the evening the following morning. Standing heat lasts an average of 18 hours, although there is some variation.

Breeding a few hours before ovulation results in the highest number of live sperm cells present when the egg arrives in the Fallopian tube to be fertilized, as previously discussed in the reproduction section.

Once a large percentage of cows are coming into heat and high-quality semen and a good heat-detection system are available, the only remaining factor is the actual breeding of cows. The first step should be to attend a good AI school. The essentials of storing and handling semen, the thawing procedures, and the process of insemination are taught by AI organizations or are given as short courses at state agricultural colleges. Because of the expense involved in the equipment and semen, and the potential for disaster by an untrained inseminator, the technique of insemination will not be attempted here.

Some general idea of AI methods can be given, however. First of all, semen must remain frozen at extremely cold temperatures ($-196°C$ or $-384°F$), which necessitates a liquid nitrogen insulated tank. The tank is opened only when absolutely necessary, and the semen ampules (tiny bottles) are exposed no longer than 9 to 11 seconds when making a selection for insemination.

Once the ampule is selected, it must be thawed out, which takes 8 to 10 minutes in an ice bath or a thaw box, to prevent shock to the live sperm. The semen must not be thawed for more than 1 hour and must be maintained in the appropriate manner until used. Various AI organizations have different techniques, equipment, and instructions, which are important to follow.

The semen is then deposited in the appropriate spot (usually through the cervix) with a thin tube, which is guided into the reproductive tract by feeling with one hand using a rectal palpation technique. After insemination, records are kept on each cow to make sure she is settled. If she returns to heat, in 21 days, she will be inseminated again. Thus, it is obvious that accurate records and identification are an important part of any AI program.

Recent advances in heat synchronization techniques (making all cows come into heat at one time) will result in more efficient use of AI in beef herds. With correct procedures, a large percentage of the cows can be bred at one time. Techniques and products are expected to be on the market in the near future that will allow the farmer to treat his cow herd by simply feeding them a synchronization additive and then breeding all of them within a specified number of hours after the material takes effect, or in some cases after the material is withdrawn. In such a program, management will become even more critical.

In summary, a successful AI program involves four areas:

1. Management of the cow herd must be arranged to identify all cows, develop good handling facilities, establish a short breeding season (preferably 60 days), provide proper nutrition, allow an adequate interval from calving to the next insemination, and establish a good herd health program.

2. Good semen must be obtained from a reputable supplier using the bull or bulls of your selection.

3. A heat-detection system must be developed, all cows checked at least twice daily, and cows bred approximately 12 hours after standing heat.

4. The herdsman has the option of inseminating cows himself after taking a good AI training course or hiring a competent technician.

8

Routine Procedures — Cattle

CASTRATION

Preparation of the animal for castration may be done by a variety of methods, including throwing with a rope, casting with a squeeze chute or tilting chute, or simply flanking to the ground. The preferred method is using a squeeze chute with a dropside plate, allowing exposure of the bottom half of the animal. One back leg is tied back on the side on which you are operating, and the procedure is done in a standing position.

It is recommended that a mild disinfectant such as iodine solution, betadine, or even soap and water be used to prepare the site by scrubbing the dirt and debris away. The standard technique is to grasp the base of the scrotum between the thumb and the forefinger and stretch the scrotum downward. With a sharp blade (preferably sterilized), cut off the bottom one-half of the scrotum (see Figure 8-1). In weaning calves, the testicles will usually drop down on their own accord.

Older animals may have a tough membrane (tunic) encapsulating the testicle. This membrane can be slit with a knife, allowing the testicles to drop below the scrotum. Younger calves may not drop the testicles, in which case the free hand is used to force them down through the incision. The testicles should be pulled out or severed with a scraping motion as high up on the spermatic cord as possible in order to sever both the cord and the vessel. A scraping cut is better to prevent unnecessary bleeding. Especially on older or fully mature animals, which are apt to have more bleeding, it is wise to use an emasculating instrument designed to crush the cord close to the body, a fraction above where the cord is severed. The Burdizzo method may be used on larger animals to prevent excessive bleeding (see Figure 8-2). The spermatic cord is crimped, and the Burdizzos are left in the crushing position for

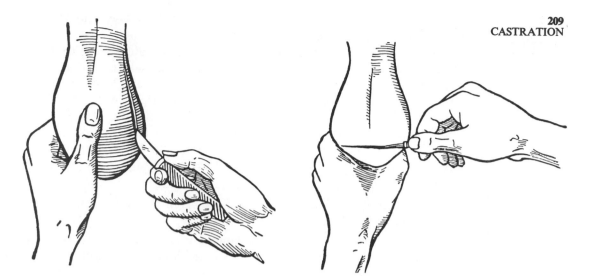

Figure 8-1. Castration with a knife is done either with a side incision or by cutting off the bottom one-third of the scrotum to remove the testicles.

a few seconds before removing. The spermatic cord is then severed with a knife just below the crimped area.

If the bull is castrated with a knife, any fat or extraneous tissues remaining in the scrotum should be pulled out with the fingers to assure a clean wound that will drain evenly. Collected pools of blood can cause abscesses if fatty tissues are left in the scrotum. The wound should be treated, especially in fly season, with any general stock salve or wound dressing.

Watch larger mature animals for the first few hours after castration for excess hemorrhaging, which could cause a bleeding death. In the event excessive bleeding does occur, the animal should be restrained and the cord pulled out and tied off with a suture.

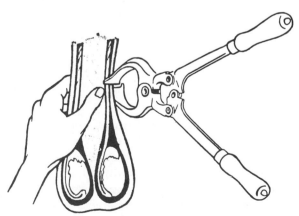

Figure 8-2. The Burdizzo or bloodless method of castration showing the proper position of the spermatic cord in the jaws of the instrument.

The use of the Burdizzo method (Figure 8-2) is very effective as a method of castration and is bloodless. It is effective if used properly and if the anatomy of the male reproductive system is fully understood. Feel for the spermatic cord high up in the scrotum, push it to one side, and squeeze with only a portion of the Burdizzo, which crushes the cord and leaves an imprint deep in the scrotum without breaking the skin. The purpose of the Burdizzo is to crush without cutting. The instrument should be left in the closed position for a couple of minutes before removing. Repeat the operation on the other side. The Burdizzo method is a simple procedure, but it is very easy to make a mistake if you are not familiar wth the procedure. The points to remember are:

1. The cord must be in the head of the instrument when clamped. This is determined by feeling.

2. Each side of the scrotum is clamped in a separate operation; never clamp the entire scrotum straight across even though the Burdizzo head is broad enough to do so, because the cords will be severed and all of the tissue below will be killed, allowing the scrotum to die and slough off. Clamp as little tissue from the scrotum as is needed.

3. Each side should be clamped at a slightly different level to assure that the blood supply to the scrotum is not cut off. This allows the testicles to degenerate but provides for a constant blood supply to the scrotum.

The elastrator is another device used in castration that operates by expanding a very stout rubber band with an instrument that allows it to be placed over the scrotum. Once the elastrator is removed, the rubber band contracts to a tiny circle, cutting off all blood circulation to the scrotum, allowing the entire system to lose its blood supply, die, and slough off. Some people still use the elastrator, but this author does not recommend it for the reasons of personal preference and because infection often occurs in such a traumatic situation. The knife or Burdizzo is considered much more humane and effective.

Any castrated animal should be watched for several days for excessive swelling or infection. If either are noted, treatment should proceed with the appropriate antibiotic, and the scrotum should be drained.

DEHORNING

Very Young Animals

A very young calf will have buttons where the horns will eventually grow, and for the first two or three months these buttons will be removable. The most effective way to remove the buttons is with an electric dehorner, a round-type iron with a hole in the center, which burns around and through the horn button, killing the germinal layer from which horn growth occurs. It may be necessary and advisable to clip the hair around these buttons for effective control. This can be done at 2 to 3 weeks of age or during the time of castration if that operation is done in the early stages of life.

Dehorning spoons are also used to scoop out the buttons mechanically. There are several different sizes of spoons to accommodate the various sizes of buttons.

The Barnes's dehorner is very effective in removing the buttons because as it scoops out the area, it gets down into a portion of the skull to insure complete removal of horn tissue so that regrowth is not likely. The Barnes's method, followed by an electric dehorner to cauterize the wound and kill any horn tissue, is highly recommended.

Weanlings

The Barnes's dehorner (a mechanical type) may be used for removing horns up to two or three inches in diameter at the base. However, some animals may have horns that are large enough to justify the use of a Keystone dehorner. Strength is needed in these situations, and the larger dehorners offer the best leverage and advantage. A head gate or squeeze chute is also recommended on large weanling calves. Restraint is the key to doing a good job of dehorning. You should get a good solid $\frac{1}{4}$ in. of hair around the horn when dehorning. It is also advisable to cauterize with a hot iron or use a hemostat to remove bleeding vessels. Cauterization is preferred. The wound should also be coated with a suitable dressing.

Mature Cattle

Mature cattle should definitely be dehorned with the larger dehorners because of the obvious force needed to do a good job. The dehorning should be deep enough to remove all of the horn if possible. In most cases, this will open the sinuses into the head, in which case the time of year will have an effect on healing. If it is hot weather, flies and maggots are a possibility and should be watched. If it is cold weather, there may be the possibility of sinus inflammation. Therefore, it is important to pick the time of year with the least flies and also to select a day that will be dry and suitable for working cattle without undue influence from the weather. After dehorning, the wound should be cauterized because mature cattle bleed rather readily, and the area should be coated with a fly-repellent antibiotic ointment.

BRANDING AND IDENTIFICATION

Branding is done for the purpose of determining ownership and individual identification.

Fire Iron Branding

The fire iron is the oldest and most popular form of branding, and dates from the days of the early cattle empires. The technique has changed very little except for the method of heating the irons. A fire iron is made of iron normally $3\frac{1}{2}$ to 4 in. high to produce a legible brand. Butane heaters have replaced the old campfires or wood fires to produce a standard red-hot iron that will produce a readable brand. The hair should be clipped if the branding is done in the wintertime and if the hair is very long. Otherwise, the fire brand will usually do a good job with little or no preparation. The animal should be restrained because jumping around could smear the brand. Hold the red-hot iron in one spot without moving until it burns about half-way through the hide (the hide is about $\frac{1}{4}$ in. thick).

Figure 8-3 gives an illustration of systems of coding numbers for individual identification brands. The biggest advantage of the system outlined in the illustration is that only one straight-bar branding instrument is required. Various combinations of straight lines are used to code numerals from 1 to 9.

Besides the convenience of needing only one tool, brands produced using this system are usually much clearer. The curved figures of numbers like 0 and 8 often produce difficult-to-read brands.

Your system of numbering animals should be as simple as possible, while still permitting easy identification. Generally not over four numbers and letters are recommended; three are even better.

A popular method of coding represents the year of birth as the first number. The numbers following it represent the number assigned to the particular animal. For example: 599 means the 99th animal born in 1975. If over 100 animals are to be coded, it is advisable to use a letter to represent the second 100 and so on: 5A33 means the 133rd animal born in 1975; and 5B1 means the 201st animal marked in 1975.

For commercial producers the year of birth designation is not so important. This can be kept on records. Thus, up to 234 animals can be coded using only one alphabetical letter and one number, for example, A3. If another letter is added to the end of the code, for example, A3C, approximately 6000 animals can be coded. More animals can be coded if the positions of numbers and letters are switched.

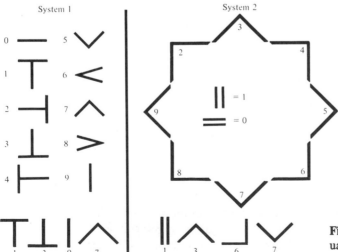

Figure 8-3. Coding systems for individual identification brands.

With the advent of computerized testing and recordkeeping procedures it becomes necessary to plan your coding system so that it is compatible with the computer. This is a good practice even though it may not presently be a concern.

Freeze Branding

Freeze branding is a new method of branding that has received widespread attention but not great acceptance because of the peculiar equipment and sophisticated techniques needed to make it operable. It is a painless method, but one that requires special copper irons kept in dry ice or liquid nitrogen to produce a temperature low enough to cause freezing of the tissues when it is applied. The surface of the hide must be prepared by clipping and cleaning with alcohol to remove any of the body oils. The freeze brand should be held firmly on the animal for 30 seconds. The frozen tissue causes little or no pain but it takes about 3 months before the brand shows up. White hair grows back in the brand area, making it easily read for identification if it is on a dark-haired animal. There are obvious limitations for use on light-haired cattle.

Acid Branding

Some special preparation is needed for acid branding, mainly removing debris and clipping the hair. A special acid paste is used to dip a brand in and apply to the desired spot. The acid works as a chemical reaction to produce a brand similar to fire branding.

The acid paste is very easy to smear and is messy to work with. For this reason it is usually used only as a supplementary form of branding or in small herds where equipment is restricted.

Ear Tattooing

The ear should be cleaned of any wax, and a large flat area selected that appears pink in the middle of the ear. Ink should be smeared on this area first; then the tattoo device with the appropriate letters or numbers should be applied, creating the punctures through the first application of ink. After the tattoo device is removed, ink should be reapplied and the area rubbed in well to assure complete penetration and a clean tattoo. It takes a little time to do this right, but the result is easy to achieve, and a beautiful, clear, permanent form of identification results.

Ear Notching

Ear notching is used primarily in the western open-range states for ownership identification. Many variations and combinations such as two notches on the bottom of the left ear, right ear tipped, etc., are used to identify ownership. Notches on the bottom or the top of each ear can be arranged in a great number of ways. Some owners get so involved with a distinctive notch arrangement that little of the original ear is left, but many western cattlemen are used to reading ear notches and find them highly appropriate for their type of operation. Figure 8-4 illustrates the standard ear markings and the name of each.

Neck Chains

Neck chains work well as individual identification in combination with a brand, for herd or ownership identification, but are not a permanent method and have disadvantages such as falling off and getting broken. There have also been cases of cattle that tangle their neck chains in brush or trees, causing severe injury to themselves, or in extreme cases, death.

Horn Branding

Horn branding works very well for those animals that are to remain with their horns intact. However, the brand is necessarily restricted to a very small size that is hard to read. After a period of several years, these brands also tend to degenerate and have to be redone because of normal horn growth.

Ear Tags

Ear tags are very popular, and the advances made in them have endeared them to cattlemen throughout the United States. They stay in the ear well, and about the only disadvantage is when the ear tag is placed too high; this allows hair to grow over the number, making it difficult to read.

DRENCHING

The procedure to follow in drenching is first to grasp the head or use nose tongs to maneuver the mouth in the right position so that the dose gun can be inserted along the top of the tongue. Care should be taken not to ram

Crop --------------

Overslope ----------

Underslope --------

Swallow fork -------

Steeple fork -------

Oversharp ---------

Undersharp --------

Split ------------

Bit, under or over ---   **Figure 8-4.** Terminology of standard ear markings.

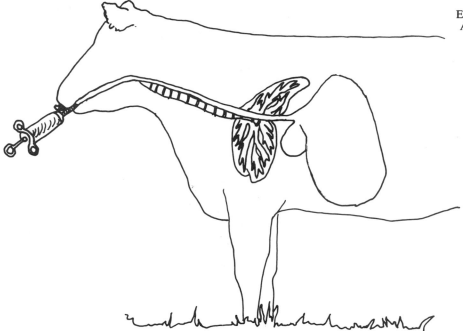

Figure 8-5. The drenching gun must be positioned properly and the head held in the right position to prevent forcing liquids into the lungs and causing pneumonia.

the tip of the dose gun into the palate or soft tissue, causing drench material thus injected to form an abscess that will have to be lanced, drained, and treated with antibiotics. Give the dosage slowly so that the animal has time to swallow to prevent overflow into the lungs, which could create pneumonia (Figure 8-5). Dose guns come in different sizes depending on the length of tip. A 6 in. tip is considered ideal to minimize the potential damage to the palate, yet be long enough to do the job. See Table 6-3 for drenching materials.

EAR IMPLANTS AND GROWTH STIMULANTS

The normal sanitary procedures apply in the case of implants. The ear should be cleaned and sterile needles used to insert the implant. The main point to remember is to place the implant just under the skin of the ear (subcutaneously) rather than into the lower depths of the ear. Implants are usually recommended to be placed on the backside of the ear. Keep extra implant pellets handy because crushing of the implant is a common occurrence.

At this point, little can be said about the future availability of specific materials listed below. Federal agencies will continue to monitor carcasses for the possibility of residues, so you should strictly follow all label restrictions and withdrawal times listed on the product you use. The recommendations, restrictions, and usages listed below are subject to change.

MGA

Melengestrol acetate (MGA) is a feed additive designed for feed-lot heifers and is available to feeders in either liquid or dry-feed supplements. Although MGA is a hormone, it is a progestational compound, whose effects differ from the estrogenic activity of other growth stimulants.

MGA acts to increase rate of gain, improve feed efficiency, and suppress heat in finishing heifers. Rate of gain is improved an average of 10.3%, feed efficiency by 6.5%. Since heat periods are suppressed, less activity in the lots is also a benefit.

Heifers that have reached sexual maturity show good response to MGA; those that are not ready to cycle show little benefit. Similarly, MGA has no appreciable effect on steers, bulls, or on spayed or pregnant heifers.

Current regulations specify 0.25 mg to 0.5 mg per head per day in the feed. MGA-supplemented feeds must be withdrawn at least 48 hours prior to slaughter. It is not approved for feeding with antibiotics. Since MGA is available only in feed form, its usefulness in other than dry-lot situations is limited.

Synovex

Synovex is a hormone implant that comes in two preparations: one type for heifers and the other for steers. Synovex-H for heifers contains the hormones testosterone and estrodiol. Synovex-S for steers contains the hormones progesterone and estradiol. The hormone preparations are contained in small pellets, which are implanted in the ear. One cartridge containing eight pellets should be used for each animal.

Regulations require at least 60 days between implanting of Synovex and slaughter. It is not recommended for animals kept for breeding.

Ralgro

Ralgro is a growth-stimulating implant that overcomes many of the common objections since it does not contain a hormone. Ralgro is made from an extract of corn mold and can be used for both steers and heifers. Since it is not a hormone, there are none of the side effects that sometimes occur with other implants. Ralgro implants apparently last for at least 100 days. Some tests indicate they may be effective even longer. Implanting once at the beginning of the finishing period should be sufficient.

The approved level of implantation for all ages of steers and heifers is 36 mg (three pellets). A withdrawal time of 65 days between implanting and slaughter is required.

Rumensin®

Rumensin is the trade name for the compound Monesin, sold as a beef feed additive. This material is not properly a growth stimulant since it acts differently than other compounds. By affecting fermentation in the rumen, Rumensin alters the relative proportions of fatty acids produced, causing the animal to utilize feed more efficiently.

Rumensin is cleared as an additive for feed-lot steer and heifer rations. A rate of 20 grams per ton is used for feeding periods of less than 60 days, 30 grams for longer periods. On the average, Rumensin improves feed efficiency by 10%, but has little or no effect on rate of gain in feed-lot situations. There is no withdrawal time, and the material can be fed up to the day of slaughter. It should be fed only to beef cattle; it may cause death if fed to horses.

Rumensin is not cleared for use with other feed additives, but it can be used in conjunction with ear implants.

Under pasture grazing conditions, where energy intake is limited by the animal's ability to consume forage, improved feed utilization from Rumensin allows cattle to gain faster. The material is expected to receive clearance for use in grazing situations.

Antibiotics

On the average, a 3% to 4% increase in weight gain and feed efficiency can be expected from antibiotic feeding.

The greatest benefit from antibiotic feeding is demonstrated when cattle are first starting on feed or have been under stress. There is a continued low-level response throughout the feeding period. In addition to the added production, a reduction in liver abscesses and other disease-control advantages result from antibiotic feeding.

HOOF CARE

Range cattle normally have no problem with hoofs growing too long except for the incidence of founder (see Chapter 6), because hoofs wear off in the normal process of grazing, especially in rocky territory. If, because of soft ground or low-lying areas, cattle should need some attention to cutting back of the hoofs, nippers are recommended rather than spending time using sanders, rasps, or more refined equipment.

Show cattle are often kept on soft bedding and are not walked as much as they should be; because stances are often in need of correction, hoof care is much more important on the circuit. A tilt table is recommended to save the back of the handler as well as to provide comfort to the animal. In the event a tilt table is not available, a squeeze chute is a second choice. One foot at a time is tied up, allowing the hoof nippers to cut back the extra growth, and a rasp is used to finish up the job for a neat appearance. Usually the nippers are used to cut back the tips only $\frac{1}{4}$ to $\frac{3}{4}$ in., avoiding the soft tissues of the quick that could cause bleeding and a tender foot. Maximum use of the rasp instead of the nippers will avoid injury.

A heavy-duty sander used with a tilt table works well. Take precautions not to get into the quick and to keep the sander moving. If you should stay in one spot too long, friction burns and tenderness can result.

DIPPING AND SPRAYING

The only precautions needed in dipping and spraying are to follow the directions exactly. If too strong a solution is mixed, toxicity problems may result. If too weak a solution is used, it does no good.

Dipping vats are still widely used across the South and West, and no problems are generally associated with their use as long as they are filled to the proper level.

Spray rigs do an excellent job if the pressure is sufficient. The only precaution to be taken using them is to refrain from spraying directly into eyes, nose, or mouth of cattle. Spraying should proceed from the top of the back to the bottom, so that full coverage and complete saturation are assured. See Table 6-4 for specific recommendations on products for external parasite control.

9

Herd Management of Beef Cattle

COWS

The references made in this section apply to cows that are permanent members of the herd, those that stay on the ranch for the normal lifetime of production.

Vaccination Program

Anthrax. Anthrax should be included in a vaccination program unless economic conditions dictate a minimum of protection and a choice has to be made. In this case, anthrax would not be considered one of the absolute necessities of vaccinations. However, if it is a reasonably risky area, anthrax vaccination should be considered. Give as small a dosage as possible. Vaccines come in 2 cc, 5 cc, and 10 cc vials. The smaller dose is recommended for the least traumatic effect.

Leptospirosis. In the past, only one or two types of leptospirosis have been recommended to be included in a vaccination program. This is a very dangerous disease and has spread widely in the past with a broad variety of organisms creating the problem. It is suggested that annual vaccination be undertaken, especially in the South. Use at least a three-way vaccine that covers *L. pomona*, *L. harjo*, and *L. grypothyposo*.

Redwater. A vaccine for Redwater is recommended twice a year along the coastal areas but only where Redwater is known to be a problem.

Blackleg. Blackleg vaccination is not normally needed in adult cows past two years of age. In the case of registered or very expensive animals, it may be worth considering for safety's sake. At least a three-way vaccine is recommended, and a seven-way vaccine as previously discussed (see Chapter 6) is even better.

220
HERD
MANAGE-
MENT
OF BEEF
CATTLE

Vibrio. Yearly vaccination for *Vibrio* is recommended in areas where outbreaks are common. This is one subject you need to discuss with your veterinarian because some vaccines have had a good protection history and others have been extremely doubtful. Your veterinarian can give you up-to-date information on brand name vaccines and their effectiveness in your area.

Anaplasmosis. Because of the current controversy over the effects of the anaplasmosis vaccine, it is not recommended that you vaccinate mature cows except in the case of an outbreak and then only on the advice of your veterinarian.

Shipping Fever (Parainfluenza$_3$, PI$_3$). It is not necessary to concern yourself with Shipping Fever in a closed herd. However, if cattle are to be stressed, worked, and moved some distance, these are the precipitating factors that bring about the disease, and a vaccine should definitely be given.

Deworming and Parasite Control

External. Backrubbers are efficient and economical. Material for use in the backrubbers is available locally in a wide variety, any of which will do a good job. If you do not use the back-rubbing method, it is suggested that cattle be sprayed every 6 to 8 weeks and watched closely during the winter for signs of lice. A pour-on insecticide for grub control and lice retardation can be effective: use in October; repeat in January or February.

Internal. Deworm with one of the broad-spectrum materials such as Thiabenzole, Levamisol, Ruelene, Tramisol, etc., twice per year during the spring and fall. Alternate the deworming material each 6 months to obtain best results, and if flukes are a problem, an additional drench with hexachlorethane is recommended.

Breeding Season

Flushing. Ten days prior to the breeding season, feed 5 lb of corn and cob meal or some high-energy grain per head per day. This is recommended to be continued for 30 days or until conception has occurred; then the diet should be restricted. Cattle in good condition should merely maintain their weight during pregnancy.

When to Palpate. Palpation should be done 60 to 90 days after the bulls have been taken out, in order to detect the "loafers" and to get maximum efficiency in reproduction.

How to Palpate. The principle involved in palpation is to insert a hand in the rectum of a cow and feel through the wall of the rectum for signs of pregnancy. Care should be taken to use a sterile, lubricated glove to protect man and animal from infection. Rectal detection can be done by competent experienced people as early as 60 days or less. However, the optimum time for palpation with a high degree of certainty is 60 to 90 days.

The question most often asked in rectal palpation is, "What are you feeling for?" There are certain landmarks that help to orient the person doing the palpation, in order to make a valid evaluation. The first point of reference could be the forward slope of the pelvis. Immediately forward of the pelvis one should be able to pick up the cervix (see Figure 9-1).

To the inexperienced breeder, it may help to describe the cervix as something approaching the size and feel of the neck of a Coke bottle. Follow the cervix to the swollen horn of the uterus. This will usually be to the right of center regardless of which horn contains the fertilized egg, since the rumen occupies most of the area to the left of the center line. Recall that the developing fetus is floating in a fluid that acts as a shock absorber; therefore, one should not expect to feel anything resembling an animal but rather something floating inside a protective membrane. It might be helpful to describe this sensation as the dribbling of a basketball. By gently pushing against the membrane with a dribbling motion, the bouncing ball (the calf) will return because of the tendency of the fetus to float to the top much like a block of wood would float inside a balloon filled with water. With proper training, one can detect this sensation at 60 days, and as the pregnancy continues and the fetus develops, the task becomes easier.

Time of Year to Breed. The actual breeding season will vary greatly depending on the type of environment in which you live. In all cases, however, the breeding season should be one time during the year for a 3-month period in order to group your calves during a 90-day calving season. The optimum time of the year varies with the part of the country, but January, February, and March in the South are considered the best time for calves to hit the ground. This gives them the opportunity to be at an age to utilize more of the summer and fall pastures because of advanced growth and age. Since the weather is mild in the South, this is entirely feasible. In the northern parts of the United States, calving is usually arranged for the early spring (April, May, and June; or March, April, and May) because the severity of the winters would rule out survival of the very young calves, especially if cows are somewhat undernourished.

Bull Selection for First-Calf Heifers. Most problems associated with calving are found in first-calf heifers. It is recommended that the type of bull be selected to breed to the heifers with this thought in mind. Angus or some other small breed is recommended in order to keep the first-calf weight down as low as possible. Some breeds, such as the Scotish Highland, are noted for producing an extremely small calf and are used in many parts of the northern United States for this purpose.

Special Health Problems

Cattlemen should keep an eye out for mastitis, which can occur prior to or just after calving. Cuts and abrasions on teats should be of concern because of the obvious reluctance of the cow to allow her calf to nurse. In

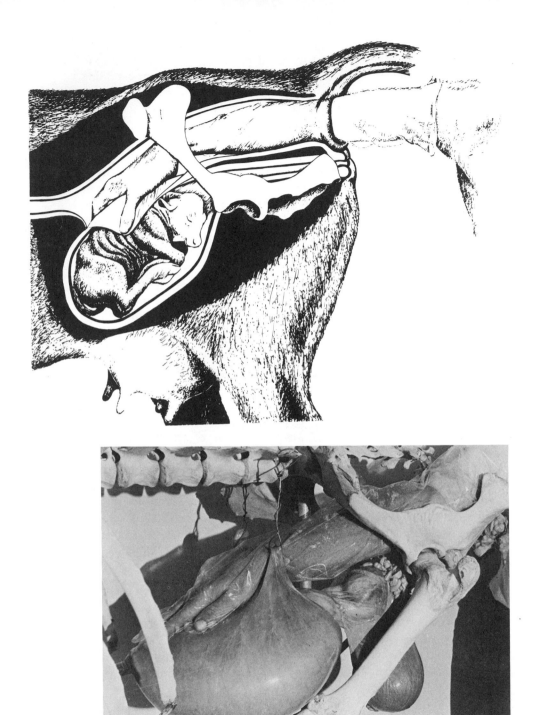

Figure 9-1. Simulated palpation of the swollen uterus with a 90-day fetus. Note the position in relation to the skeleton. (From Blakely and Bade, *The Science of Animal Husbandry*. Reston, Va.: Reston Publishing Company, Inc., 1976)

some cases, cuts are serious enough to cause a cow to kick a calf off completely. Prolapses occur both before and after calving. Vaginal tears also should be watched for during and after calving, as these could need immediate medical attention. Rectal and vaginal fistulas (tears in the wall between the rectum and the vulva) occur with regularity and allow fecal material and urine to filter into the tissues, causing infections. Retained placentas and calf malpresentations are other special problems of concern. All of these possibilities should be kept in mind and immediate attention should be given.

Most of the problems that you can solve with little or no help are covered in Chapter 7. Ask your veterinarian for advice on any problem that you lack the knowledge or skill to take care of.

Pasture Management

Rotation. The primary reasons for rotating pastures are to provide cattle new grazing areas and to give the grass a chance to recover. Rotations also are very effective in controlling parasites by removing cattle to a clean area and allowing a rest period long enough to break the cycles in areas from which they have been removed. Rotations may vary from months to weeks or even days. One extreme example to give an indication of the imaginative systems that have developed is the confining of 100 cows on 100 acres by dividing the pasture into 6-acre blocks using electrical fencing. The cows are moved every 3 to 5 days depending on pasture and weather conditions. This allows the maximum intensive grazing with the minimum length of time for cattle to be on the ground. A light harrow or spring-tooth plow is used on the pasture immediately after removing the cattle, in order to break fecal masses so as to control parasites and promote better pasture growth.

The most practical rotation appears to be 30 days on one pasture before moving to a new area and allowing for at least 30 days before returning. Some annual rotations are also recommended, such as cattle the first year, sheep or swine the second year, and cropping the soil the third year before cattle are returned. This gives maximum rotation and rest of the soil in order to control parasites as well as to produce maximum grazing and fertility.

Fertilization and Parasite Control. Fertilizing of the pastures should be done according to soil type and soil tests. Grass production is directly related to nitrogen applications, and phosphorus and potash applications are related to proper nutrition and skeletal development as previously discussed in the nutrition section.

Parasite control in the pasture can be accomplished more readily through rotations, especially lengthy rotations, and should definitely be considered if intense concentration and grazing are a part of the program.

Improving pastures through the use of grasses and legumes for your area is definitely a part of good management and sanitation. Lush growth prevents cattle from grazing so close to the ground that parasite eggs are

224
HERD
MANAGE-
MENT
OF BEEF
CATTLE

picked up. Legumes in a rotation will add nitrogen to the soil in addition to serving as a barrier to parasite development and continuation.

BULLS

Conditioning of bulls prior to breeding season should be a matter of feeding adequately in preparation for the breeding season. This has been covered giving specific recommendations in Chapter 5. A good nutrition program ensures top-notch physical health and rules out a deficiency of some essential element at the time of fertility testing.

In general, adequate nutrition is supplied by pasture with a minimum amount of grain or high-energy feed supplement. Breeding seasons usually take place during the spring so that most requirements will be met by pasture.

A vaccination program for the bull will be similar to that for the cow with a few exceptions. It is not recommended that the bull be vaccinated for brucellosis. In the case of anaplasmosis, bulls would be vaccinated; cows would not. In areas where Redwater disease is a problem, bulls and cows would both be vaccinated.

Parasite control, external and internal, is the same as for the rest of the herd. One possible exception is that bulls are more physically difficult to handle, and this is a case where injectable anthelmentics may be of advantage.

REPLACEMENT HEIFERS

Vaccination Program

A planned health program for replacement heifers is necessary so they can be properly immunized prior to joining the herd.

There are six diseases causing either abortion or infertility in cattle for which there are currently vaccines available. These diseases are: brucellosis, leptospirosis, vibriosis, IBR (Red Nose), PI_3 (parainfluenza$_3$), and BVD (bovine virus diarrhea.) In some parts of the country, Blackleg and Redwater disease are disease problems not of an abortive or infertility nature but rather of general concern to the cattleman.

Brucellosis. Although the incidence of brucellosis has been greatly reduced by the National Eradication Program, a small number of herds are still infected, and vaccinations are still being carried out. Vaccination should be done when the young heifer calves are 3 to 6 months of age.

Leptospirosis. Leptospirosis vaccination should be accomplished 30 to 60 days before the replacement heifers are to be bred. Follow the advice of your veterinarian as to which species of *Leptospira* are found in your area and should be included in your vaccination program. Use at least a three-way vaccine that covers *L. pomona*, *L. harjo*, and *L. gripothyposo*.

Vibriosis.   Vibriosis vaccine is administered 30 to 60 days before breeding. The organism *Vibrio fetus* (which causes abortion) is transmitted to females from infected bulls during breeding; so it is important to immunize the heifers.

IBR (Red Nose).   Since IBR is very common and vaccination is not recommended on pregnant animals, it is advisable that heifers be vaccinated 30 to 60 days before breeding.

PI$_3$ (Parainfluenza$_3$).   It has been concluded that PI$_3$ may be an important cause of abortion in cattle. Vaccination for this disease is now being included in many cattlemen's vaccination programs as a precautionary measure.

BVD.   Occasionally, unfavorable reactions follow the use of modified live virus BVD vaccines. The risk of these vaccines should be weighed against the possibility of losses resulting from BVD infection before a decision is made about using them. Consult your veterinarian concerning the need for this vaccine in your area.

In summary, a vaccination program can be scheduled for heifers by vaccinating for brucellosis at 3 to 6 months of age. At 30 to 60 days before breeding, leptospirosis, vibriosis, IBR, PI$_3$, and BVD vaccines can be injected. Leptospirosis and vibriosis are recommended to be repeated annually at 30 to 60 days prior to breeding. Brucellosis is a single vaccination for the life of the animal.

Other Practices

With the exception of the special nutritional needs (flushing) discussed in Chapter 5, heifers are handled at the same time as the rest of the herd for parasite control, pregnancy testing, etc.

BABY CALF MANAGEMENT

The First Twenty-Four Hours

When a calf is born in a normal presentation and without difficulties, the navel should be dipped into iodine—if the calf is born in confined quarters. If it is born in an open-range situation, one that is not overcrowded, then the iodine is not necessary.

Make sure the baby calf nurses within 15 minutes after birth if possible, in order to consume the colostrum milk that contains the antibodies to protect it against disease. Colostrum can also be collected from high-producing cows that have lost their calves; it should be stored in a deep freeze for later emergency use.

In areas where viral scours are a problem, Scour-vac Reo oral vaccine should be given for protection against this type of scours. If viral scours are

226
HERD
MANAGE-
MENT
OF BEEF
CATTLE

suspected, collect fecal samples from 6 to 8 calves within 4 hours of the start of scouring; then freeze the samples and submit them to your veterinarian for diagnostic laboratory tests.

Baby calves may also be injected with a combination vitamin ADE material. This is optional but has proven beneficial in many areas, especially in colder climates.

The baby calf may be tagged with an ear tag for identification, castrated, and dehorned with a horn paste to prevent horn growth. This will be the easiest time to do these operations since a baby calf offers no resistance, but many cattlemen prefer to wait until weaning.

There may be cases of abandonment of calves. In this situation, the baby calf should be fed colostrum milk from another cow, or use colostrum that has previously been frozen. After 3 or 4 days of colostrum consumption, the calf may be switched to a nurse cow or one that has lost a calf.

Birth to Weaning

Most calves are placed on pasture by at least 2 months of age, if not born on pasture. If branding and castrating were not done at birth, this is a good age to do these procedures. A two-way Blackleg (*C. chauvoei*, *septicum*) may be given at this time if Blackleg is a problem in your area.

Calf herd vaccination for brucellosis may be given to heifers at 3 to 6 months of age; never beyond 10 months.

If calves are worked 30 days prior to weaning, the vaccination program may include Pasteurella bacterin (multocida and hemolyticum), IBR, PI$_3$ (parainfluenza$_3$), and grub treatment (if before October 31).

At weaning, if the calves have been vaccinated 30 days previously, the second injection of Pasteurella may be given along with a four-way Blackleg vaccine (if determined to be needed). Steers and heifers may also be implanted at this time with such products as Ralgro or Synovex.

If calves are worked only at weaning, a typical vaccination program would be a combination of IBR and leptospirosis. Four-way Blackleg (*C. chauvoei*, *septicum*, *sordelli*, and *novyi*) is also recommended in many areas. Grub treatment, if before October 31, can be initiated at this time, and implants may be used. If calves are to be shipped any distance or if they are headed for a feed lot, Shipping Fever vaccines and/or a preconditioning program needs to be considered in the management plan.

Parasite control usually will not be a major problem in calves if the herd has been properly treated according to a herd health plan, but calves may also receive individual treatment as previously recommended.

For an easy checklist, a condensed version of month-by-month activities is given in Table 9-1.

Table 9-1. Beef Cow Management Calendar

Month		Health	Nutrition	Management
Spring Calving	*Fall Calving*			
January	July	Watch for abortions, spray for lice.	Provide shelter or increase energy level of ration.	Provide 5 gal of water per day per cow.
February	August	Watch for foot rot, vaccinate cows with *Clostridium perfringens* to prevent some type of scours in calves when born.	Keep nutritional level as outlined for December.	Check pregnancy exam records to know calving dates. Implant with Ralgro when calves are 2 wk of age.
March	September	Get ready for calving; provide clean, dry calving facility. Know how to calve cows.	Provide a minimum of 9 lb TDN before calving and up to 16 lb after calving. Feed and manage first-calf heifers and old cows from rest of herd.	Record birth dates, separate nonpregnant cows, identify calves. Castrate and implant.
April	October	Identify difficult calving cows on your records.	Plan pasture program.	Purchase sires for this year's breeding program. Make final selection on heifer replacements. Castrate calves when implanting.
May	November	Fertility check bulls, vaccinate open cows for vibriosis, IBR, and leptospirosis 30 days prior to breeding. Vaccinate for BVD.	Watch for grass tetany. Feed MgO_2 0.5 oz day/head.	Start breeding heifers, one cycle before cows; castrate and dehorn calves (45 days old).

227

Table 9.1 (*Continued*)

Spring Calving	Fall Calving			
June	December	Get ready to use AI. Natural breeding one bull (fertile) for 25 cows.	Provide creep rations; pasture should carry cows.	Creep feed.
July	January	Vaccinate all calves over 3 months of age for Clostridial group (Blackleg, etc.). Vaccinate heifer replacements with Strain 19 at 2–6 mo of age.	Check pastures for poisonous weeds	Consider weaning if pasture is short.
August	February	Check on pinkeye and treat.	Plan winter feed supply.	Remove bulls. Re-implant calves.
September	March	Watch for grass tetany. Check on foot rot and cancer eye.	Watch supplementary crops for frost damage. Include MgO^2 in feed.	Plan calf program, wean.
October	April	Pregnancy check cows, treat for external parasites, worm calves, and treat calves for grubs.	Turn cows into stalks.	Cull cows, back tag all cows going to slaughter.
November	May	Vaccinate calves for IBR and PI_3 (BVD) and clostridial group. Repeat Pasteurella.	All calves should be weaned. Provide mineral mix for cows.	Select replacement heifers, permanently identify calves.
December	June	Check cows for abortion, heat periods, and parasites.	Check feed supplies and cows' winter rations.	Feed first-calf heifers separately from older cows.

Source: John B. Herrick, *Feedstuffs*. (Minneapolis, Minn.: Miller Publishing Company, 1977). Reprinted by permission.

Dairy Cattle

10

Nutrition of Dairy Cattle

SPECIALIZED DAIRY NEEDS

The ruminant anatomy and physiology are covered in Part 2 on beef cattle. Digestion and rumination are the same for dairy as for beef cattle.

Still, there are important practical differences between feeding dairy cows and beef cows. Dairy breeds have been selected for centuries for maximum milk production. This heavy milk production, especially during early lactation, places a great deal of physiological stress on the animal at a time when she is also expected to prepare for rebreeding. For this reason, dairy herd nutrition is a very crucial issue. If the cow is unable to handle the stress of milk production, reproductive performance will probably be the first to suffer, followed by other health problems.

Dairy cows require considerably more feed nutrients than other cattle. During periods of heavy lactation it may be physically impossible for a cow to consume enough feed to produce at her maximum. Bulky, low-quality forages will complicate this problem even further. Thus, feeding of high-quality roughages supplemented with concentrate feeds should be the basis of dairy cow nutrition.

You can approximate the total daily feed consumption of a dairy cow by the following formula: 2% of body weight plus 33% of milk production (4% fat-corrected milk). As an example, a 1200 lb cow producing 60 lb of 4% milk daily will eat about 44 lb of dry matter daily.

Table 10-1 gives a summary of the fat-soluble vitamins needed in dairy rations and their functions. Table 10-2 summarizes mineral requirements in the dairy ration, including functions, deficiency symptoms, recommended minimum and maximum levels, and feed sources for dairy cattle.

Table 10-1.   Summary of Fat-Soluble Vitamins in Dairy Rations

Vitamin	Function(s)	Deficiency signs and associated problems	Common feed sources for Dairy Attle
A	Essential for normal vision; cellular function; and maintenance of epithelial linings of respiratory, reproductive, and digestive tracts.	Night blindness; skin problems; blind, dead, or weak calves; reproductive problems.	Sources of carotene: green, leafy forages; hays; haylages (little weathering); unfrosted corn silage; synthetic A; vitamin premix; fish liver oil.
D	Normal bone growth and development; absorption of calcium and phosphorus; mobilization of calcium and phosphorus.	Rickets, osteomalacia.	Sun-cured forages; fish liver oils; synthetic premixes.
E	Antioxidant; associated with selenium.	Oxidized flavor in milk; muscle problems; white muscle disease; cardiac muscle abnormalities.	Alfalfa; germ of cereals; wheat germ oil; cereal grains; synthetic premixes.
K	Required for blood clotting.	Moldy sweet-clover disease; hemorrhages.	Green, leafy forage. Ample amounts normally are synthesized in the digestive tract.

Source: University of Minnesota. *Feeding Dairy Cattle.* Bulletin No. 218.

Water

Water is required by lactating dairy cattle in very large amounts and should always be available, free of contamination from bacteria or high nitrates and sulfates.

Milk contains about 87% water, and cows will normally consume about 4 to 5 lb of water per lb of milk produced. Cows will drink from 12 to 25 gallons of water during a day.

Feedstuffs

Legume and Grass Mixtures for Hay and Low-Moisture Silage. Legumes and grass mixtures are excellent sources if harvested and stored properly. When grain intake is limited, cows may consume $2\frac{1}{2}$ to 3% of their weight as forage dry matter.

Important considerations in legume and grass mixtures are the cutting date and stage of maturity. Legume and grass silage should be put up at 30 to 40% dry matter in a bunker silo, 40 to 50% in a concrete or stave silo, and 50 to 60% in an oxygen-limiting silo.

Hay should not be bailed or stacked until dry matter content is at least 80%. Otherwise heating and molding can develop.

Corn and Sorghum Silage. Corn and sorghum silage should contain nearly 50% grain for an excellent source of energy. This feed must be supplemented with protein and minerals to be balanced for high milk production.

To attain maximum yields, corn should be harvested for silage when it has reached physiological maturity: kernels are fully dented, and cells at the base of the kernel (when dissected) are black. Dry matter content should be about 35%.

Small Grain Silages. Oats, barley, wheat, and rye can be used for silage. They should be harvested in the boot stage to early milk stage for high crude protein content. Peas can be included with oats to increase protein content. These crops should be wilted to 60% moisture before ensiling.

Green Chop. Harvesting feeds by field chopping rather than by grazing and feeding has the advantage of reducing field losses. However, cutting every day can be a problem during wet weather.

Forage Evaluation. A precise value can be obtained through chemical analysis for dry matter content, crude protein, and crude fiber to better balance rations and to achieve maximum milk production. It is best to obtain haylage and silage samples at the time of ensiling. This material should be refrigerated during storage, before analysis, to prevent deterioration or change in chemical composition. A quart of material should be sent for testing. Periodic checks should be made during the season, especially if the material in the silos is in "layers" or if different crops were used. Straw, stover, and poor-quality roughages may be used sparingly in "salvaging" situations.

Table 10-2. Summary of Minerals in Dairy Rations

Mineral	Function(s)	Deficiency signs and associated problems	Recommended minimum and maximum levels	Feed sources for dairy cattle
Calcium (Ca)	Bone and teeth formation; blood clotting; muscle contraction. .12% in whole milk.	Rickets; slow growth and poor bone development; easily fractured bones; reduced milk yield; milk fever is a disturbance of normal calcium metabolism.	Minimum level is .55% for young calves; .4% for growing heifers; .4% to .75% for lactating cows depending on production level.	Alfalfa and other legumes; ground limestone; dicalcium phosphate; steamed bone meal.
Phosphorus (P)	Bone and teeth formation; P is involved in energy metabolism, part of DNA and RNA; .09% in milk.	Fragile bones; poor growth; low blood P (less than 4–6 mg/100 ml); depraved appetite—chewing of wood, hair, and bones; poor reproductive performance.	Minimum level is .42% for calves; .3% for growing heifers; .3% to .5% for lactating cows.	Monosodium, monoammonium, and dicalcium phosphates; steamed bone meal; oil seed meals; cereal grains; grain byproducts.
Sodium (Na)	Acid-base balance; muscle contraction; nerve transmission.	Craving for salt; reduced appetite; if very severe: incoordination, weakness, shivering, and death.	Minimum level for salt is .25% for young cattle and .45% for lactating or dry cows.	Common salt.
Chlorine (Cl)	Acid-base balance; maintenance of osmotic pressure; manufacture of hydrochloric acid in abomasum.	Craving for salt; reduced appetite.	(See above)	Common salt.
Magnesium (Mg)	Enzyme activator; found in skeletal tissue and bone.	Irritability; tetany; increased excitability.	Minimum level is .07% for young calves; .16% for growing calves and dry cows; .20% for lactating cows.	Magnesium oxide; forages.
Sulfur (S)	Needed for rumen microbial protein synthesis especially when nonprotein nitrogen is fed; found in cartilage, tendons, etc.	Slow growth; reduced milk production; reduced feed efficiency.	Minimum recommended level is .20%; levels above .35% may reduce feed intake.	Elemental sulfur; sodium and potassium sulfates; protein supplements; legume forages.
Potassium (K)	Maintenance of electrolyte balance; enzyme activator; muscle function; nerve function.	Decrease in feed intake; loss of hair glossiness; lower blood and milk potassium.	Minimum recommended level is .80%.	Legume forages; potassium chloride; potassium sulfate.
Iodine (I)	Synthesis of thyroxine.	Big neck in calves; goitrogenic substances may cause deficiency.	.5 ppm for adult cattle; .25 ppm for young cattle. Toxicity signs may appear at 50 to 200 ppm. Signs include excess salivation, watery nasal discharge, coughing. Safe levels are 20 ppm for young cattle; 50 ppm for adult cattle.	Iodized salt or trace mineralized salt.

Element	Function	Deficiency Symptoms	Requirement/Toxicity	Source
Iron (Fe)	Part of hemoglobin; part of many enzyme systems.	Nutritional anemia.	100 ppm in dry matter is recommended level. Safe level for cattle appears to be 400 to 1000 ppm depending on form of iron.	Forages; grains; trace mineralized salt.
Copper (Cu)	Needed for manufacture of hemoglobin; coenzyme.	Severe diarrhea; abnormal appetite; poor growth; coarse, bleached, or graying haircoat; osteomalacia.	10 ppm in dry matter is recommended level. Cattle can safely tolerate 100 ppm. Toxicity signs include jaundice, liver damage, and death.	Widespread in feedstuffs; trace mineralized salt.
Cobalt (Co)	Part of vitamin B_{12}; needed for growth of rumen microorganisms.	Failure of appetite; anemia; decreased milk production; rough haircoat.	Minimum level is .1 ppm of dry matter; 10 to 20 ppm is upper level. Signs of toxicity include reduced feed intake and body weight; emaciation; weakness; anemia.	Trace mineralized salt.
Manganese (Mn)	Growth; bone formation enzyme activator.	Delayed or decreased signs of estrus; poor conception.	Recommended level is 40 ppm for cattle. Maximum safe level is 1000 ppm. Excess interferes with iron metabolism and may induce hypomagnesia.	Widely distributed in feeds; trace mineralized salt.
Zinc (Zn)	Enzyme activator; wound healing.	Decreased weight gains; lowered feed efficiency; skin problems; slow healing wounds; listlessness.	Minimum level is 40 ppm. Maximum safe level is not more than 500 ppm for young cattle and 1000 ppm for cows.	Forages; trace mineralized salt.
Fluorine (F)	Not known if it is essential for ruminants; has been shown to be essential for laboratory animals.		Maximum safe level is 30 ppm. Severe reduction in feed intake; stiffness in legs; enlarged bones. A problem with high fluorine phosphates.	Rock phosphate mineral.
Selenium (Se)	Functions with certain enzymes. Associated with vitamin E.	White muscle disease in calves. Retained placenta (not clean).	Minimum level is .1 ppm. Maximum safe level is about 3 to 5 ppm. Toxicity shown by alkali disease or blind staggers; lameness; sloughed hooves.	Oil meals; alfalfa; wheat; oats; corn; amount varies with content in soil.
Molybdenum (Mo)	Part of the enzyme xanthine oxidase.	Loss of weight, emaciation; diarrhea.	Maximum safe level is 6 ppm. Signs include emaciation; intense liquid diarrhea; weakness, stiffness; hair color changes.	Widely distributed in feeds; deficiency is rarely a problem.

Source: University of Minnesota. *Feeding Dairy Cattle.* Bulletin No. 218.

235

Grains. Energy is the main nutrient contribution from grain. Rolling, crimping, cracking, or grinding increases the digestibility of grain, especially if it is coarse-textured. Finely ground grain can lower digestibility and milk fat percentage and can cause rumen acidosis. Pelleted grain increases palatability and intake.

Corn and Cob Meal. Corn and cob meal contains 10% less energy than shelled corn, but the added fiber aids in maintaining the fat tests and keeping cows on feed.

Shelled Corn. Because of the caloric content of shelled corn, good management is necessary to obtain maximum consumption without causing digestive disturbances.

Oats. With about 85% of the energy content of shelled corn, oats add fiber and bulk to a grain mix and help maintain rumen function.

Barley. Barley should be added gradually if used in large amounts. Rolling will improve palatability. If the barley is finely ground, it shouldn't make up more than 50% of the grain ration.

Wheat. Wheat is not often used in dairy rations but is acceptable in amounts of less than 50% of the grain ration.

Protein Supplements

Soybean Meal. Soybean meal is generally the most common and economical vegetable protein supplement available in the United States. It contains between 46 and 50% protein.

Whole Soybeans. Ground whole soybeans can be included in dairy rations. The maximum amount should not exceed 20% of the grain mix. Cows should be adjusted to them gradually to avoid scours or going off feed. The raw beans contain the enzyme urease, which releases ammonia from urea. For this reason, NPN (synthetic urea) and raw beans should not be used together.

Cottonseed Meal. Cottonseed meal is available throughout the southern states and other cotton-producing areas of the world. Cottonseed meal is somewhat lower in protein than soybean meal, but it makes an excellent supplement.

Linseed Meal. Linseed meal is a product of the flax industry. It is a good protein supplement and is used in fitting cattle for show or sale because it adds shine to the haircoat.

Urea. Urea is an NPN (nonprotein nitrogen) compound containing about 45% nitrogen, a protein equivalent of 281%. Some guidelines to successful utilization of urea are as follows:

1. Feeds that are most successfully supplemented with urea are high in energy, low in protein, and low in natural urea. Drought-stricken corn silage

made from heavily fertilized corn may contain considerable natural NPN, and urea should not be used in this case.

2. Maximum amounts of urea to feed are 1% in the grain mix, .5% in corn silage (10 lb/ton), or .4 to .5 lb urea per head per day. Higher levels can be toxic. Urea should be limited in the early period of lactation.

3. If cattle have not been fed urea previously, a 7 to 10 day adjustment period in which the urea is gradually increased will help to maintain feed intake and production. A mixture of 56 lb of ground shelled corn, 7 lb of urea, and 37 lb of soybean meal are equivalent to 100 lb of soybean meal in total energy and protein equivalent. This mixture can be substituted for soybean meal. It should not be used for top-dressing, grain, or silage because of possible bitter feed taste and feed refusal.

Byproduct Feeds

Brewer's Grain. If you are located near a brewery, wet brewer's grain may be obtained at a reasonable cost. It contains about 80% water, requiring large amounts to be fed to obtain substantial intake of dry matter. Cattle should be adjusted to it gradually. It is high in protein and a fair source of energy.

Wheat Bran. Wheat bran is included to add bulk and fiber to a grain mixture. It is relatively high in protein and phosphorus; it improves ration palatibility; and it functions as a laxative.

Beet Pulp. Beet pulp may be obtained in plain form or as molasses beet pulp. It is high in energy, adds digestible fiber and bulk, improves palatability, and can make up 30% of the ration dry matter.

Whey. Both dried and liquid forms of whey are available in most cheese-producing areas. Dried whey can be mixed in grain mixtures at 10% levels. Dried whey can also be added to the silo at filling time at a rate of 20 to 100 lb per wet ton of forage. Liquid whey can be offered to cattle on a free-choice basis. It should not be over 36 hours old because it will become acidic, and cattle will not drink it. Flies can be a problem if strict sanitation is not insured.

Molasses. Cane and beet molasses supply energy and are used primarily to improve the acceptability of the ration. Limit the amount to 5 to 7% of the grain mix (10% in pelleted feeds) to avoid undesirable rumen effects.

FEEDING THE DAIRY HERD

Dairy Cow Nutrition

Nutrient requirements vary with the stage of lactation and gestation. Four feeding periods can be defined in feeding the dairy herd.

Period 1: Early Lactation. (70 days after calving—peak milk production). Milk production increases rapidly, peaking at 4 to 6 weeks after calving. Increasing the grain 1 to 2 lb per day after calving will increase nutrient intake while minimizing off-feed problems and acidosis. Excessive levels of grain (more than 65% of the total dry matter) must be avoided since fiber level in the total ration should be above 15% (13 to 17% range) to maintain rumen fermentation. Top-dressing natural protein can help meet protein needs if it is not possible to feed complete rations. Extra protein may be needed during this peak period. One pound of soybean meal (or equivalent) for each 10 lb of milk over a 50 lb base of milk production is a safe guideline. If urea is used, it should be limited to .4 to .5 lb per day.

Low peak production and ketosis problems occur when the nutrient levels are not met. If grain intake is increased too rapidly, or if it is too high, problems such as off-feed, acidosis, and displaced abomasum are possible.

Period 2: Peak Dry Matter Intake. (the second ten weeks after calving —70 to 140 days, declining milk production). Cows should be kept at peak production as long as possible. Grain intake can reach $2\frac{1}{2}$% of the cow's body weight. Forage intake (dry matter basis) should be at least 1% of the cow's body weight to maintain ruminant function and to meet fat test. Feeding beet pulp, corn and cob meal, and/or molasses can encourage cows to eat high levels of grain and will maintain rumen digestion. If urea is used, it should be limited to .4 lb/cow/day.

Potential problems during this period include a rapid drop or decline in milk production, low fat tests, a lack of heat signs, and ketosis.

Period 3: Mid to Late Lactation. (140 to 305 days after calving—declining milk production). Most cows have few problems during the third phase. You should guard against wasteful grain feeding to low producers in this declining period. Match grain intake to milk production. Cows that lose weight in early lactation should be fed extra nutrients to replace body reserves at this point, because cattle are most efficient while lactating. Do not wait until cows are dry to rebuild body condition. This is the period of time best suited to putting back the weight previously lost in the efficient milk production phase. Young cows should receive additional nutrients for growth (two-year-olds about 20% more; three-year-olds about 10% more).

Period 4: Dry Period. (45 to 60 days before the next lactation). Although nutrient requirements are not high, the fourth period is a critical stage for dry cows. Improper feeding during the dry period can adversely affect milk yield in the next lactation. The amount of grains fed during the dry period will depend on forage quality and type. Limiting feed may be necessary ($1\frac{1}{2}$% body weight as corn silage dry matter, use of corn stalks or straw, etc.). Some grains should be fed 2 weeks before calving to establish the rumen microflora that digest grain. Calcium and phosphorus needs must be adequate but avoid excessive calcium intakes (over 100 gr per day) and provide minimum phosphorus needs (40 gr per day). The calcium to phosphorus ratio should be approximately 2:1. Supplemental vitamins A and D, injected or fed, can improve calf survival, increase colostrum level of vitamins, and lower retained placenta and milk fever if the feed sources are low or deficient. Trace minerals, especially iodine and cobalt, should be supplemented.

Potential problems in this period include milk fever, displaced abomasum, and fat cow syndrome.

Based on the period feeding approach, Tables 10-3 and 10-4 contain suggested grain and protein guidelines. Sample rations based on the period feeding concept are listed in Table 10-5 for legume, grass, and corn silage forage-based rations.

CALF NUTRITION

Amount to Feed, Feeding Frequency, and Age of Weaning

A prime consideration in raising a calf is to provide adequate dry matter for growth. For an 80 to 100 lb Holstein calf, 1 lb of dry matter daily from milk or milk replacer is adequate from birth to weaning at 4 weeks. Estimate the dry matter percentage in the liquid diet and dilute as necessary in relation to the total volume offered the calf (see Table 10-6).

Table 10-3. Amount of Grain to Feed by Periods (1400 lb Cow, 4% Milk)

	PRODUCTION ABILITY OF THE COW (LB)[a]			
Average daily 1st period:	50	60	80	90–100
LACTATION TOTAL:	10,000	12,000	15,000	18,000
Period of lactation		*Grain-to-milk ratio*		
1. (1st 10 weeks)	1:4	1:3	1:3	1:3
2. (2nd 10 weeks)	1:4	1:3	1:2.5	1:2.5
3. (Last 24 weeks)	1:4	1:4	1:3	1:3
4. (Dry, 6–8 weeks)	3–4 lb daily	4 lb daily	4 lb daily	6 lb daily
Total grain (approximate)	3000 lb	4000 lb	5000 lb	6000 lb

Source: University of Minnesota. *Feeding Dairy Cattle*. Bulletin No. 218.
[a]Ratios based on 100% dry matter basis, grain containing 80% TDN and forage 60% TDN.

Table 10-4. Protein Levels of Total Rations During Four Periods
of Lactation

	PRODUCTION ABILITY OF THE COW		
Average 1st 10 weeks:	60 lb	80 lb	90 lb
Lactation total:	12,000 lb	15,000 lb	18,000 lb
Period		*% of ration dry matter*	
1. (1st 10 weeks)	16	19	20
2. (2nd 10 weeks)	13	15	16
3. (Last 24 weeks)	12	12	12
4. (Dry, 6–8 weeks)	9	9	9

Source: University of Minnesota. *Feeding Dairy Cattle*. Bulletin No. 218.

Table 10-5. Sample Rations for Cows in Various Feeding Periods with Various Forage Types and Combinations

TYPE OF FORAGE	PERIOD 1[a]	PERIOD 2[a]	PERIOD 3	PERIOD 4
Legume forage				
Alfalfa hay (lb)	22	29	29	22
Grain mix (lb)	41	33	19	6
Oats (lb)	580	630	660	630
Sh. corn (lb)	1180	1280	1300	1300
44% supp. (lb)	200	60	0	0
Dical. (lb)	20	10	20	50
Trace mineralized salt and vit. (lb)	20	20	20	20
Corn silage limited hay				
Alfalfa hay (lb)	6	6	6	6
Corn silage (lb)	45	63	63	45
Grain mix (lb)	36	27	14	2
Oats (lb)	465	460	460	650
Sh. corn (lb)	1000	935	900	1300
44% supp. (lb)	480	550	585	0
Dical. (lb)	20	25	30	30
Limestone (lb)	15	10	5	0
Trace mineralized salt and vit. (lb)	20	20	20	20
Legume ($\frac{1}{2}$)				
Corn silage ($\frac{1}{2}$)				
Alfalfa hay (lb)	11	15	15	11
Corn silage (lb)	30	40	40	30
Grain mix (lb)	38	29	16	4
Oats (lb)	520	540	580	660
Sh. corn (lb)	1075	1095	1200	1300
44% supp. (lb)	360	325	185	0
Dical. (lb)	15	20	0	0
Monosod. phos. (lb)	0	0	15	20
Limestone (lb)	10	0	0	0
Trace mineralized salt and vit. (lb)	20	20	20	20
Grass				
Grass hay (lb)	22	29	29	22
Grain mix (lb)	42	34	21	7
Oats (lb)	550	575	635	655
Sh. corn (lb)	1113	1170	1265	1300
44% supp. (lb)	290	210	60	0
Dical. (lb)	10	10	5	0
Limestone (lb)	17	15	15	25
Trace mineralized salt and vit. (lb)	20	20	20	20

Source: University of Minnesota. *Feeding Dairy Cattle*, Bulletin No. 218.

Notes: Production: Period 1 = 90 lb, Period 2 = 80 lb, Period 3 = 50 lb; fat test = 3.8% all periods and 1300 lb cow.

Dry matter levels: hay = 90%; corn silage = 33%; and grain = 88%.

Forage content (100% DM): alfalfa = 16% CP (crude protein) and 33% CF (crude fiber); corn silage = 8% CP and 26% CF; and grass = 12% CP and 37% CF.

[a]The amount of feed indicated meets the cow's needs. Cows may not be able to consume the indicated amounts in periods 1 and 2.

Table 10-6.   Dilution Rate for Various Liquid Diets for Calves Fed Once or Twice Daily

Type of milk	% Dry matter	ONCE DAILY FEEDING[a] IN-GREDIENT + WATER = LB DRY MATTER ...lb/feeding daily	TWICE DAILY FEEDING[a] IN-GREDIENT + WATER = LB DRY MATTER ...lb/feeding daily
(Ingredient)			
First milk colostrum	28	3.5 + 3.5 = 1.0	2.0 + 2.0 = 1.1
Pooled excess			
colostrum	16	6.0 + 0 = 1.0	3.0 + 1.5 = 1.0
Whole milk,			
Holstein	12	7.0 + 0 = 0.8	4.0 + 0.0 = 1.0
Milk replacer	88	.8 + 5.0 = 0.7	0.5 + 3.5 = .9

Source: University of Minnesota. *Feeding Dairy Cattle*, Bulletin No. 218.
[a] Use 75 to 80% of these amounts for Jersey or Guernsey calves.

Many calves have been weaned successfully at 3 to 4 weeks of age. Only healthy calves that won't be subjected to stresses such as extreme cold conditions should be weaned before 4 weeks. Also, calves weaned at this earlier age should be offered a palatable calf starter feed containing slightly more protein than normal (about 18%). Calves should be consuming at least 1 lb of starter feed daily prior to weaning.

Preventing Calf Scours

A number of management practices encourage the outbreak of scours in small calves. Avoid the following conditions if at all possible:

1. Overcrowding—Provide 24 to 28 sq ft of bedded area or about 20 sq ft of building floor space for calves raised in confined, elevated stalls.

2. Inadequate ventilation, wet stalls, and overfeeding.

3. Low resistance—Vitamin A, D, and E supplements given in oral or injectable forms immediately after birth may be helpful.

4. No first milk colostrum—About 40% of the calves born receive insufficient colostrum to be protected. Therefore you should see that calves consume it as soon as possible after birth (preferably within 15 minutes). A minimum of 2 quarts for a Holstein and 3 pints for smaller breed calves is recommended. It is important for calves to get sufficient quantities of colostrum in order to receive the antibodies that will protect them against disease.

5. Dirty Utensils—Clean the feeding utensils thoroughly after each feeding, and store them upside down to drain all water out.

Early detection of sickness and prompt corrective action are important to prevent scours (see section on scours in Chapter 6 for recommended treatment).

Starter Rations

A good quality, palatable calf starter should be offered at about 3 days of age and certainly no later than the tenth or twelfth day. Calf starters should be fed until calves are about 12 weeks of age. Intake should be limited to about 3 or 4 lb per calf each day. Commercial calf starters do an excellent job. Table 10-7 gives some examples of home-mixed rations that produce equally good results.

Table 10-7. Example Calf Starter Rations

INGREDIENTS	RATION[a]					
	A	B	C	D	E	F
Corn, coarse grind	50	39	54	44	34	24
Oats, rolled or crushed	35		12	22	34	24
Barley, rolled or coarse grind		39				
Beet pulp, molasses						20
Corn cobs, ground					15	
Wheat bran		10	11			
Soybean meal	13	10	8	26	15	25
Linseed meal			8			
Molasses, liquid			5	5		5
Dicalcium phosphate	1	1	1	1	1	1
Trace mineral salt	1	1	1	1	1	1
Vitamin A (I.U.)	200,000	200,000	200,000	200,000	200,000	200,000
Vitamin D (I.U.)	50,000	50,000	50,000	50,000	50,000	50,000
Total (lb)	100	100	100	100	100	100
Protein (% of DM)	16	16	16	20	16	20
Fiber (% of DM)	6	5	5	5	11	9

Source: University of Minnesota. *Feeding Dairy Cattle*, Bulletin No. 218.

[a]Rations A, B, and C recommended for calves weaned after 4 weeks of age and receiving forage.

Ration D recommended for calves weaned before 4 weeks and receiving forage.

Ration E recommended for calves weaned after 4 weeks and not consuming forage.

Ration F recommended for calves weaned before 4 weeks and not receiving forage.

HEIFER NUTRITION

Rearing the Calf from 12 Weeks to One Year

Pasture can be used successfully in the feeding program for young heifers, but it should not be expected to supply all the nutrients for calves in this age group. A grain mix and some stored forage are desirable for young calves on pasture. Trace mineralized salt and a calcium-phosphorus supplement can be offered on a free-choice basis if not adequately supplied in the grain mix. Grain should be limited to about 4 lb, or no more than 5 lb, per day, depending on forage quality. This is to keep down excessive fatness, which can result in breeding problems and fatty tissue in the udder.

Table 10-8 gives examples of grower rations for 300 to 400 lb calves.

Table 10-8. Grower Rations for 400 lb Calves

Ration 1

6 lb alfalfa-grass hay, free-choice (16–18% CP*)
4 lb grain mix (9.8% crude protein)
    1500 lb coarsely ground shelled corn
     455 lb rolled or ground oats
      20 lb trace mineral salt
      20 lb monosodium phosphate
       5 lb vitamin premix

Ration 2

5 lb alfalfa-grass hay, free-choice (12–16% CP*)
5 lb grain mix (12.8% crude protein)
     900 lb rolled barley
   1000 lb rolled oats
      55 lb dry molasses
      20 lb trace mineral salt
      20 lb dicalcium phosphate
       5 lb vitamin premix

Ration 3

5 lb grass hay, free-choice (10–14% CP*)
5 lb grain mix (10.9% crude protein)
   1800 lb corn and cob meal
    100 lb soybean meal
     55 lb dry molasses
     20 lb trace mineral salt
     20 lb dicalcium phosphate
      5 lb vitamin premix

Ration 4

6 lb corn silage (8–9% CP*)
3 lb grass hay (12–14% CP*)
4 lb grain mix (17% crude protein)
   1000 lb coarsely ground shelled corn
    655 lb rolled or ground oats
    300 lb soybean meal
     20 lb trace mineral salt
      5 lb limestone
     15 lb dicalcium phosphate
      5 lb vitamin premix

Source: University of Minnesota. *Feeding Dairy Cattle*, Bulletin No. 218.

*CP = crude protein.

Feeding Program for Heifers One to Two Years of Age (To One Month Before Calving)

Heifers should gain 1.5 to 1.8 lb per day. The rations in Table 10-9 indicate the amounts to feed when various forage and grain combinations are offered to 700 lb heifers. Trace mineral salt and a calcium-phosphorus supplement are advised on a free-choice basis.

Animal size is a more important factor than age in influencing development of the reproductive tract. Most Holstein heifers seldom show estrus (heat) before reaching 600 lb. Holstein heifers can be bred to freshen at 22

Table 10-9. Rations for 700 lb Heifers That are Gaining 1.5 lb per day

Ration 1	Ration 5
42 lb corn silage (33% DM)	7 lb alfalfa hay
1 lb grain mix	20 lb corn silage
	2 lb grain mix
160 lb corn and cob meal	1940 lb corn and cob
1705 lb 44% supplement	35 lb monosodium phosphate
98 lb dicalcium phosphate	20 lb trace mineral salt
12 lb limestone	5 lb vitamin premix
20 lb trace mineral salt	
5 lb vitamin premix	

Ration 2	Ration 6
50 lb sweet-corn cannery silage (20% DM)	7 lb grass hay
5 lb grain mix	20 lb corn silage
	3 lb grain mix
1274 lb corn	1314 lb shelled corn
425 lb oats	438 lb oats
247 lb 44% protein supplement	211 lb 44% supplement
10 lb dicalcium phosphate	8 lb dicalcium phosphate
19 lb limestone	4 lb limestone
20 lb trace mineral salt	20 lb trace mineral salt
5 lb vitamin premix	5 lb vitamin premix

Ration 3	Ration 7
28 lb oat silage	15 lb alfalfa hay
2 lb grain mix	3 lb grain mix[b]
1960 lb corn and cob	955 lb barley
5 lb limestone	1000 lb oats
10 lb dicalcium phosphate	20 lb trace mineral salt
20 lb trace mineral salt	20 lb monosodium phosphate
5 lb vitamin premix	5 lb vitamin premix

Ration 4	Ration 8
15 lb grass hay	20 lb corn stover (stalkage)
5 lb grain mix	3 lb grain mix
1975 lb corn and cob meal[a]	1100 lb corn and cob meal
20 lb trace mineral salt	865 lb 44% supplement
5 lb vitamin premix	20 lb trace mineral salt
	10 lb dicalcium phosphate
	5 lb vitamin premix

Source: University of Minnesota. *Feeding Dairy Cattle*, Bulletin No. 218.
[a]Could substitute barley-oats (50–50 mixture).
[b]Could substitute corn and cob meal.

months, and weigh 1100 lb if fed and managed properly. Overconditioning and late breeding should be avoided.

RATION FORMULATIONS

Because of the complexities involved with milk production and the changing stages of lactation, the science of ration balancing is extremely critical and should not be undertaken by the amateur. Although a generalized discussion of the basics of nutrition is given in Part 2 on beef cattle, it is recommended that the dairyman take a specialized course in dairy nutrition and work with an extension agent, and/or have his rations computerized.

The computerized dairy ration balancer program is available to dairymen, veterinarians, feed dealers, and agri-business firms in many parts of the United States. The computer quickly and accurately balances the dairy ration for energy, protein, calcium, and phosphorus. Forage testing results and customized feeding programs can be utilized through the use of forms usually obtainable from local extension directors. The forms are mailed in, and a feeding program and recommendations are received by return mail. This method is highly recommended as the computer is able to make thousands of decisions, many of which could save the cost of the service.

11

Reproduction in Dairy Cattle

The basics of reproductive physiology for all cattle have been discussed previously (see Chapter 7, Reproduction). Only specific reproductive peculiarities that apply to the dairy animal are covered in this chapter.

DETECTION OF HEAT

Detecting heat is the first step in getting cows to breed. Failure to detect estrus in cows soon after calving is very largely responsible for delayed first services, which of course leads to longer calving intervals and reduced income. Losses result from reduced milk production, fewer calves born, and increased feed needed for pregnant replacement cows.

Some goals that should be set in any herd are a 90% detection of all heat periods, a $12\frac{1}{2}$ month calving interval, $1\frac{1}{2}$ services per conception, and 70% of the cows settled on the first service.

The common signs of estrus (heat) are:

1. Cows that stand when mounted by other cows provide the most reliable sign of heat.

2. Occasionally a cow that is doing the mounting is the one that is in heat, but that is rare. Checking records will help to determine if she is in heat.

3. Many cows in heat will have a clear mucous discharge on the tail or pinbones, or on the vulva hair. The vulva may be slightly swollen. Blood on the tail may also be seen, which indicates that the cow was probably in heat 48 hours previously and should be checked again in about 18 days.

4. Hair knocked off of the top of the rump and over the pinbones is another sign of heat. This is due to the cow's being mounted by other cows; because of the weight of the other cow, the area over the tailhead and pinbones is scraped. The breeding record is all-important here, checking when

the cow was last in heat, when she last had a calf, etc. to give you an idea of her true reproductive cycle.

5. Other signs include bawling, restlessness, excessive walking, off-feed, and in general a cow that seems to be irritated and not her normal self. These signs are usually seen in a very early stage of heat. The other cows sense the excitement and many sniff at the cow exhibiting estrus. Almost 90% of the cattle in heat can be detected by close visual observation.

When do cows return to heat after calving? Most cows' ovaries start to cycle again shortly after calving, with the first ovulation in normal cows occurring after about 17 days. However, approximately 75% of these cows will not show any outward signs of heat during this first ovulation. It is usually another 18 to 20 days to the first observed heat, which occurs 34 to 35 days after calving. Most cows should have come into heat within 45 days after calving. If this is not the case, an examination by a veterinarian should be performed. The key to detection of heat is observation. It takes a trained eye and frequent observation of the cattle. This observation should be done when nothing else is going on. Animals that show only slight signs of heat are not going to be detected if the only time they're checked is when they're being fed or when they're being driven up to the holding area for milking. They need to be observed when they are peaceful and quiet. Usually, it's a good idea to have one person responsible for checking heat. The best times are thought to be early in the morning, at noon, and in the quiet of evening after milking.

Heat periods vary in length, from 12 to 18 hours on the average. There are several types of heat. They are usually classified in four categories: (1) strong signs of heat for a long period of time; (2) strong signs of heat for a short period of time; (3) weak signs of heat for a long period of time; and (4) weak signs of heat for a short period of time. It's very easy to miss those animals that are showing very weak signs of heat for only a short period of time if they're not observed at least three times a day.

The exact time to breed cows is another important consideration, especially with the practice of artificial insemination and a small amount of semen. Usually, if the reproductive tract is in good shape (normal delivery with no complications), a cow can be bred within 50 days or so after calving with little reduction in fertility. However, if there are any signs of infection, these should be cleared up before she is bred. Since dairy cows are usually in heat for 12 to 18 hours and ovulate 10 to 14 hours after the end of heat, accurate heat detection is valuable in determining the best time to breed. The life of the egg following ovulation is approximately 6 to 10 hours. Sperm can live in the reproductive tract for approximately 24 hours, although it takes 4 to 6 hours after deposition of the sperm before it can fertilize the egg. The sperm needs to be present when ovulation occurs for the best conception rate. Therefore, we want to breed these cows some 8 to 10 hours after they are first observed with signs of heat. This would be near the end of the standard heat period. According to the rule of thumb, cows observed in standing heat during the morning should be bred late the same day, and cows observed in standing heat in the afternoon should be bred the following morning.

Figure 11-1 shows the best breeding period in relation to the beginning of standing heat. Note that breeding should take place a few hours before ovulation occurs. Since the time of egg release cannot be predicted exactly, timing of breeding should be based on the time when standing heat began. However, some cows complicate the picture by having longer or shorter heat periods. The average duration of a heat period is 18 hours, but it can range from 3 to 28 hours. For good results, cows that do not fit the normal pattern may need to be bred a few hours earlier or later than usual.

Records are indispensable in a good breeding program. Records should include all heats, even those as early as 2 weeks after calving. This will assist your veterinarian in evaluating reproductive problems if he is called upon for consultation. Many record forms are available. One type is illustrated in Figure 11-2. This includes everything from calving records to mastitis, a complete production and health record in one source, usually a loose-leaf type of folder with a page for each cow. Entries should include heat dates, breeding dates, calving dates, bull bred to, and pregnancy exams, as well as any treatment the cow has received. Perhaps the biggest help from records is in improving your ability to anticipate heat periods. Close observation when the cow is due to be in heat will increase the chance of detection. Also, records reduce the chance of the cow not being bred because someone thought she hadn't been fresh long enough. Records also help detect failure to cycle or erratic cycles sooner, so that treatment can begin quickly. Check your records every morning.

There are several aids for detecting heat. One of them, of course, is a spotter, "Gomer," or teaser bull. This is a bull that has been surgically rendered incapable of settling a cow but still has all the natural native instincts and will follow and point out the cows that are in heat. There are also some mechanical devices. One is a chinball marker, which uses a device that resembles a big ball-point pen. It straps under the chin of steers or teaser bulls. Mounted cows are marked with the dye. Another device used is a dye indicator that is cemented to the rump of the cow. When the other cows ride her, the pressure releases a red dye, which marks her tailhead.

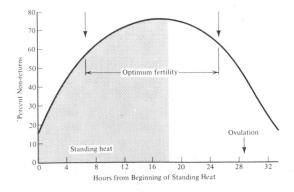

Figure 11-1. Optimum time to breed during standing heat.

DHIA-205 LIFETIME HISTORY OF INDIVIDUAL COW

12-72   Start this record on the heifer calf at birth and maintain for the lifetime of the animal.

Index No.		
Barn Name		

Identification Numbers

Cow Name		Reg. No.		Tattoo No.	
		Ear-tag		Birth date	
Sire				Breed	
Dam				Dam's Index	

←—— Place printed identification label here ——→

IOWA STATE UNIV., STATE AGRICULTURAL EXTENSION SERVICES AND UNITED STATES DEPT. OF AGRICULTURE COOPERATING

Sketch markings or attach picture.

Heifer Record

(List all treatments and conditions prior to first freshening of this heifer.)

Date	Condition	Remarks	Date	Condition	Remarks
	Calfhood vaccination				

Type and Management Traits

(Complete this section after heifer has freshened and information is available.)

Milking Speed	Fast	Average	Slow
Disposition	Quiet	Nervous	Ornery
Ketosis, Milk Fever	None	Light	Severe
Mastitis	None	Some	Chronic
Udder Edema	Light	Moderate	Severe

Outstanding qualities:

Main faults:

Classification	Date	FS		DC	B	M	St	Hd	FE	Bk	Rp	HL	Ft	FU	RU	US	Qy	Tt	Mc

Purchased from _____ Date _____ Price _____

Date left herd _____ Reason _____

Sold to _____ Price _____

Figure 11-2. A DHIA form for recording a complete lifetime history of a cow. These records may also involve a system of color-coded signal tabs for quick observation of herd reproductive status. Black tabs denote month of calving; blue tabs, month of first breeding after calving; green tabs, month to be turned dry; red tabs, any abnormal reproductive occurrence.

Jan.	Feb.	Mar.	Apr.	May	June	July	Aug.	Sept.	Oct.	Nov.	Dec.	Index	
												Name	

Breeding and Calving Record

Date Calved	Heat Dates	1st Service	2nd Service	3rd Service	4th Service	Sire used	Confirmed Pregnant	Date Calved	Sex of Calf	Eartag No or Disposal
(heifer)										

Reproductive Problems

Date	Condition	Treatment

Mastitis and Other Problems

Date	Condition	Treatment

249

ROUTINE VETERINARY EXAMINATIONS

After heat detection and complete recordkeeping, the next most important thing in a breeding program is routine veterinary examinations of the reproductive tract of all nonpregnant cows. You should establish an examination schedule in advance, so that it's set up on a routine, preferably monthly basis, where the veterinarian and the dairyman know exactly when the visits are scheduled. In very large herds, examinations may need to be done more than once a month, whereas in smaller herds of less than 40 cows, examinations every 6 weeks may be sufficient. Cows that have to be examined should be corralled prior to the veterinarian's visit. Also, the animal's reproductive life record and monthly heat periods, etc. should be available so that the veterinarian can better determine individual peculiarities. It's important to identify animals to be examined. Be alert for the special attentive needs of the individual.

As discussed in Chapter 7, any cow that has had a retained placenta for more than 3 or 4 days should have special attention by the veterinarian. It is important that you do not attempt to remove the retained placenta because cotyledons may be torn and bleeding can occur.

Cows that are fresh from 25 to 40 days should be examined prior to breeding to make sure the reproductive tract is free of gross infection and is undergoing involution at a normal rate. This also gives you a chance to pick up problems like cystic ovaries.

Cows with an abnormal or cloudy discharge generally should be examined to determine the source of infection. Any discharge that contains pus is abnormal. Usually there is a strong odor along with it. Cows that have had some type of abnormal reproductive event (difficult births, aborted or mummified fetuses, etc.) should be examined.

Cows with abnormal heat or heat cycles should be examined. The normal estrous cycle is usually 18 to 23 days. Individuals that vary from this (frequent cycles or prolonged intervals) are production problems. Cows not showing heat 45 to 60 days after calving should also be examined for cystic ovaries, infected uteruses, etc. Early discovery leaves time for correction of the problem without getting behind in production.

Cows bred 35 to 60 days that have not returned to heat should be examined for pregnancy, and cows that were palpated prior to 60 days should be checked a second time at 60 to 90 days to be sure they have not aborted without detection.

Normal examination by a veterinarian would include examination of the vulva with a speculum light. Swollen lips may indicate vaginitis. Slight pimples or pustules inside the vulva indicate granular vaginitis. The condition of the vagina and the vaginal walls should be checked for possible infections or adhesions from previous calvings or injuries at breeding time. Also, the cervix should be examined for infections of the outer opening, double cervix, adhesions, tears, and patency.

The uterus should be examined, first, for possible pregnancy, then for tone, size, abnormal masses (which may indicate tumors or mummified fetuses), and pus in the uterus.

The Fallopian tubes and oviducts are checked for size and viability. Occasionally, adhesions can be detected, due to long-standing pyometras or endometritis (uterine infections). The ovaries should be checked for normal size and consistency to detect follicles, cysts, or pathological conditions (indicated by enlargements).

INFERTILITY AND CAUSES OF INFERTILITY

Metritis or Endometritis

Metritis is an inflammation of the lining of the uterus. It may be due to a retained placenta, but it can occur for other reasons. Usually it shows up 1 to 10 days following calving. The cause is frequently uterine inertia or a flaccid uterus, followed by infection with bacteria.

Clinical signs are loss of appetite, fever of 103° to 105°, decreased milk production, and a thick, cloudy vaginal discharge (often with pus). Severely affected animals may go down and die.

Localized treatment of the uterus with systemic broad-spectrum antibiotics and intravenous electrolytes is recommended. Dextrose (if the condition has deteriorated) and estrogens may be advised by the veterinarian.

An endometritis (inflammation of the very thin endometrial lining of the uterus) often follows a metritis or retained placenta. This is frequently the result of physical damage from calving difficulties, such as twin births, premature births, abortions, or very difficult births. It is very difficult to diagnose even by rectal palpation. Often there is not even an abnormal vaginal discharge. Cattle usually cycle normally but don't conceive.

Treatment consists of localized uterine antibiotics, or stimulants like weak solutions of tamed iodine. Estrogens in the uterus, or intramuscularly, are recommended along with the antibiotics.

Delayed Uterine Involution

A delayed uterine involution is commonly seen in older high-producing dairy cows. It is often associated with difficult births, twins, abortions, etc. It may occur following metritis or genital tract infection. The clinical signs are lack of estrus or repeat breeding. Treatment is the same as for endometritis.

Pneumovagina or Air in the Vagina (Wind-Suckers)

Pneumovagina is found in older cows when the cervix and the uterus extend forward over the brink of the pelvis. The vulva is then pulled forward into the pelvis. This condition results from tears or lacerations of the vagina caused during calving. Clinical signs are air-sucking of the vagina after urination, defecation, or getting up; a reddened, sometimes ulcerated vaginal wall; usually vaginal discharges; and urine retained in the vagina along with fecal material and other contaminants, which adds to the problem. This results in poor conception rates. Treatment is directed towards correcting tears and lacerations by surgery, use of antibiotics, and rebreeding after approximately two heat periods.

Pyometra (Pus in the Uterus)

Pyometra is associated with retained corpus luteum (see Chapter 7 on beef cattle reproduction). Causes are abnormal calving, uterine infections, retained placentas, and incomplete uterine involution. Occasionally pyometra will follow conception and a mummification of the fetus. Insertion of the breeding pipette into a pregnant uterus can also trigger pyometra.

Clinical signs are a failure to exhibit heat and large amounts of pus in the uterus (usually 45 to 90 days after calving). This material can be detected by rectal palpation. Occasionally you will notice pus escaping through the cervix and to the tail and around the vulva.

Treatment includes ridding the cow of the corpus luteum by manual removal or with the use of drugs. Treatment should be done by a veterinarian, someone who knows what he is doing because of the danger to the cow. The uterus is flushed, along with manual massage, to push out as much of the infection as possible.

The animal's breeding life may be ended if diagnosis and treatment are not prompt. Pyometra can lead to permanent infertility, caused by hormonal disturbances, such as cystic ovaries. The condition may also cause early embryonic death, uterine infection, and weak or silent heat periods.

Palpation and ovary checkups may allow the veterinarian to determine when a follicle is ready, and the cow can be bred by manual manipulation.

ARTIFICIAL INSEMINATION (AI)

The subject of artificial insemination from the female side was covered in Chapter 7. Now it is necessary to discuss the male side of artificial insemination, as it is extremely important in dairy operations. The bull has a tremendous impact on production progress in the dairy herd. Since 70 to 100% of all heifers born must be saved for replacements in the breeding herd, the bull may contribute 90% or more of the genetic makeup of your herd in four generations.

The overwhelming importance of milk and butterfat production per animal in dairy herd profit demands that these two traits receive top priority in any breeding and sire selection program.

There are other factors of economic importance to consider. Studies show that cows with high first-lactation production typically stay in the herd longer, and low production is responsible for 40% of the cows culled annually.

The cow's feet and legs, pelvic region, dairy character, and mastitis
resistance are all important to a long, productive, and profitable life. When selecting semen it is wise to consider traits of the bull and his daughters or other close relatives in his pedigree. Look for high production first and then the body and mammary system traits that allow a longer life.

The primary limitation is that the more traits on which you base selection, the slower the progress for any one given trait. For instance, if you are selecting for milk production but decide to add equal selection for one other trait, you slow progress in improving the first trait (milk production) to about 70% of what is possible. If you select for three or four traits, the progress slows down correspondingly. You should select highly heritable traits that will give you the best return on each dollar invested. Those traits for which you might expect significant improvement have high heritability values. Table 11-1 gives heritability estimates for the different traits of economic importance in dairy breeding and production.

Artificial insemination offers the greatest possible improvement for individual cows. Therefore, the old method of keeping a bull on the farm is to be discouraged. The tool that has really made the big difference between the economics of natural versus AI service is the dairy herd sire summary now available for most AI bulls. This summary gives you the true genetic value of each bull and the amount of improvement you can expect.

The *predicted difference* (PD) of a sire is a measure of his transmitting ability to his daughters. The value given is the expected production difference between his daughters and their herdmates in herds with average production for the breed. This difference is obtained by comparing the sire's daughters with other animals that freshened during the same period of the year, with the production figures adjusted for age and geographic region of the country.

Table 11-1. Heritability of Dairy Cow Traits

Trait	Heritability value (%)
Length of teats	75
Percent butterfat content	55
Disposition (temperament)	40
Diameter of teats	35
Udder attachments	
Fore udder	30
Rear udder	16
Milk production	25
Butterfat production	25
Dairy character score	25
Final type score	25
Mastitis resistance	25
Speed and ease of milking	24
Mammary system score	20
Size and shape of udder	14
Feet and legs	12

The figure itself is based on the breed average production; so if your herd is above or below the breed average, your actual predicted difference would vary. A rule of thumb is for every 1000 lb of milk your herd differs from the breed average, you should change the predicted difference figure given by 100 lb. If you are above the breed average, you would subtract 100 lb from the predicted difference given; but if below, you would add 100 lb.

Applying this rule of thumb, you can see that more rapid progress can be made with high PD bulls in herds that are below the average production for the breed than for those that are above the average production. For example, a herd that is producing 2000 lb higher than the average would need a bull with a PD of plus 200 lb of milk just to stay even. The same bull used in a herd 2000 lb below the average would be expected to improve production by approximately 400 lb per annual lactation period in his daughters.

The repeatability figure for a sire is a statistical measure and tells you approximately how much you can depend on the particular bull to transmit the given amount of production improvement shown. It is based on the number of daughters on which records have been kept, the number of herds they were in, and the number of records kept per daughter being used in this daughter–herdmate comparison. The greater the number in each of these categories, the more reliable the predicted difference of the bull will be. A repeatability of 70% or greater is considered high, although some popular, well-proven bulls can reach 99%. A repeatability of 30% or less is considered low.

When using the predicted difference and repeatability figures, you should balance them out in your herd breeding program. Select bulls with high predicted differences—certainly not bulls with low negative predicted differences. Depend on bulls with high repeatability. At least 70% of your herd should be bred to bulls with 70% or higher repeatability.

You can use bulls with less than 30% repeatability for up to 10% of your herd, but use several bulls rather than just one. This improves your chance of getting high-quality offspring, while giving young bulls a chance to prove themselves. The other 20% of your herd can be bred to bulls with between 30% and 70% repeatability figures.

Your bull selection program may vary somewhat according to the specific needs of your herd and other management factors. However, these general guidelines should be followed in most herds:

1. Breed 70% to 80% of your herd including heifers to proven bulls shown to be reliable in increasing production. Use bulls with at least a 500 lb improvement for milk production, and a repeatability of at least 70% for Holsteins—60% for other breeds.

2. Pick a few sires with the highest PD and select from among them the bulls that can improve one or two traits that are most in need of improvement in your herd.

3. Breed at least 20% of your herd to carefully selected young sires that are in the process of being proven.

OPTIMUM REPRODUCTIVE MANAGEMENT

255
OPTIMUM
REPRO-
DUCTIVE
MANAGE-
MENT

The optimum calving interval is $12\frac{1}{2}$ to 13 months. Recommendations on achieving this goal have already been discussed from a reproductive standpoint. However, management of the cow near the end of lactation has an equally important function in her health, well-being, and future production.

A dairy cow needs a rest from lactation to rejuvenate milk-producing cells in her udder. Milk production with no dry period has been shown to drop to 75% of normal. During the third lactation, research has indicated production drops still further to about 62% of normal.

The length of the dry period should be neither too long nor too short. Short dry periods will not optimize production in the following lactation, while long periods are needless and reduce total production.

Most cows should be dry for a period of 6 to 8 weeks. Many dairymen shoot for an 8-week period and average about 7 weeks. Without good records, it's easy to misjudge when a cow should be turned dry; so consult your books.

Drying up can be done in several ways. Your goal should always be to dry up as rapidly as possible without causing injury to the udder. When milking ceases, pressure in the cow's udder stops milk secretion, and the remaining milk is eventually absorbed. The faster the transition, the better for the cow.

For most cows, the best drying up method is to remove the cow from the milking herd, eliminate grain feeding, and feed limited forage and water for 2 or 3 days. Then stop milking abruptly. Her udder should be watched closely for 2 to 3 weeks. High producers may require several milkings to relieve udder pressure before they completely dry up without attention.

Udder infusion of all cows at the last milking with an approved dry cow-mastitis treatment is recommended by most researchers. Treating only selected cows is not advisable unless a herd maintains a low cell count. One study showed that half of all cows have some infection at drying up, and if left untreated, the level of infection increased to 60% during the dry period. Most new mastitis infections occur during the first 2 weeks of the dry period.

Always practice extreme sanitation after treating dry cows. Dip the teat after each treatment. Check udders daily, especially during the first few weeks after drying up. Monitor health and body conditioning and watch cows that are close to calving.

Facilities for dry cows make managing easier. Moving cows out of the milking herd aids in drying up and also reduces milking time since dry cows don't enter the milking barn. Separate facilities also permit you to feed a controlled ration. Exercise during the dry period is important. Free access to pastures and lots helps maintain good muscle tone and adequate blood

Table 11-2. Dairy Cow Disease Control

Disease/Causes	Signs	Prevention	Treatment	Withholding Period
Mastitis: *Streptococci ssp.* *Staphylococci ssp.* *E. coli* *Others*	Increase in somatic cell count. Abnormal milk. Swelling—fever in mammary glands of toxic animals.	A complete program. Use Somato-Staph for prevention of staph ssp. infections. Use teat dipping after milking and dry cow treatment.	Depends on type of organism involved and sensitivity testing. Intramammary or intravenous routes give best results. Oral feeding of drugs not recommended.	Withhold milk from market for 96 hours after treatment. Withhold treated cow from slaughter for 30 days.
Cowpox: *Virus*	Sensitive teats and udder. Lesions start out as a papule, then to a vesicle, followed by a pustule and scab.	No treatment to destroy virus. Avoid bringing the virus in with herd replacements. Do not use sponge to wash udder; use recommended teat dip after milking.	Antibiotic ointments after milking to keep down secondary infections.	None
Winter Dysentery: *Virus?* *Never isolated.*	Diarrhea lasting for 3–6 days, usually in stabled herds.	Must be differentiated from virus diarrhea, coccidiosis, and salmonellosis.	Sulfonamides.[a] Antibiotics.[a]	
Ketosis: *Metabolic*	Off feed, milk production down.	Propylene glycol 0.25–0.50 lb/head/day beginning 2 weeks after freshening. Continue for 6 weeks.[c] Sodium propionate twice daily continuously for 6 weeks after calving.	Propylene glycol 0.25–1 lb/4–16 fl. oz/head/day for 10 days.[b] Sodium Propionate 0.5 lb twice daily for 10 days.	None
Milk Fever: *Metabolic*	Uncoordination. Animal down before or after freshening.	20 million units of D2 daily in two equal feedings for 5–7 days before calving.	Calcium products.[a] IV.	None

Disease: Cause	Symptoms	Prevention	Treatment[a]	Treatment[b]
Grass Tetany: *Hypomagnesemia*	Nervousness, staggering, convulsions, and death.	Usually occurs on fresh, succulent, well fertilized forage. Magnesium oxide 0.5–1 oz/head/day.	Magnesium sulfate, IV. 200 ml of 25% solution.	None
Johne's Disease Paratuberculosis: *Mycobacterium, paratuberculosis. Laboratory confirmation necessary.*	Chronic diarrhea.	No vaccine available. Test: remove reactors. Hygenic program for calf raising, separate from adult herd.	Temporary treatment from symptomatic treatment but no complete cure.	None
Vibriosis: *Vibrio fetus*	Repeat services.	Vaccination of females and bulls prior to breeding. Use of artificial insemination. Untried bulls on virgin heifers.	None	None
Leukosis: *Not known, virus suspected. Laboratory diagnosis necessary.*	Enlarged lymph nodes.	Prohibiting sale of animals for breeding purposes. Prevention of infected animals going into noninfected herds.	None	None
Displaced Abomasum: *Suspect calcium imbalance; high concentrate rations.*	Fetid diarrhea, off-milk production.	High roughage diet.	Replacement by surgery or manipulation.	None

Source: John B Herrick, *Feedstuffs.* (Minneapolis, Minn.: Miller Publishing Company, Ref. Issue, Vol. 49, No. 30, 1977), p. 85. Reprinted by permission.
[a]As prescribed by a veterinarian.
[b]Follow manufacturer's recommendations.

circulation. If cows are kept in stanchions, turn them out for a few hours each day.

CALVING .

Difficulties at birth and recommended procedures have been previously discussed in the beef cattle section (Chapter 7). These same precautions and procedures apply to dairy cattle as well.

SPOTTING PROBLEMS

A few simple observations made daily will enable you to spot reproductive problems or indications that an abnormal condition is developing. You should be on the lookout for the following abnormalities. Think of this as a checklist to monitor each cow daily for a few simple telltale signs of impending disaster. Although your checklist may be expanded, the following observations can be a good start:

1. Any type of discharge from the vulva.

2. High tailheads. This may indicate cystic ovaries or nymphomania.

3. Changes in attitude or temperament of individual cows. Bellowing or pawing the ground, if not a common characteristic of the individual, should be regarded as a sign of hormonal imbalance or some type of pain.

4. Any downward breaking of the udder, which indicates hormonal problems or injury.

5. Repeat breedings, assisted by records, can indicate reproductive problems.

DISEASES

Although diseases have been discussed in detail previously (Chapter 6), the following information (Table 11-2) gives a brief description, plus signs, preventive methods, and treatment for the specific diseases of dairy cattle. Withholding periods are also noted to give added emphasis to the dairyman's problems of complying with government controls. Although of a general nature, the information is considered to be an excellent guide to detection and, in some cases, to correction. As always, if a problem exists that is beyond your capabilities, do not hesitate in calling for assistance. Speed is especially essential in treating disorders of dairy cattle if you are to maintain the high health and production required of an economically sound dairy production system.

12

Mastitis Control

Mastitis is an inflammation of the udder. Estimates of the average annual economic loss from mastitis in dairy herds in the United States are as high as $133 per head ($1.3 billion nationally). These losses are due to decreased milk production, cost of medical treatment, lower sales due to milk withheld from treated cows, and replacement costs for animals culled from the herd because of mastitis and low production.

A mastitis problem herd may be defined as:

1. Being in danger of being downgraded because of high somatic cell counts exceeding 1.5 million/ml (1–1.5 million is approaching unacceptable standards).

2. Having a high rate of clinical mastitis.

3. Having a high rate in the California mastitis test (CMT) in the 2 and 3 range. Over 30% reaction on tests on individual quarters of the udder is very high; 21 to 30% reaction also indicates an above-average problem.

4. Having a poor production rate and a high culling and replacement rate due to mastitis.

TYPES OF MASTITIS

Mastitis disease may be classified according to clinical signs into three groups: (1) acute clinical, (2) clinical, and (3) subclinical.

Acute Mastitis

The acute clinical animals represent about 1% of all the cases and are characterized by systemic signs such as fever, depression, weakness, loss of appetite, reduced milk production, abnormal milk, and possibly one or more swollen quarters.

Clinical Mastitis

Clinical cases usually indicate some form of abnormal milk such as clouding, flakes, blood, or other visible abnormalities. Systemic signs are usually absent, but the udder may be swollen, hardened, or sensitive. Clinical cases make up about 24% of all mastitis infections.

Subclinical Mastitis

Subclinical mastitis represents approximately 75% of all the cases. These are not apparent to dairymen unless special tests are used for detection. However, there is a significant decrease in milk production and an increase in somatic cell counts from these infections.

ORGANISMS CAUSING MASTITIS

Infectious bacteria and other microorganisms are usually involved, including streptococci, staphylococci, coliforms, pseudomonas, bacilli, yeasts, and mycoplasma. It is estimated that over 95% of all the mastitis cases are caused by either strep or staph organisms. Approximately 50% of all cows have mastitis organisms present in one or more quarters.

Streptococcus organisms that could cause mastitis generally depend on direct or indirect transmission from cow to cow. The strep organism is found in the udder of a cow, where it lives in the milk. It does not invade milk-secreting tissue. Although it may cause clinical mastitis, it usually does not develop resistance to antibiotics and, therefore, can be eliminated from a dairy herd by antibiotic treatment. However, unless management practices are followed to prevent the spread of new infection, little or no improvement in the overall mastitis situation will result.

Staphylococci are readily available in the environment and can be easily transmitted to the udder. These organisms usually enter the mammary gland through the teat canal. An entry is aided by injury or other factors affecting the teat. Staph organisms can be found practically everywhere: on the skin, in the nose and throat of humans and animals, on the floors and bedding, and on milking equipment. Even without the aid of an injury or lowered resistance, staph organisms can invade healthy secreting tissues. They are frequently resistant to antibiotics and other drugs. There are less of the highly inflamed or acute clinical cases with staph than with strep. Therefore, staph organisms are a major cause of chronic mastitis or subclinical mastitis, which results in a slow but permanent wasting away of milk-producing udder tissue. Staph infections are rarely satisfactorily eradicated by treatment during lactation. However, after milking, teat disinfection will reduce the rate of cross-infection from one cow to another. Good management with treatment at the last milking prior to drying up will also minimize the severity of infection. Milking techniques and sanitation will strongly influence the teat canal and its ability to act as a barrier against the mastitis-producing organisms.

A relatively new form of mastitis is coming from dairy herds that are bedded in sawdust and is a result of infection by klebsiella organisms. If this becomes a problem, dairymen should switch to another type of bedding or disinfect or sterilize sawdust. Some researchers have controlled klebsiella mastitis by dumping a shovel full of lime on top of the sawdust in the back of each stall once a week. In other herds where this has been done, it was not satisfactory; so paraformaldehyde pellets were tried and were reported to be helpful.

Also, a new vaccine developed by Michigan State University has been clinically impressive. Vaccination needs to be repeated at 6-month intervals.

MASTITIS PREVENTION AND CONTROL

In order to control any mastitis problem, the problem must first be defined. One of the best methods at this time is the CMT (California mastitis test). The monthly use of a "cowside" test, such as the CMT, is an excellent tool to indicate the quality of milking that is being done. A dairyman can usually catch an upward trend of somatic cells before the situation gets out of hand. Done routinely and over a period of years, the CMT results tell a dairyman where he has been, where he is now, and in what direction the mastitis situation of his herd is heading.

The test is simple and economical (about 1¢ per test), and it detects the mastitis while it is still in the subclinical stage, not visible to the naked eye. The test is based on the degree of reaction between the test reagent and a component of the white blood cells in the milk (white blood cells are produced by the body as a result of the infection). The greater the mastitis infection, the more white cells present, and the more of this reactive substance there will be to react with the CMT agent. A jell-like substance is formed as a result of the reaction. The amount and consistency of this substance are in direct proportion to the number of white cells in the milk. The reaction is scored as either "negative," "trace," or "one," "two," or "three." "Three" represents a strong jell formation, one that tends to adhere to the paddle.

Foremilk is first drawn from each quarter into the separate cups of a four-cup plastic paddle. The paddle is then tilted so that only $\frac{1}{2}$ teaspoon of milk is left in each of the cups. An equal amount of test reagent is added to each cup; the paddle is then rotated to mix the reagent; and the milk and color changes as well as jell formation are observed within 10 to 15 seconds after mixing. Milk from a normal quarter remains liquid and flows freely. A moderate reaction is shown by the formation of a jell that is fragile and breaks into small masses or clumps. Milk samples that form a jellylike mass that actually clings together and is not broken up as the paddle is rotated indicate severe infection. Milk from badly infected quarters also shows a deepening of the purple color of the milk reagent mixture. Interpretation is a little more difficult than running the test; it takes a little time and effort to learn to interpret this test properly, but once accustomed to procedures, it goes very rapidly and is very accurate. When all lactating animals are tested and records are kept for each monthly test, you can expect to receive the following benefits:

1. Early detection of inflammation, so that more expensive laboratory testing for cultures to detect specific organisms involved is needed only on inflamed quarters; treatment can be made promptly and effectively; udder damage is minimized; and milk losses are reduced.

2. Milking order can be based on test results. This is a very important practice in preventing the spread of the infection.

3. Indication of when treatment may be needed, and whether treatment has been effective.

4. Indication of when to dispose of an animal.

5. Better service from a veterinarian because he knows the history of the udder health.

There are some factors that can confuse the results and can cause inaccurate CMT test results. These include:

1. Rapid changes in feeding program, especially from roughage to pasture.

2. Very early colostrum and late lactation.

3. Leaving the milker on too long.

4. Excessive or fluctuating vacuum on milking machines.

5. Injury to the udder.

6. Periods of estrus.

Selection is an important part of mastitis prevention. Cows with a very pendulous, very large udder tend to be much more susceptible to mastitis than cows with smaller, more compact, well-hung, or well-supported udders. There will be more chance of damage from cuts, stepping on the teats, bruising, chapping, dragging in the mud, and organism entry through the teat canal. Also, these types of udders tend to break down, the milking machines don't fit as well, the cows are very often "hard milkers," and often they don't let down their milk as easily as other cows. All of these factors contribute to causing mastitis. You can eliminate a lot of these problems by careful selection of replacement heifers and by culling of problem cows.

Another area of control is the milking techniques. Proper stimulation of the milk letdown can result in a dramatic increase in milk production each year. Preferably, the udder should be washed by using a warm-water spray and gently rubbing with your hand. A device for metering sanitizing solution into the water as it is sprayed is ideal. Following this washing, the udder should be dried with a single-service paper towel. If a spray is not available, it may be necessary to use two buckets, one with the washing solution and the other with a sanitizing solution. After washing, a single-service paper towel should be used to apply the sanitizing solution. Dry the udder with paper towels. The sanitizing solution should contain approximately 200 ppm chlorine or 25 ppm iodofor.

Milk two or more streams from each teat into a strip cup before attaching the milker. This is important in removing bacteria from the teat canal. Also, it provides the last opportunity for inspection of the milk quality before applying the milker.

If the cow has been properly stimulated, a heavy flow of milk should begin as soon as the milking machine is applied. Milk quickly and thoroughly and then remove the unit. When milk flow ceases, hold down on the milker unit momentarily to remove any milk still in the gland cistern. It is impossible to remove all of the milk in the udder. Shut off or break the vacuum before gently removing teat cups.

After each cow is milked, the teats should be dipped in a disinfectant solution of either chlorine, iodine, or chlorhexadene. In very cold weather, the teats should be dried with a paper towel to remove any excess solution before letting the cows outdoors. It's also a good practice to avoid hand stripping if possible and to wash and disinfect your hands after handling an infected cow. Good milking techniques require close attention. Don't attempt to do other chores while milking.

The milking machine itself is also very important in mastitis control. A poorly maintained milking machine or an improperly used machine is a major cause of udder irritation and will lead to infection. Low vacuum, fluctuating vacuum, overmilking, and a failure to stimulate milk letdown before applying the milker are all likely to contribute to mastitis infection. Correct operation of the milking machine is prescribed in the milking machine owner's manual. The machine should be routinely serviced twice a year. However, the owner's manual also advises you to check certain components daily and weekly.

Medium to narrow bore inflations that do not crawl as the udder is milked have resulted in less mastitis. Inflations must be in good repair, and should be clean and highly elastic to provide adequate massage and to reduce spread of infection. Alternating sets of inflations weekly with one week of use, a special cleaning, and then a week of rest is recommended. Upon removing a set of inflations for the milking units, fat droplets can be removed by boiling in a 5% lye solution (one 13 oz can of lye to 2 gallons of water for 30 minutes). Upon removal from the lye solution, rinse, and then scrub the inflations in a hot solution containing milkstone remover. The inflations should then be rinsed again and should be stored dry until exchange with the set of inflations in use. The service life of an inflation is 1200 to 1500 cow milkings, after which all inflations should be replaced.

One practice that can really help eliminate mastitis problems is close observation and treatment of dry cows. Cows should be observed regularly for mastitis during the dry period. If one or more quarters appear abnormal, the cow should be milked out, and all quarters should be treated with an antibiotic in a long-lasting base. A teat dip should always be used after each milking and after each intramammary infusion. Current research recommends treatment of all cows at the time of drying up. Infusion of an antibiotic of high potency and a long-lasting base into all quarters at the last milking prior to drying up is indicated. This recommendation is justified because old infections are more easily and effectively attacked at this time, at a minimum cost; and most of the infection occurs in the first 2 days to 2 weeks after the drying up period. If the herd has a low somatic cell count, treatment may be limited to those cows with a history of mastitis. Dry cow treatment in the herd should be followed until the cell count and the bulk milk drop below 600,000 for at least 3 months. After that level has been maintained for 3 months, treat only those quarters showing a CMT 2 or 3 score during the last month of lactation and only those cows having a history of mastitis. Culture tests may be used to select quarters for treatment. Treatment of selected dry cows will not protect untreated cows against new infections that occurred in the early days of the dry period. Remember when treating dry cows that poorly administered treatments under unsanitary conditions can do more harm than good; so always use complete sanitary procedures.

Feeding is also important in mastitis control. No particular feed or ration will cause mastitis, but feed may have an indirect effect. Bacteria are present in the udder, and a sudden change in ration may indirectly contribute to mastitis by upsetting the cow's general condition. More cases of mastitis are noted when cows go to pasture in the spring or when certain silages or green forages are fed. It is very important that a definite milking order and a definite milking time be established. In the milking order, heifers should be first, clean cows second, cows with suspected udder inflammation next, and infected cows last. This may be difficult to do in modern milking parlors, but it is one of the most effective means of preventing the spread of mastitis through the herd. The CMT can help in establishing the milking order. In large herds, it may be possible to group cows according to the status of infection.

Mastitis may be lowered as much as 50% when raising replacement heifers as compared with purchasing the replacements. Raise calves in individual pens or stalls until they are old enough to be weaned from milk or milk replacers and are no longer likely to suck one another. If you must purchase replacements, give purchase preference in the following order: open heifers, bred heifers, young heifers, and older cows. If you purchase a mature cow, your chance of buying an infected cow is better than 50–50.

Also, it is important to provide good safe housing. Good ventilation without draft assures a dry, more sanitary environment, and prevents chilling of the udder. Free stalls provide comfort and protection. Stalls should be well-maintained, and sharp curves at the rear of stalls should be avoided.

TREATMENT OF MASTITIS

Treatment depends on the type of organism(s) involved. Sensitivity testing of the samples determines the organism or organisms that are causing the problem and allows selection of the most effective antibiotic against the organism(s). In collecting samples, the dairyman must remember that all surfaces outside the cow contain large numbers of microorganisms. Neither the milk nor the sample container should touch any of these surfaces. Clean, disinfect, and dry the cow thoroughly before collecting the sample. The teats should be disinfected with alcohol solution, cleaning the far teats first and then the near teats. Samples should be taken in sterile plastic bags or tubes. Remove the first two streams of milk before taking samples. Ice them immediately and transport them to the laboratory within 24 hours. If samples must be held over 2 days or more, freeze them and keep them frozen until delivery to the lab.

A list of the various organisms causing mastitis and the anitbiotics that have been found most often to be effective against them is given below.

1. *Streptococcus agalactia*—cloxacillin and penicillin.

2. Other strep organisms—cloxacillin, erythromycin, neomycin, and penicillin.

3. Staphylococcus—cloxacillin, erythromycin, lincomycin, neomycin, novobiocin, penicillin, and tetracyclines.

4. The coliforms—dihydrostreptomycin, neomycin, and polymixin B.

5. Pseudomonas—polymixin B alone or in combination with neomycin.

6. Yeast organisms—Never use antibiotics. Treatment is generally ineffective. These animals should be culled and you must correct faulty management.

7. Mycoplasma—There is no effective treatment available. Anti-inflammatory drugs, such as hydrocortisone and prednisolone, may be helpful when administered in conjunction with antibiotics for acute mastitis cases or in various stages of clinical mastitis; but their use should be discontinued at least 24 hours before antibiotics are stopped. Also, undesirable effects can occur under certain conditions, and these drugs should be used only under direction of the veterinarian.

Drug residues in milk are very important. Improper use of antibiotics will cause illegal residues, and the FDA will withdraw them from the market if such residues are found. The individual dairyman is responsible for preventing this from occurring, so that the effective drugs can be kept on the market and can be utilized. It is extremely important, therefore, to read the label on the medication. All mastitis medications must list a specified period of time after treatment during which milk must be withheld from market. The dry cow treatments all have a long milk withdrawal time (4 to 6 weeks) after treatment. Therefore, only cows that are dry for more than a month from calving can be treated. The dry treated cows cannot be slaughtered within 2 months of treatment. Again, the dairy industry cannot let the meat become adulterated with antibiotic residues. Otherwise we would not have effective drugs to use against mastitis. Several drugs have been removed from the market already. Our task is to see that no more are lost.

13

Maintenance of Dairy Equipment

The modern milking machine is a device designed to extract milk without causing injury or discomfort to the teats of the cow. The vacuum extraction is achieved (on the average milking machine) by providing a flexible sleeve (liner) within a metal teat cup. Utilizing pressure changes, the sleeve alternately collapses and expands to produce the desired results.

COMPONENTS OF A MILKING MACHINE

Most of the milking machines in the United States may be divided into the following basic components:

1. Teat cup—A liner (inflation) is used inside a metal cup so that a replaceable, inexpensive surface may provide comfort to the cow and protection to the cup. This also allows for adequate sanitary measures to be taken, in order to meet standards for the wholesomeness of milk.

2. Claw—The claw is a collecting chamber, of which there are several types.

3. Pulsator—The pulsator is a mechanical device responsible for the rhythmic contraction cycles, creating an alternate collapse and expansion of the liners in a cycle that normally ranges from 40 to 60 pulsations per minute.

4. Vacuum device

Collecting Systems

Most milking machines are the same except for the different types of collecting systems, which are outlined below.

Bucket Plants. In bucket plants the milk flows directly to a container placed near the cow. These systems are very stable but require a great deal

266

more labor than the more recent systems on the market. Small dairymen still find the bucket plant desirable because of lower initial expense.

Recorder Jar. The recorder jar may be located below or above the udder level. In the overhead type, the elevation of the milk may cause some reduction in milking volume and rate.

Pipeline System. There are basically three types within the pipeline units.

1. The first type consists of a unit in which all the vacuum is supplied from the milk pipeline itself. This is the least desirable of the pipeline systems.

2. High line—A separate air line is provided for pulsators in this setup. However, this type may allow milk to move in "clusters" and can cause interunit infections.

3. Low line—A milk line, in this instance, runs below the cow's udder, giving greater stability and producing little damage to the cow or the milk.

SANITATION AND CLEANING

Clean dairy equipment is essential to wholesomeness of milk and to human acceptance and consumption. Grade A classification of milk requires that sanitation be extremely well controlled. Sanitation is also necessary in order to hold down the major problem in dairy production, mastitis.

There are two types of cleaning, regardless of the form of machine milking involved: (1) the routine cleaning after milking, which is done manually or through circulation of a chlorinated solution; and (2) the removal of accumulated deposits.

The factors contributing to the production of a clean surface may be categorized as follows:

1. Water hardness and alkalinity—Water that is high in mineral deposits causes a buildup of calcium and other mineral sediments because of a reaction with hot water. Most hard or alkaline waters are high in minerals and may require a water softener before top-notch sanitation procedures may be observed in a dairy.

2. Concentration of detergent—Too weak a cleaning solution does not do the job, while an overabundant concentration may leave behind deposits that could contaminate milk.

3. Temperature of rinse and wash—The first rinsing is very important in cleaning out the entire milking system. The water should not be too hot because it denatures proteins in milk, causing them to stick to surfaces. However, the water should be warm enough to dissolve some of the fatty substances such as butterfat. Therefore, a rinsing with warm, but not hot, water is the first step.

Second, hot water (maintain 130° F) with an alkaline detergent has proven to be effective as a cleaning agent. It is difficult to maintain 130° F unless you start higher than that; so the normal recommendation is to use 160° F in order to maintain the required 130° F. The detergent will vary from dairy to dairy because of the quality of water used. Use a detergent that has proven to be successful under your conditions and with your water. You should seek help through the extension service or a factory representative to select the proper material for your cleaning operations. Cleaning should also be done with a brush in every place possible, followed by a thorough rinsing. Add 1 oz of acid detergent per 5 gallons of water in the rinse. This acid detergent rinse is necessary to neutralize the alkaline detergent soap cleaner. Through neutralization, deposits are kept to a minimum, or are kept from forming, and are allowed to be washed away in the rinse.

4. Mechanical action—In the cleaning of the accumulated deposits, several factors need to be considered. In addition to the physical action of scrubbing, other procedures can assist in doing a first-rate job. For example, fat melts at 95° F; so it is important to use an alkaline cleaner and some heat to remove the greasy formations that develop in the milk transports. Mineral deposits, however, respond best to acids. Thus, an acid rinse is helpful in reducing this type of formation. Proteins are usually best cleaned by hand brushing or through circulation of chlorine through the system.

Despite all of these precautions, accumulated deposits sometimes develop over a period of time and must be removed. The following steps are helpful in developing a method of removal.

1. Use equal parts of chlorinated alkaline cleaner, hot water, and liquid chlorine to remove fat and protein.

2. Apply a full-strength acid detergent directly to mineral accumulations, or soak in one part acid detergent to three parts water at 135° F for 10 to 15 minutes.

3. An alternate procedure for removal of fat protein and mineral deposits is to wash alternately with chlorinated alkaline detergent (1 oz per gallon of water at 130° F) and an organic acid detergent (one part to three parts of water at 145° F); then rinse in acidified water (1 oz per 5 gallons of water).

All items should be drained and stored properly for drying. Before they are used again, they should be sanitized by at least a 1 minute exposure to a solution of 150 to 200 ppm hypochlorite at 75° F or more.

Iodophors (at least 25 ppm concentration) can serve as a substitute for the above sanitation procedure but may cause off-flavors in milk at concentrations lower than the hypochlorite solution.

The care of the rubber parts of the milking machine are extremely important. This is one place where a dairyman should not be conservative. Problems with mastitis and lack of sanitation occur more frequently here due to defective parts than in any other area of the milking system. Liners should be washed after each milking, stored dry between milkings, and rotated. A rotation using two sets of liners for each unit is recommended. You should alternate use of liners for one-week periods. The set that is not in use should be boiled in 5% lye solution (one 13 oz can of lye per 2 gallons of water) and rinsed; then scrubbed in a hot solution containing milkstone removers (1 oz of organic acid detergent per gallon of water). The liners are then rinsed and stored dry for a one-week rest period, to be rotated at the end of that time with the other set.

MECHANICAL PROBLEMS IN MILKING MACHINES

Problems in the milking machine can usually be divided into the following areas:

1. Inadequate vacuum or fluctuation—The causes of inadequate vacuum pressure are usually a pump that is worn, too small or plugged lines, a sticking vacuum regulator, worn belts, and/or air leaks. However, the main cause of inadequate vacuum pressure is usually too many units on a line. Do not exceed the limits of your systems.

2. Vacuum level too high—If the vacuum level is to high, it is most often due to a sticky regulator. The regulator should be cleaned and oiled often.

3. Pulsators too fast or slow—Check the pulsators and adjust them to the manufacturer's recommended rates (usually 40 to 60 pulsations per minute) at least twice yearly.

4. Ballooned, cracked, or blistered inflations (liners). Inflations should be changed at regular intervals. Do not hesitate to buy new ones if there is any suspicion of problems due to age or condition.

Selection and maintenance of the proper equipment and adherence to a strict sanitation program are the keys to management of high-producing cows and excellent quality milk.

14

Herd Health

BABY CALF MANAGEMENT

Birth

Calves should be housed in a box stall that has been disinfected between calves. Make sure the baby calf consumes colostrum milk within the first hour after birth, preferably within the first 15 minutes in order to receive the antibodies from the dam's milk. Many dairymen prefer to leave the new calf with its dam for 48 to 72 hours.

The navel should be dipped in a solution of tincture of iodine. Repeat this treatment on days two and three.

Leave the calves in individual stalls for the first month; then remove them to small groups, ten or less, of about the same age.

Suggested Vaccination Program

See your veterinarian for specific vaccination suggestions in your area. Although recommendations will vary, the following vaccinations are generally recommended:

1. At 3 to 6 months of age—Blackleg and brucellosis (heifers only).

2. At 4 months of age—IBR (Red Nose), PI$_3$.

3. At 6 to 8 months of age—BVD.

4. At 4 to 6 weeks prior to breeding—Revaccinate for IBR, BVD, and PI$_3$. A three-way leptospirosis vaccine may also be given at this time if needed.

5. After first calving—Repeat IBR, BVD, and PI$_3$.

270

Calf Scours. Calf scours that occur during the first ten days of life are usually the result of an infection of *E. coli*. Calves should be removed from all milk and/or replacers and given only water and electrolytes for three to six feedings. Systemic antibiotics should be given to keep down secondary infection. A culture may be needed to determine the specific type of organism involved if scours is a big problem on the farm. As the feces start to firm up, slowly replace the milk diet, starting with a dilute solution and working up to about 1 gallon of liquid per calf per day. Severe cases of scours may require intravenous injections of electrolytes; this should be done by a veterinarian. For specific recommendations of electrolyte therapy and home treatment that you may be capable of, see section on Scours in Chapter 6.

If scours occur in later life, the cause may usually be traced to salmonella infections brought about by overfeeding.

Navel Infections. In the event a preventive dipping of the navel in iodine was not done, or if a unique case of navel infection does occur, the signs will be listlessness, high temperature, and a hot, thickened, hard navel cord. Such an infection may require a sensitivity culture to determine the type of organism involved and the specific antibiotic needed to combat it.

Respiratory Diseases. Diseases of the respiratory tract are very common in baby calves due to stress, overcrowded conditions, poor ventilation, wet and unsanitary stalls, and a poor-quality milk replacer.

The pasteurella organism and the viruses of BVD, IBR and PI$_3$ are most commonly involved.

The signs are rapid breathing, coughing, elevated temperature, and perhaps associated diarrhea (scours).

Massive doses of antibiotics and electrolyte therapy are recommended.

Feeding is very important in the prevention of scours and the resulting respiratory diseases brought on by stress and weakness. Proper feeding and reduction of stress are the keys to healthy young calves. A high-quality milk replacer (20% protein, 10 to 20% fat, and lactose or dextrose as an energy source) is required in order to provide the high nutritional requirements of the baby calf. A calf should consume about 1 gallon per day, divided into two feedings. This keeps down the incidence of scours and prevents the build up of respiratory disease possibilities.

MILKING HERD

Reproduction and herd management from a reproductive standpoint have been discussed previously in Chapter 7. The same philosophy will prevail in dairy cattle with the following exception; that is, very few vaccines or deworming agents can be used in a wet herd because of the possibility of milk contamination. Treatment must be left to the dry cow period, or vaccination must be immediately after calving before the cow goes back into the milking herd.

SPECIAL PROBLEMS IN THE MILKING HERD

Behavior

The social order is very well defined in dairy cow herds, and it is important for the dairyman to recognize that there is a social order that ranges from the timid cow to the "boss" cow. Some timid cows may be so harrassed that they do not even get sufficient quantities of water. Attending to their needs with special watering facilities and care will pay dividends in milk production.

Because of the social behavior of cows, it is normally recommended that dairy herds be limited to groups of 100 as the maximum size. Some research indicates that smaller herds (100 or less) have shorter estrous cycles because of less social stress and disorder, especially among young cows.

Foot Rot

Foot rot (see Chapter 6) can be a big problem in dairy herds and should be watched very closely.

DRY HERD

Protein and energy feed should be adjusted to the dry cow's needs in order to prepare her for the next lactation (see Chapter 10, Nutrition).

Injections of vitamins A, D, and E are often recommended by some veterinarians, particularly in adverse climates. The dry period is the time to give these injections.

This is also the time for preventive vaccine programs. As a general recommendation, vibrio, leptospirosis, anthrax, and Redwater will need to be considered in areas where they have been a problem.

Deworming with a general agent such as thiabendazole (see Internal Parasites, Chapter 6) is recommended at this time.

BULLS

Since artificial insemination has taken over most of the reproductive chores in the United States, bulls will be kept on most farms only to breed problem cows or for special size considerations in breeding young heifers.

A vaccination program for bulls will, in general, include anaplasmosis, Redwater, leptospirosis, and anthrax. Bulls should be dewormed twice yearly with a general product such as thiabendazole. They should be fertility-checked at least twice annually.

4

Swine

15

Nutrition of Swine

THE DIGESTIVE SYSTEM

Because a hog is a monogastric (simple-stomached) animal and is reputed to be a glutton, most stockmen have the mistaken opinion that a hog can balance its own ration if turned loose with all the ingredients that might be needed. A student once asked his professor why it was not possible just to give a hog all he wants to eat of the various nutrients and let him balance his own ration. The professor's answer was, "If the hog is smarter than you are, let it balance the ration. If you are smarter than it is, then you balance it. But don't underestimate the hog." This is an indication that hogs are quite well adapted to balancing their own ration due to their natural inclination to eat what the system craves under wild conditions. However, in domestic swine, man has so modified the diet and environment that it is impossible for the hog to root out a nutritionally balanced diet. If it does find food to fill its requirements, the diet may be severely out of balance from an economical standpoint. For example, a hog will eat a tremendous amount of peanut meal if given the opportunity, simply because the meal appeals to its taste buds; however, only a small amount of this would be needed to satisfy the animal's protein requirements, and the rest would be wasted. So you must manage the feed ingredients for an economical balancing of the ration, but also be very sharp if you are to outdo the hog from a nutritional standpoint.

The first step in understanding feeding requirements of any animal is to be aware of the anatomy and physiology of the digestive system. Figure 15-1 shows an artist's conception of the various parts of the swine's digestive plumbing. You will note that it is a very simple arrangement, and because of this there are some very definite requirements, such as high concentrate rations, that make for specific management techniques.

275

The digestive system begins with the *esophagus*, which is where the food initially passes after being chewed well and mixed with saliva before swallowing. The esophagus leads to the *stomach*, which is responsible for serving as a storehouse for food and also for mixing certain acids and gastric juices to begin the digestive process. The small intestine then follows from the stomach. There are three distinct sections of the small intestine from an anatomical standpoint, but physiologically they all act as points of absorption for carbohydrates, proteins, fats, minerals, vitamins, and water. For the purposes of our discussion, we can simply refer to this mass of the digestive system as the *small intestine*. The next portion of the system is the *cecum*, which is the same as the appendix in humans. It is simply a blind pouch and has no real function. As in humans, a hog can do without the cecum, and no serious complications arise if it is taken out. Also, as in humans, occasionally food does get compacted in this area and creates a condition much like an appendicitis in humans. The remainder of the digestive system is the *large intestine*, which simply serves as a storehouse for waste products and to reabsorb water after most of the absorption has taken place in the small intestine.

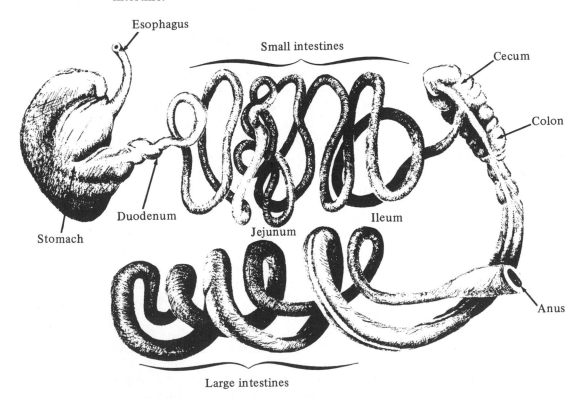

Figure 15-1. The monogastric digestive system. (From Blakely and Bade, *The Science of Animal Husbandry*. Reston, Va.: Reston Publishing Company, Inc., 1976)

This very "simple-stomached" animal has specific requirements because of this digestive system. It is important to recognize that it is the very simplicity of the digestive arrangement that is the key to feeding problems.

THE KEY TO FEEDING

Because of the lack of a rumen or the ability to regurgitate, the hog must be fed food or feeds that have three characteristics—if the maximum production and efficiency are to be achieved:

1. Low Fiber—Less than 5% fiber is the normal rule for any swine ration. Although alfalfa hay is quite often used in a swine ration, or alfalfa leafmeal, it is used at 5% or less. Alfalfa is added for protein, minerals, and bulk (in order to supply the necessary vitamins to a ration at an economical level). Alfalfa leafmeal is especially high in vitamins and minerals. Higher roughage levels may be used to purposely control weight in sows. Alfalfa is also used as a bulk additive to produce a laxative effect in sows just prior to or just after farrowing.

2. B Vitamins—Because a hog does not have the fermentation vat and the vast resources of rumen bacteria, it has to have B vitamins supplied in the ration for normal health. In the case of cattle, B vitamins are manufactured in the rumen by bacteria. Since the hog is a simple-stomached animal, it lacks the bacteria to manufacture these B vitamins in time to be reabsorbed. (*Note*: Some B vitamins are formed in the large intestine but are not absorbed.)

3. Quality Protein—There are ten essential amino acids that must be in the diet of swine. For this reason, SBM (soybean meal) or a mixture of vegetables and animal protein supplements are almost always included in a swine ration in order that the proper amino acids are supplied. It is not unusual for a swine ration or supplemental protein product to contain up to three or more protein sources. For instance, soybean meal (a vegetable source), tankage (an animal source), and bonemeal (another animal source) are quite often used to make up a protein supplement to be added to a grain product for a swine ration.

Although this list may seem an oversimplification of the requirements of swine, it is adequate for the layperson to know that a ration that contains low fiber, a high level of B-vitamin supplementation either from natural or synthetic sources, and a quality protein source will meet the minimum requirements for all swine.

NUTRITIONAL DEFICIENCIES

The signs of nutritional deficiencies can be broken down into the following main areas of concern.

Mineral Nutrition

Mineral nutrition is generally regarded to be of greatest concern, including, in order of importance, calcium, phosphorus, iron (and copper), magnesium, manganese, iodine, sodium and chlorine, zinc, and selenium.

1. Calcium is probably the most needed mineral in swine rations, and if deficient in hogs (Figure 15-2), can create a lameness as well as a gradual deterioration of the hindquarters. You may recall that a lack of calcium in other animals produces rickets, but in swine the early signs are not quite as severe from the standpoint of a deterioration of skeletal development. It is more a condition of lameness and brittle bones because swine develop so rapidly. Long-term deficiencies will produce ricketlike signs particularly in the ribs. Therefore, the skeletal development may seem relatively intact, but there is an obvious weakness in the hindquarter with the animal losing proper muscle function. Bone meal, ground limestone, dicalcium phosphate, or ground oyster-shell flour are common ingredients added to the ration in order to prevent this deficiency.

2. Phosphorus is needed for proper skeletal growth and development (see Figure 15-3). The deficiency signs are quite similar to those for lack of calcium, providing a form of rickets that includes weak legs and crooked leg

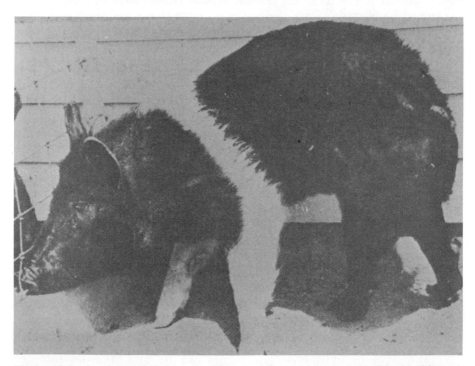

Figure 15-2. A calcium-deficient pig. This pig will soon lose control of its hind legs. A deficiency of calcium often results in rickets; an excess results in parakaratosis. (*Photo courtesy of H. D. Wallace, University of Florida*)

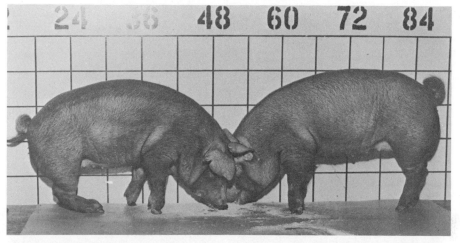

Figure 15-3. A typical phosphorus-deficient pig. Leg bones are weak and crooked. The pig on the right received the same ration, except the ration was fortified with calcium phosphate to supply adequate phosphorus. (*Courtesy of M. P. Plumlee and W. M. Beeson, Purdue University*)

bones. While it is not as obvious in swine as it is in other animals, a phosphorus deficiency does create some skeletal changes, although not as severe as the rickets previously discussed in cattle. Steamed bone meal or monocalcium phosphate and dicalcium phosphate are good sources of phosphorus.

3. Iron and copper may be lumped together because of the similar need for both of these minerals in the normal blood functions in swine. Hemoglobin utilizes both iron and copper in order to carry oxygen through the blood system of the animal. If either of these ingredients is missing from a ration, an anemia may develop (Figure 15-4), resulting in a pounding of the heart of baby pigs that is so loud that it may be audible to the swine herdsman upon picking up affected pigs. Since it makes a thumping sound, the disorder is most often referred to as "baby pig thumps." The condition is simply an attempt by the heart to overreact and pump more blood faster through the system in order to deliver oxygen to the cells. The most effective anemia treatment and/or preventive in this case is to add iron and copper to the ration, or to inject iron dextran at 1 to 3 days of age and again at 3 weeks of age. The level of injection is usually 100 mg per pig for the first injection and 50 mg for the second. Copper deficiency is rare because of its presence in natural ingredients. However, excessive levels of iron may increase copper requirements.

4. Magnesium deficiency has been documented in swine; it produces muscle twitching, a staggering gait, and a noticeable weakness in the pasterns. Magnesium is necessary for normal muscle reactions and for equilibrium in the hog. For this reason, practical rations usually have small levels of

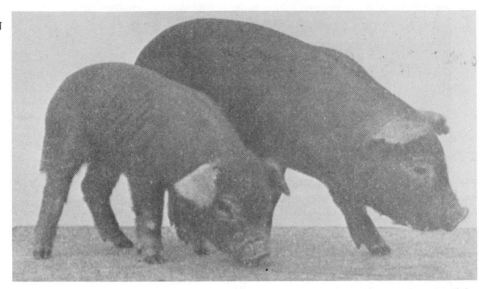

Figure 15-4. Anemic pig on the left is from the same litter as the pig on the right. Anemia can be caused by a lack of iron or copper in pigs. It is most often a result of low iron consumption and may be prevented by the administration of supplemental iron and/or copper. (*Photo courtesy of H. D. Wallace, University of Florida*)

magnesium added to them, making the possibility of a deficiency rather remote because of the very small requirement. However, the deficiency does occur in nature as well as in the feed lot.

5. Manganese is normally not a problem, but deficiency signs have been produced under experimental conditions (Figure 15-5). The occurrence of manganese-deficient pigs has been noted, and the signs include pigs that are born very weak and with a poor sense of balance. Since this is a rare occurrence, manganese is not usually of concern to the average stockman. It

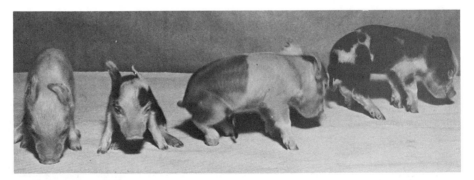

Figure 15-5. Litter from sow fed 0.5 ppm (0.23 mg/lb) of manganese. The pigs showed weakness and poor sense of balance at birth. (*Courtesy of M. P. Plumlee and W. M. Beeson, Purdue University*)

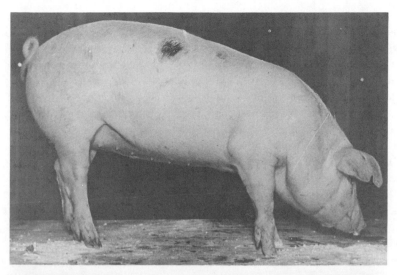

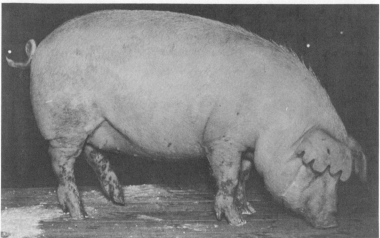

Figure 15-6. A 132-day-old gilt fed 40 ppm (18 mg/lb) of manganese since she weighed 8.5 lb (top). A littermate gilt (bottom) started at 8.5 lb and 132 days old was fed 0.5 ppm (0.23 mg/lb) of manganese. Note increased fat deposition due to low manganese diet. (*Courtesy of M. P. Plumlee and W. M. Beeson, Purdue University*)

is known that a minor deficiency can lead to poor production through increased fat deposition (Figure 15-6).

    6. It is well-documented that iodine is needed in swine rations. If it is not available, the condition of goiter (a swelling of the thyroid gland in the neck area) is evident. Sows that are deficient in iodine may develop goiter, and their offspring may be stillborn or born hairless, weak, and small. The best source of iodine for preventing this disorder is iodized salt, which can be either added to the ration or fed free-choice.

7. Sodium and chlorine are perhaps the most needed minerals in a swine ration, and both of them are supplied through the use of sodium chloride or common table salt. However, the addition of salt should be watched very carefully because unlike the ruminant digestive system, any simple-stomached animal has a relatively low tolerance to salt, and if you should make a mistake in the decimal point and get too much salt in a ration, it could create some severe problems such as diarrhea or a lack of appetite. Swine have a minimum salt requirement of .2% of the ration, but as a practical rule, .5% is the accepted guide for the layman if he should decide to mix some of his own rations. The upper level definitely should not be exceeded because of the possibility of producing a salt poison syndrome if the pigs are restricted on water intake. However, if no salt is supplied in any form, it could produce a condition characterized by a depraved appetite and an unnatural chewing of wood and foreign objects, as well as extremely poor growth.

8. Zinc is now known to be an essential mineral, especially in those areas of the country where zinc deficiencies exist in the crops or in the soils from which the crops are grown. Zinc is needed for normal growth and health, but its most obvious deficiency sign is a condition known as *parakaratosis* (Figure 15-7), also referred to as *swine dermatosis*. This is a condition that has been noted over the past two decades as an extremely

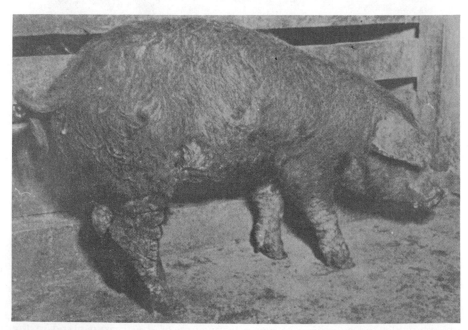

Figure 15-7. A hog suffering from parakaratosis. Zinc will prevent this condition; excess calcium may cause it, so it is important to have adequate levels of zinc and the proper balance of calcium. (*Courtesy of H. D. Wallace, University of Florida*)

severe skin disorder. The skin becomes thickened, rough, and flaky. Generally this affects all areas of the pig's body.

The functions of zinc are not fully understood, but it is known that it is connected in some way with normal skin function and body growth. It is also known that high levels of calcium and phosphorus—if accidentally added by mistake to a ration—can bring on a deficiency of zinc even though the zinc is at the proper level. This indicates a relationship between zinc, calcium, and phosphorus. For this reason, it is very important to have a trained nutritionist develop your swine rations, especially if any exotic changes are to be made in mineral supplementation. It is quite common to add zinc to a ration in quantities higher than normally needed in those areas where parakaratosis has been noted to be a problem. Levels as high as 450 mg per pound have been fed without any toxic side effects, although 75 to 125 mg per pound are normal supplement levels.

9. Selenium is an essential mineral element, and data are available to show that feeding practical-type rations formulated from ingredients grown on low-selenium soils may result in a selenium deficiency. Although the function of selenium is not completely understood, it is known to be closely related to that of vitamin E. The most striking signs of a selenium deficiency are sudden death and muscle and liver necrosis.

The total selenium level needed in practical diets is a minimum of .10 mg per kg (0.1 ppm in total diet). Levels above 5 to 8 mg per kg (5-8 ppm) of diet are toxic.

Although deficiency signs are not acute, a lack of adequate selenium reduces production and creates a brownish yellow discoloration of fat tissue, a waxy degeneration of muscle tissue, and edema (accumulation of water in the tissues). Reduced pig survival and reduced milking ability have also been shown in selenium-deficient sows. Because of the close association of selenium with vitamin E, some manufacturers have begun using selenium or vitamin E, or both, in their supplements. It is not a major consideration in most cases, but it is receiving more attention as confinement feeding operations and farrowing houses develop. Reliance on a completely enclosed production system and more purified diet supplementation in the future may cause an increased awareness of the need for selenium and/or vitamin E.

Vitamin Deficiencies

Some vitamin deficiencies exist in swine at a higher level of incidence than in other animals because of the lack of bacteria to manufacture the necessary vitamins.

Fat-Soluble Vitamins. Fat-soluble vitamins are vitamins A, D, E, and K. Each of these could be deficient in a ration, and all are normally supplied in either a natural source such as alfalfa leafmeal or in synthetic form through a supplement made especially for swine rations.

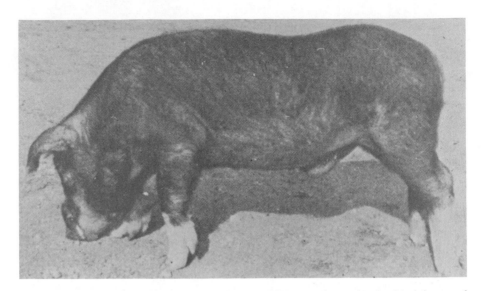

Figure 15-8. A hog deficient in vitamin A exhibits weakness in the hind legs and curvature of the spine (lordosis). Many swine rations have inadequate levels of vitamin A. (*Courtesy of H. D. Wallace, University of Florida*)

1. Vitamin A (Figure 15-8) is necessary for the prevention of lameness or stiffness in the joints and, as in cattle, for normal reproduction. A deficiency may cause the same kind of muscular incoordination, lameness, swollen joints, and night blindness as previously discussed for other species. Pregnant sows often give birth to pigs that are extremely weak, and these offspring may never fully recover—if they live at all. The cause of many pigs being born dead, deformed, or blind may be traced back to a vitamin A deficiency in the sow (see Figure 15-9). However, a supplementation of concentrate is generally in excess of requirements, making signs rare in the United States.

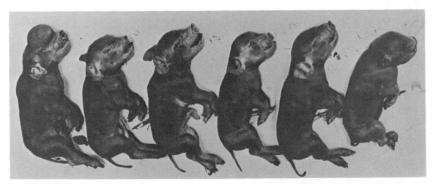

Figure 15-9. Vitamin A deficiencies in sows can result in abortions, weak pigs, water on the brain in pigs as shown at the extreme left, and other abnormalities. Vitamin A is often deficient in swine rations. (*Photo courtesy of Fred Hale, Texas A & M University*)

2. Vitamin D is associated (Figure 15-10) with calcium and phosphorus and is normally needed for proper skeletal growth and development. Although vitamin D is not required if animals are in direct contact with sunlight, it is a very common occurrence for swine to become deficient in vitamin D because of the system of production in which swine are housed for most of their lives, especially in the northern climates. The chief deficiency signs of vitamin D are enlarged joints, weak bones, and pigs that walk on their front knee joints rather than standing on their feet and pasterns. This is the form in which rickets usually shows up in swine. A deficiency of phosphorus or calcium could produce similar deficiencies, but vitamin D is normally the most suspected culprit. The best natural source of vitamin D is any sun-cured forage, which is another reason for including alfalfa products as bulk in gestation rations; but alfalfa is not recommended for grower-finisher or lactation-starter rations. Synthetic sources of vitamin D are also available at very cheap rates and should be used according to directions.

3. Vitamin E is known to be associated with selenium and reproduction in most animals, and swine are no exception. Apparently vitamin E from natural sources is quite sufficient to meet the animal's needs if selenium levels are adequate. However, spoilage, storage, high temperature, and rapid drying of grain may reduce natural vitamin E levels.

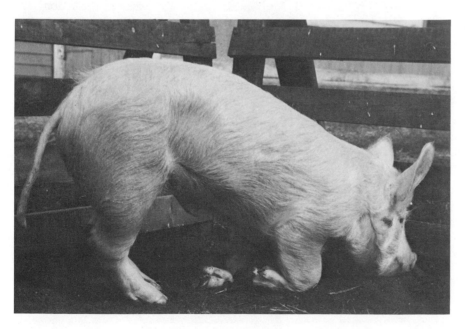

Figure 15-10. Vitamin D deficiency. The pig shown above developed rickets, caused by a lack of vitamin D. However, this pig responded to vitamin D supplement in the diet and recovered normal functions. (*Photo courtesy of J. M. Bell, University of Saskatchewan, Canada*)

4. Vitamin K is needed in order to produce the proper blood-clotting factor when swine are injured through cuts, abrasions, or bruises. A deficiency of vitamin K can cause unstoppable internal bleeding, hemorrhages under the skin, bleeding into the intestinal tracts, or, in young pigs, navel cord bleeding, all resulting in death. However, vitamin K deficiency is a very rare occurrence in swine. Moldy foods, improper storage, and high storage or drying temperatures may cause destruction of vitamin K or lack of absorption leading to deficiency signs.

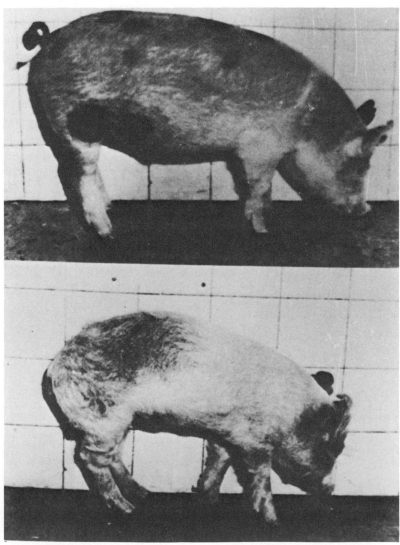

Figure 15-11. Niacin deficiency. The pig shown at top has received adequate niacin. The pig at the bottom has not. The difference in growth and condition is due to the addition of niacin in the diet containing 80% ground yellow corn. (Reprinted by permission from *Nutrient Requirements of Swine*)

Water-Soluble Vitamins. The water-soluble vitamins are generally referred to as B vitamins. There are ten of them that appear to be essential to swine nutrition. However, since some of the signs have only been produced artificially, we will be concerned only with those vitamins that have been seen under natural conditions: niacin, pantothenic acid, riboflavin, and vitamin B_{12}. These vitamins may be supplemented in synthetic commercial form, vitamin premix, or natural sources. Assuming the availability of synthetics of the vitamin in question, we will cover only natural products.

1. Niacin has been demonstrated to be necessary for normal health and skin development. If there is a deficiency (Figure 15-11), it usually shows up chiefly as lesions on the skin known as "pig pellagra" and severe diarrhea. The gut, particularly the colon, has severe thickening, with layers of dead tissue attached causing a blackish gray discoloration. Feed may be attached to this material and be difficult to remove. Natural sources used for niacin supplementation to prevent this condition from occurring are distiller's dried solubles, condensed fish solubles, and alfalfa leafmeal. However, under most circumstances niacin levels are met entirely with synthetic niacin supplementation. This is because of the wide range of niacin availability in common rations.

2. Pantothenic acid (Figure 15-12) has a function in swine for proper muscle and nerve development and activity. This is a classic deficiency sign in swine and is more evident in this species than in any other farm animal. The affected hogs walk with an uncoordinated motion and kick their hind feet up in a very stiff unnatural fashion, which has been related to the style of

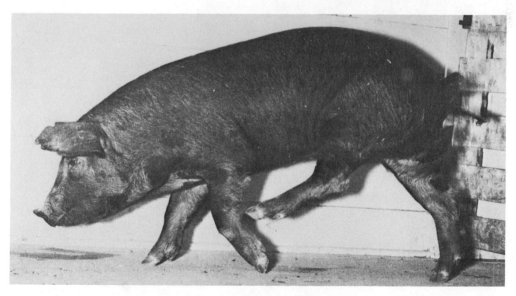

Figure 15-12. Pantothenic acid deficiency. Locomotor incoordination ("goose-stepping") was produced by feeding a ration (corn-soybean meal) low in pantothenic acid. (Reprinted by permission from *Nutrient Requirements of Swine*)

marching used by the Russian soldiers of today. This is referred to as "goose-stepping" and has been quite widespread in the past when hogs were not fed proper rations. In addition, hair loss, poor growth, lack of appetite, and diarrhea have been seen with this deficiency. The best source of pantothenic acid is dried brewer's yeast, dried whey, and alfalfa leafmeal.

3. Riboflavin is needed for normal growth and reproduction. The most obvious deficiency signs in swine are crooked legs, lameness, diarrhea, anemia, and slow growth (Figure 15-13). There are indications that reproduction and lactation are lowered in deficient sows. The best sources of riboflavin are any milk products, and for this reason dried skimmed milk has been a part of many rations.

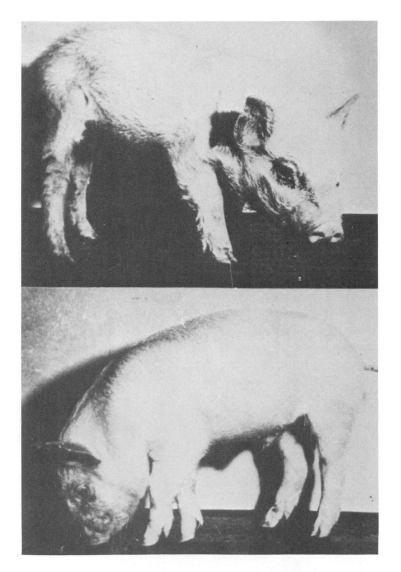

Figure 15-13. Riboflavin deficiency. The pig at top received no riboflavin. Note the rough coat, poor growth, and dermatitis. The pig at bottom received adequate riboflavin. (Reprinted by permission from Nutrient Requirements of Swine)

Table 15-1. Experimentally Induced Signs Of Severe Dietary Deficiencies In Swine

Deficiency	Slow or Interrupted Growth	Reduced Feed Intake	Poor Hair and Skin Condition	Lameness and Stiffness	Weakened Bone Structure	Diarrhea	Impaired Breeding-Gestation	Offspring Dead or Weak at Birth	Other (Footnotes)
Energy	X							X	1
Protein level	X	X	X				X		2
Protein quality (essential amino acids)	X	X	X				X		2
Essential fatty acids	X	X	X						3
Calcium	X	X	X	X	X		X		4
Phosphorus	X	X		X	X		X		5
Potassium	X	X	X						6
Sodium	X	X							7
Magnesium	X	X	X	X	X				8
Iodine	X	X	X				X	X	10
Iron	X	X	X						11, 12
Copper	X		X	X	X				12, 13, 14
Zinc	X	X	X	X	X				15
Selenium	X	X				X			16
Vitamin A	X		X	X	X		X	X	17
Vitamin D	X			X	X				18
Vitamin E	X	X							16
Vitamin K	X								19
Thiamine	X	X					X	X	20
Riboflavin	X	X	X			X	X	X	21
Niacin	X	X	X			X	X		22
Pantothenic acid	X	X		X		X	X	X	23
Vitamin B$_6$	X	X	X						12, 24
Choline			X				X	X	25, 26
Vitamin B$_{12}$	X		X				X		12
Biotin	X	X	X	X					27

Source: University of Florida. Based on National Research Council information.

Footnotes:
1. Reduced fat deposition.
2. Poor feed efficiency.
3. Loss of hair, scaly, dandrufflike dermatitis, especially of feet and tail.
4. Rickets; reduced serum calcium and tetany in severe cases.
5. Reduced inorganic blood phosphorus.
6. Decreased feed efficiency; cardiac impairment.
7. Depraved appetite.
8. Hyperirritability and tetany; weak pasterns.
9. Reduced skeletal growth; increased backfat; irregular estrus.
10. Pigs hairless at birth? goiter.
11. High mortality in young pigs; susceptibility to disease; thumps.
12. Anemia.
13. Lack of rigidity of leg joints; hocks excessively flexed; forelegs crooked; use of forelegs impaired.
14. Lowered elastin content of arterial wall.
15. Severe dermatosis; parakeratosis.
16. Liver necrosis, brownish yellow discoloration of adipose tissue, waxy degeneration of muscle tissue, edema, sudden death.
17. Increased cerebrospinal fluid pressure, incoordination, weakness, and paralysis.
18. Rickets; enlarged joints; weak bones.
19. Blood-clotting time prolonged, hemorrhage, hyperirritability.
20. Slow pulse; low body temperature; flabby heart.
21. Crooked legs; stillborn pigs.
22. Occasional vomiting; foul-smelling feces; pig pellagra.
23. Incoordinated, wobbly gait (goose-stepping), stiff-legged.
24. Epilepsylike fits; slowing of growth after first convulsion.
25. Lack of coordination; improper rigidity of joints; fatty liver; renal glomerular occlusion; tubular epithelial necrosis.
26. May be associated with spraddled-leg condition at birth.
27. Spasticity of hind legs; loss of hair; dermatosis; cracks in feet.

4. Vitamin B_{12} is necessary in swine for normal growth, lactation, and appetite. Deficiency of B_{12} is not often seen in the field. The use of tankage, meat scraps, distillery byproducts, and dairy byproducts is widespread to prevent a deficiency of vitamin B_{12}. Pigs can synthesize some vitamin B_{12} in their lower gut and therefore may be able to obtain B_{12} by eating their manure.

Although this has been a very sketchy discussion of the nutritional requirements of swine, it is felt that the various situations covered are more than the average stockman is likely to encounter. It is doubtful that any swineman will ever see all of these conditions, but they have been included in order to give some basic knowledge in the event an unusual condition is noted. Under current feed production procedures, most vitamins are added in synthetic form to meet the animal's requirements, with the natural levels used as insurance against a problem. Table 15-1 gives a condensed version of the worst things that could go wrong under an extreme deficiency condition.

RATIONS

Cookbook Methods

Since the balancing of rations for monogastric animals requires a great deal of nutritional expertise and added capital to maintain inventories of all needed ingredients, it is not recommended that the average stockman start from scratch in developing a ration. The cookbook method of balancing is therefore recommended for those who would like to utilize some of their own

Table 15-2. Ration Suggestions (Rations Using Premixed Commercial Supplements)

	18% starter		16% grower		14%finisher	
Grain (corn or milo)	50	60	42.5	38.5	66.5	62.5
Cereal grain (oats, barley, wheat)	16.5	12	35	35	15	15
35% supplement	33.5			21.5		17.5
40% supplement		28	17.5		13.5	
Alfalfa leafmeal			5.0	5.0	5	5
	100 lb	100 lb	100 lb	100 lb	100 lb	100 lb
	14% gestation				16% lactation	
	Dry lot		On pasture			
Grain (corn or milo)	78.5	76.5	78.5	82.5	42.5	38.5
Cereal grain (oats, barley, wheat)					35	35
35% supplement		18.5	21.5			21.5
40% supplement	16.5			17.5	17.5	
Alfalfa leafmeal	5	5			5	5
	100 lb	100 lb	100 lb	100 lb	100 lb	100 lb

Source: Blakely and Bade, *The Science of Animal Husbandry* (Reston Publishing Company, Reston, Virginia, 1976), p. 214.

home-grown grains, plus a commercially prepared supplement that will contain sufficient vitamins and minerals to meet the animal's needs. Such a cookbook suggestive tabulation is given in Tables 15-2 and 15-3. The 35% supplement and 40% supplement refer to commercial products that are available from most feedstores. These supplements contain 35 to 40% protein plus the essential vitamins and minerals normally required. Either of these supplements added to the corn, milo, oats, barley, or wheat, plus the recommended amounts of alfalfa leafmeal where suggested, should produce excellent results without worrying about balancing. Do not "short" the use of supplement during times of high feed costs or some deficiencies or poor performance may occur. Always follow label instructions.

Feeding Systems

Feeding of swine can be divided into feeding systems and suggested rations and management techniques within these systems.

Simplified versus Complex Ration. Swine rations are becoming more simplified today than formerly. A simple corn-soybean ration properly supplemented with minerals and vitamins is considered by many to be the standard for comparison. On the other hand, feed companies because of large-volume buying of ingredients and computerized ration balancing can develop more sophisticated rations based on least-cost calculations. A complex ration is used by some feed companies in order to juggle ingredients while maintaining the best price structure without affecting guaranteed minimum contents and performance of the ration. There may be occasions when a commercial feed company can provide a ration cheaper than you can mix it. In this case, buy the complex ration. When using your own grains, generally the simple ration will be the less expensive alternative. If you mix your own ration, great care must be taken to get the right weight of each ingredient added and a good mixing job done before feeding the hogs.

If drugs are used in a home mix, special care must be taken in order to prevent exceeding safe residue levels and subsequent condemnation of carcasses. Swine producers have been under fire for sulfa and other drug residues found in pork. The problem often stems from a continuous accumulation of low-level drug usage in feed mixing equipment without proper cleaning procedures. The following guidelines are suggested by Dr. James D. McKean, Iowa State extension veterinarian, to guard against drug contamination.

1. Know the labeled uses, mixing instructions, and withdrawal times for all medications used.

2. Clean the mixer before use to avoid contamination with previous medications.

3. Do not exceed mixing capabilities of equipment. Premix all medications into large enough quantities for accurate weighing and mixing. Where

Table 15-3. Life Cycle Swine Feeding Program

STAGE OF CYCLE	LENGTH OF FEEDING PROGRAM	SEASON	COMPLETE RATION		LB CORN OR GRAIN/DAY	LB/SUPPLEMENT/DAY
			% PROTEIN	LB/DAY		
Boars	From time purchased at 5–6 mo of age	Summer	12–16	4–6	3–5	
		Winter	11–14	5–7	4–6	0.8–1.0
			Increase intake 1–2 lb during the heavy breeding season.			
Gilts Pregestation	From time selected at 5–6 mo until breeding at 7–9 mo of age.	Summer	12–16	4–6	3–5	
		Winter	11–14	5–7	4–6	0.8–1.0
Flushing and breeding	For 3 weeks prior to breeding (do not continue after breeding).		11–14	6–9	5–8	1.0–1.2
			Increase corn intake approximately 2 lb/day.			
Gestation		Summer	12–16	4–5	3–4	
		Winter	11–14	5–6	4–5	0.8–1.0
			Increase intake 1–2 lb last 3–5 wk of gestation if gilts appear to be too thin.			
Lactation	Wean at 3–5 wk after farrowing.		13–16	10–14	Full feed complete ration.	

Sows					
Breeding and gestation	Breed back at first heat period after weaning (flushing isn't beneficial with sows).	Summer	13–18	3–4	2–3	0.8–1.0
		Winter	12–16	4–5	3–4	
	Increase intake 1–2 lb last 3–5 wk of gestation if sows appear to be too thin.					
Lactation	Wean 3–5 wk after farrowing.		13–16	12–16	Full feed complete ration.	
Pigs						
Milk replacer	Use only if weaned before 3 wk and feed until pig weighs 12 lb.		20–24		Full-feed complete ration.	
Starter	Use as a creep feed and continue after weaning until pigs are 8 wk of age or 40 lb		18–20		Full-feed complete ration.	
Grower-finisher	From 8 wk of age or 40 lb until market weight.		12–16	Full-feed (may limit feed after 125 lb).	With free choice, corn consumption varies depending on wt of pig. Supplement intake should be approx 0.75 lb regardless of the wt of the pig.	

(Courtesy Iowa State University)

293

stationary mills are used, follow manufacturer's instructions on premixing and adding medications.

4. Establish a mixing order for all ingredients.*

5. Measure ingredients by volume or by weight. Weight measurements are most accurate, but volumetric methods will give satisfactory results when regular calibrations are made. Calibration is particularly important with stationary volumetric mills.

6. Whenever possible, mix all feeds containing medications in sequence. Then clean equipment before manufacturing unmedicated feeds. Make swine finishing or withdrawal feeds after cleanup and other nonmedicated feeds.

7. Clean out mixer after medication use by flushing with several hundred pounds of soybean or ground corn. Remove flush material and store for future medication usage.

8. Keep all medications in a well-lit storage place, with enough room to avoid cluttered storage and preserve original packages.

9. Read all labels and observe withdrawal times.

10. Periodically sample purchased premixes or supplements. Label and hold these samples until 3 months after hogs have been marketed.

11. Clean out augers, holding bins, delivery wagons, and feeders before withdrawal (nonmedicated) feed is mixed. Augers can be flushed with ground corn or other suitable flush material. Bins, wagons, and feeders can be swept out. Do not put withdrawal feeds into bins or feeders with medicated feeds.

12. If NDA-1800 drugs are used, mixing operations must conform to good manufacturing practices (GMP). Be familiar with and observe GMPs. (Additional sources of information about medicated feeds and premixes can be found in the *Federal Register* and the *Feed Additive Compendium*, Miller Publishing Co., Minneapolis, Minn.)

Complete Self-Fed Rations. Self-fed rations developed on the farm are usually made by mixing a purchased balanced supplement with ground grain from the farm. The trend is toward the use of complete self-feeding of these rations for growing and finishing pigs because this method has been proven superior to free-choice both in performance and in cost of the ration. Faster gains have been shown on self-fed rations than on limited or free-choice feeding. Table 15-4 gives grower-finisher rations intended to be self-fed.

---

*One recommended mixing order is: (a) one-half of soybean meal or supplement, (b) medication and/or vitamin premixes, (c) one-quarter of soybean meal or supplement—to flush premix into mixer, (d) mineral premix, (e) remainder of soybean meal or supplement, (f) mix thoroughly while grinding corn, (g) add ground corn and mix for 8–10 minutes, or according to manufacturer's instructions. Proper mixing is all-important. (Adapted from Dale Hull, 1970, *Argricultural Engineering*, Iowa State University.)

Table 15-4 Grower-Finisher Rations

PERCENT PROTEIN	INGREDIENTS	FOR PIGS 40-120 LB			FOR PIGS FROM 120-240 LB[a]		
		1	2	3	4	5	6
8.9	Corn[b,c]	1660-1590	1550-1450	1666-1601	1733-1658	1648-1548	1747-1667
44	Solvent soybean meal[d]	280-350	—	200-265	205-280	—	120-200
37	Soybeans, whole cooked[e]	—	390-490	—	—	290-390	—
50	Meat and bone meal	—	—	100	—	—	100
	Calcium carbonate (38% Ca)	15	15	6	15	15	6
	Dicalcium phosphate (26% Ca, 18.5% P)	23	23	4	25	25	5
	Salt	10	10	10	10	10	10
	Trace minerals	2	2	2	2	2	2
	Vitamins	10	10	10	10	10	10
	Feed additives (gm/ton)[f]	0-100	0-100	0-100	0-100	0-100	0-100
	TOTAL	2000	2000	2000	2000	2000	2000
	Calculated Analysis %						
	Protein %	13.54-14.77	14.10-15.51	14.32-15.46	12.22-13.54	12.70-14.10	12.92-14.32
	Calcium %	0.62-0.63	0.63-0.64	0.60-0.61	0.54-0.64	0.64-0.66	0.60-0.61
	Phosphorus %	0.50-0.52	0.52-0.53	0.51-0.52	0.51-0.52	0.52-0.54	0.51-0.52
	Lysine %	0.65-0.75	0.68-0.79	0.66-0.75	0.55-0.65	0.58-0.68	0.55-0.66
	Methionine %	0.24-0.25	0.24-0.26	0.25-0.26	0.22-0.24	0.22-0.24	0.23-0.25
	Cystine %	0.23-0.24	0.23-0.25	0.21-0.23	0.21-0.23	0.21-0.23	0.19-0.21
	Trytophan %	0.14-0.17	0.16-0.18	0.13-0.15	0.12-0.14	0.14-0.16	0.11-0.13
	Megabolizable Kcal/lb energy	1324-1318	1382-1391	1321-1316	1330-1324	1373-1382	1328-1321

(Courtesy Iowa State University)

Note: For pigs from 40 to 240 lb: Start with the higher level of soybean meal (lower level of corn) with lighter pigs in each group, and decrease the soybean meal (increase the corn) in 50-100 lb increments until you reach the lower level. If you prefer, one level of protein can be fed from 40 lb-240 lb with similar results as with the varying levels. In this case use a level of soybean meal and corn that is approximately the high point of the listed range for growing pigs(for example, in ration 1 you might use 1590 lb of corn and 350 lb of soybean meal). If barrows and gilts are separated, use the higher end of the range for soybean meal for the gilts and the lower end for the barrows.

[a] For pigs going to market, the level of dicalcium phosphate may be reduced by 10 lb; this provides a level of about 0.51% calcium and 0.41% phosphorus. Replacement gilts and boars should be fed the levels provided in the above rations.

[b] Ground milo, wheat, or barley can replace the ground corn. Ground oats can replace corn up to 20% of the total ration.

[c] If the ration is to be pelleted, 25-50 lb of molasses or binder can replace 25-50 lb of corn.

[d] 3 lb of L-lysine, 1 lb of DL-methionine, and 96 lb of corn can be substituted for 100 lb of soybean meal.

[e] Since the high fat content of whole cooked soybeans increases the energy content of the ration, the protein level in a ration utilizing whole cooked soybeans should be approximately 1% protein higher than a similar ration with soybean meal in order to replace an equal amount of corn.

Limit Feeding

Gilts and Sows.   Some herdsmen use bulky or fibrous ingredients added to a gestation ration to serve as a limit-feeding program. This can work successfully provided the ration is properly formulated and is fed according to the gestating animal's requirements. A few producers are feeding a gestation feed of alfalfa haylage with mineral supplementation. Corn is added to the ration when additional energy is required. Limit feeding is the most commonly used method of maintaining the proper weight of gilts and sows and to prevent them from getting too fat. Table 15-3 gives specific recommendations for feeding these females at the various stages of their development. Remember when feed is limited, additional vitamin and mineral supplementation is required to insure adequate total daily intake.

Growing and Finishing Pigs.   The use of limit feeding is questionable for growing and finishing pigs under current U.S. marketing systems. Limit-fed hogs at about 95% of full feed grow as efficiently and have leaner carcasses at slaughter than self-fed pigs. However, the added work and time to market are generally great enough to offset any advantage.

Most research findings indicate that full-feed growing and finishing pigs is the most efficient and profitable system of feeding. Table 15-4 gives examples of rations and levels of feeding for pigs from 40 to 240 lb.

Interval Feeding.   Interval feeding is actually a method of limit feeding gestating gilts and sows. In this system, females are turned in to a self-feeder for 2 to 8 hours every third day. The daily feed consumption averages approximately 4 lb per day with gilts (12 lb consumed every third day) and 5 lb with sows (15 lb every third day). Gilts and sows may not do as well as expected in cold weather under this system, and sows may overconsume in summer. Amounts eaten can be varied by the length of time feeder access is allowed. Research indicates reproductive performance with interval feeding has been essentially the same as with hand feeding or other limit-feeding methods.

Liquid Feeding.   The rate of gain is essentially the same as conventional methods. Liquid full-fed pigs have generally been slightly less efficient than full-fed pigs on dry rations. Recent work with a paste feeding method has indicated some promise but has not been properly evaluated at this point. Liquid feeding systems would appear to be more a matter of convenience and a way of keeping down dust problems.

Pelleted Complete Rations.   Pelleting of rations usually increases average daily gain by about 5% and improves feed efficiency by 10%, although the economical advantage would not justify the purchase of a pelleting machine for most farm operations. Given a choice of a commercial meal or pelleted ration at essentially the same price, the pelleted ration would be preferred.

High-Moisture Corn. High-moisture corn, substituted for dry corn on an equal dry matter basis, is an excellent form of energy. The only problems associated with high-moisture corn are (1) an improved palatability, which sometimes causes hogs to overeat corn and not eat enough supplement, thus creating a deficiency in minerals and/or vitamins and (2) the inability of young pigs (under 25 lb) to fully utilize the rations until older. Since complete ground and mixed rations using high-moisture corn cannot be stored long due to the moisture content and spoilage, a system should be developed to allow mixing of the high-moisture shell corn with a pelleted supplement on a daily basis to make this a feasible feeding program. Additions of preservatives when feed is mixed during the warm months have also been used successfully to retard spoilage.

Whole Cooked Soybeans. Research has indicated that whole cooked soybeans can be substituted in the place of soybean meal with no problems. Their use will increase the energy content and may increase feed efficiency by 5 to 10%. Whole soybeans are, however, lower in total protein, which must be taken into account when formulating the ration. The decision as to their use in a ration must be based on comparative costs with soybean meal and other protein sources and the value of soybeans on the market plus processing costs. Rarely in recent history have whole soybeans been an economical addition to swine rations. Table 15-4 gives sample rations using both whole soybeans and soybean meal.

Feeding High Lysine Corn (HLC). Lysine is one of the essential amino acids previously referred to in the protein discussion (The Key to Feeding). To make full use of high lysine corn, it must be analyzed and rations balanced according to the lysine requirement rather than the protein requirement. Savings on protein can be substantial but may be offset by poorer bushel per acre production from high lysine corn varieties. Your extension agent can help you in this specific balancing problem.

Feeding Corn Silage. Corn silage can be used successfully in the diet of the replacement gilt and in pregestation and gestation swine diets. It is not recommended for growing-finishing pigs or lactating sows because of the bulkiness of the feed. Sows and gilts will consume about 12 lb per day of corn silage, roughly three times the limit fed in a dry ration. Corn silage should be used with 1 to $1\frac{1}{4}$ lb of supplement mixture containing protein, salt, minerals, and vitamins.

The advantage to using corn silage in a ration is that lower production costs are obtained, the sow's hefty appetite is satisfied, and more nutrients are harvested per acre. The disadvantages are in the mechanics of feeding and the possibility of spoilage or abortion caused by sows consuming moldy feed. If the silage is fresh and watched carefully, this shouldn't be a problem. Make sure females are eating enough corn silage. If not, you may need to add some grain to the diet to maintain proper body condition.

16

Diseases of Swine

IDENTIFYING A SICK HOG

Swine should be observed more as a herd than as individuals because diseases affecting them generally affect numerous animals. They also should be observed while quiet, rather than when people are around working and moving them. You should be familiar with the normal habits of swine before determining what abnormal habits might be signs of impending problems.

The normal hog is a very curious mammal that will be constantly poking around and interested in observing any approach to the pen by people or other animals. A sick hog will appear listless and dull, will show a lack of curiosity, and will not be eating. If you don't hear the sound of the feed lid clanking, there definitely should be a suspicion that something is wrong.

The stool of the hog is also a good indication of difficulties. A hard stool is usually seen when body temperatures are high. Temperature elevation is frequently the result of an infective agent. A loose stool, on the other hand, is an indication of intestinal problems, infection, or poisoning. And loose, bloody stool is a possible sign of swine dysentery or whip worm infections.

Total feed consumed by the herd should be monitored. Since hogs are very fast growers, the feed consumption should always be on the increase. If for some reason there is a decrease, it is important to find out why. Quite often, this lack of appetite is a first sign of impending disease.

Hogs are very prone to several severe respiratory problems. Coughing, sneezing, drainage from the nose, temperature rise, etc., are all signs of respiratory problems, bringing about weight loss and possible death. Elevated environmental temperatures will predispose the animal to numerous respiratory problems. Because the hog does not sweat, the lungs have to take on the major responsibility for cooling the hog. An elevated temperature, whether

Table 16-1. Swine Disease Guide

BOARS

Disease / Cause	Prevention[5]	Treatment[5]	Withdrawal
	Buy boars early from herds known to be free of disease. Isolate from the swine herd for 2–3 weeks. Prior to using the boars, expose them to the females of the breeding unit 30 days before they are to be bred. This may be done by fence line contact. Have sufficient boar power, one boar for each 10 gilts to be bred in a 3-week period. Use double mating. Since mating is a learned response, spend sufficient time with the new boars in trial mating to be sure they are capable of breeding.		
Swine erysipelas: *Bacteria* *Erysipelothrix* *insidiosa*	Erysipelas vaccine,[1,3] (avirulent) Erysipelas bacterin[1,3] Oral erysipelas vaccine	Penicillin[2] Anti–swine erysipelas serum[2] Oxytetracycline injected[2]	5 days 18–22 days
Leptospirosis *Leptospira* *pomona* *grippotyphosa* *canicola* *icterohemorrhagicae* and other serotypes	*Leptospirosis*[3] bacterins Use type according to strain of leptospirosis diagnosed.	Oxytetracycline injected[2] Streptomycin injected[2] To reduce chronic carrier state of leptospirosis Chlortetracycline 200 g/ton continuously 400 g/ton at least 14 days Oxytetracycline 500 g/ton 7–14 days	18–22 days 30 days None established 5 days
Respiratory infections Pneumonia Influenza *Influenza virus* Other viruses Bacterial infection Stress from environ- mental changes	Isolate new animals. Avoid drafty conditions.	Individual treatment[2] Penicillin, injected Oxytetracycline, in- jected Herd treatment[2] Chlortetracycline or oxytetracycline in drinking water Sulfathiazole in drinking water Tetracycline in drinking water	5 days 18–22 days 1–2 days 1–2 days 10 days 4 days

Disease / Cause	Prevention[5]	Treatment[5]	Withdrawal
Arthritis and Lameness (get proper diagnosis) Bacteria Erysipelothrix insidiosa Mycoplasma hyosynoviae (gallinarum) Injuries Foot pads Hoof wall cracks	Sort for good feet and legs, good conformation.	Dependent upon diagnosis[2] Tylosin Lincocin Penicillin Antiswine erysipelas serum	4 days 2 days 5 days
Brucellosis (Bang's Disease): Bacteria Brucella suis	Buy from validated herds. Blood tests before adding animals to herd.	None	

SOWS PREGESTATION

Disease / Cause	Prevention[5]	Treatment[5]	Withdrawal
Brucellosis (Bang's disease): Bacteria Brucella suis	Buy tested animals only or from validated herds and retest before adding to the herd.	None	
Leptospirosis: (See Boars)	Vaccination 2–3 weeks prior to breeding[3]. Repeat at 6-month intervals.	Chlortetracycline 200 g/ton continuously or 400 g/ton at least 14 days Oxytetracycline 500 g/ton, 7–14 days approximately one month before farrowing. Oxytetracycline injected[2]	None established 5 days 18–22 days
Erysipelas: (See Boars)	Vaccination 2–3 weeks prior to breeding[3].	(See Boars)	

Respiratory infections Pneumonia Influenza: (*See Boars*)	Influenza during or shortly after breeding may produce a reproductive problem.		
Arthritis and lameness: (*See Boars*)	Sort breeding stock for good foot and leg conformation.		

Gestation and Farrowing

Nonspecific infections causing early embryonic death: *Bacteria* *Viruses*	Co-mingle sows and gilts. Expose them to each other 30 days prior to breeding so they will develop immunity to the bacteria and viruses that may be present in the herd. No preventive treatment is available for viral infections.		
MMA Mastitis Metritis: *Bacteria* *E. coli* *Streptococci sp.* *Corynebacterium* and other bacteria Management factors Nutritional deficiencies Unknown causes	Feed antibiotics[4] which sensitivity testing indicates would be of value in your herd. Vaccination of the sow use mixed bacterins.[3] Autogenous bacterins[3] prepared from bacteria involved in the herd problem are best. Use at 6 weeks and 2 weeks before farrowing (two injections). Vitamin E 10,000–20,000 units/ton	Streptomycin injected[2] Corticosteroids injected[2]	30 days
Agalactia: *Constipation*	Thyroprotein 100 g/ton Oxytetracycline 50 g/ton Sole ration 3 days prior to farrowing and for first week of lactation.	Mineral oil by mouth, enemas, Epsom or Glauber salts in feed or water.	None established

Disease / Cause	Prevention [5]	Treatment [5]	Withdrawal
Mastitis Metritis Hormonal deficiencies	Caution: This drug will increase the metabolic rate. Sows and gilts will become very thin unless pigs are weaned early. Not recommended for routine use. Consult your veterinarian.	See above See above Posterior pituitary extract[1]	
Atrophic rhinitis: Bacteria Bordetella bronchiseptica	Nasal swabbing is a method to aid in the diagnosis and the control of this disease. Consult your veterinarian for details	None	
Secondary invading bacteria.	To reduce carrier state from sow to pigs, use 1 lb of sodium sulfamethazine in 600 gal of drinking water 3 weeks prior to farrowing. (Many strains of Bordetella are resistant to sulfa drugs. Keep old sows in preference to gilts to reduce the amount of spread to pigs.)		10 days
Influenza Pneumonia: Influenza virus Pasteurella and other bacteria	Avoid bringing in new animals. Exposure to viruses, including eqinfluenza during gestation, may affect the baby pig before birth.	Sulfathiazole[2] in drinking water Individual treatment[2] Penicillin, injected[2] Oxytetracycline, injected[2] Tylosin, injected[2]	10 days 5 days 22 days 4 days
SMEDI Stillborn , mummified pigs Embryonic death Infertility:	Co-mingle sows and gilts 30 days before breeding. Give fence line contact with new boars. Avoid exposure of pregnant	None	

Enteroviruses *Influenza virus* *Pseudorabies virus* *Parvo virus* Hog cholera virus and other viruses which may affect the unborn pig causing early embryonic death or mummification and stillborn or weak pigs at birth.	animals to outside animals. Animals so affected usually will carry normal litters at the next breeding if not exposed to a different virus. This condition may recur in 2–3 years cycles on some farms.	None
Pseudorabies (Aujesky's disease) Virus, produces abortions, mummification of fetuses.	Bring in blood test negative animals (SN).	None
Brucellosis: *Bacteria* *Brucella suis* Abortions	(See Boars)	None
TGE Transmissible gastroenteritis: *Virus*	Vaccination of the sow twice,[1,3] 6 weeks and 2 weeks prior to farrowing.	None Avoid outside exposures during farrowing periods.
Clostridial enteritis Type C: *Bacteria* *Clostridium perfringens Type C*	Vaccination of the sow twice,[3] 6 weeks and 2 weeks prior to farrowing.	This is a disease of the baby pig which may be prevented by sow vaccination. Schedule the second vaccination as near to 2 weeks prior to farrowing as possible.
Erysipelas: *Bacteria* *Erysipelothrix insidiosa*	(See Boars) Vaccination of sow[3] can be done anytime during gestation, prefer before breeding to get maximum protection of sow.	May repeat vaccination 3–4 weeks prior to farrowing to help protect the baby pig. (See Boars)

Disease / Cause	Prevention[5]	Treatment[5]	Withdrawal
Leptospirosis: *Bacteria* *Leptospira* *pomona* *grippotyphosa* *canicola* *icterohemmor-* *rhagicae* *and other serotypes*	(See Boars) Vaccination of sow[1,3] can be done anytime during gestation. Prefer before breeding to get maximum protection. (Also see feed recommendations under Boars.)	(See Boars)	
Arthritis and lameness *(get proper diagnosis)* *Bacteria* *Mycoplasma hyosynoviae* *(gallinarum)* *Erysipelothrix* *insidiosa* *Mineral deficiencies* *Injuries* *Foot pads* *Hoof wall cracks*	Good selection practices may be an aid.	Treatment based on diagnosis[2] Tylosin Lincocin Penicillin Corticosteroids Antiswine erysipelas serum	4 days 2 days 5 days

BABY PIGS

Disease / Cause	Prevention[5]	Treatment[5]	Withdrawal
Hypoglycemia *Sugar deficiency:* *Starvation* *Chilling*	Avoid chilling. Allow pigs to nurse shortly after birth. (Don't keep the pigs away until the sow is through farrowing.)	Dextrose or dark syrup by mouth or injected intraperitoneally as dextrose, solution.	
TGE Transmissible gastroenteritis Baby pig disease: *TGE virus*	Avoid exposure. Limit people, animals, trucks on the premises. Don't bring it home from markets or your neighbors. Sow vaccination (See Sows)	No treatment is of value. Normal electrolytes[1] in water will help to replace the fluid loss in pigs. If they are over 2–3 weeks of age, you may save a few more pigs. Consult your veterinarian.	

Disease	Prevention	Treatment
Clostridial enteritis: *Bacteria Clostridium perfringens Type C*	Sow vaccination[3] to protect baby pig through colostrum. (See Sows) Clostridium Type C antitoxin at birth. This may be too late, sow vaccination preferred.	None
Pseudorabies (Aujesky's disease) Virus, produces central nervous disturbances, diarrhea, vomiting, severe death losses.	None (See Sows— Gestation/Farrowing)	None
Nonspecific diarrheas: *E. coli and other*	Before farrowing, expose the sow and gilt to manure from the farrowing house. Bacterins to the sow (preferably autogenous) may be helpful. Sanitation of the building, wash and fumigate. Wash the sow or gilt when brought to the farrowing house. They may be carriers. Allow an interval between farrowings. Consult your veterinarian for a specific program.	Early treatment (first 24 hours most important) with an antibiotic or sulfonamide drug selected by using a sensitivity test.[4] Where the problem exists, treatment at 24 hours whether scours is observed or not is a good practice.
Nutritional anemia: *Iron deficiency*	Inject with injectable iron compounds at 1–3 days of age. Inject into the muscle of the neck or under the skin of the neck or flank. Give a second injection if pigs are not starting to eat	Once anemia occurs, use injectable iron compounds. Add additional iron and copper to the creep rations.

Disease / Cause	Prevention[5]	Treatment[5]	Withdrawal
	creep feed by $3\frac{1}{2}$ weeks of age. Oral iron dosed individually twice weekly until the pigs are eating will prevent anemia, but it is a time-consuming job. Oral iron in moss or feed is a valuable aid to prevent nutritional anemia.		
Pneumonia: Bacteria Pastuerella Mycoplasma Secondary to atrophic rhinitis Drafts	Improve management, avoid drafts and chilling. Bacterins (preferably autogenous) for Pastuerella pneumonia.	Oxytetracycline[2] Penicillin[2] Tylosin[2] These drugs are to be injected. Broadspectrum antibiotics oxytetracycline or chlortetracycline fed at high levels may be valuable in secondary chronic pneumonias.	22 days 5 days 4 days
Atrophic rhinitis: Bacteria Bordetella bronchiseptica	Nasal swabbing of sows. (Consult your veterinarian about the merits and demerits of nasal swabbing.) Rhinitis-free breeding stock. Wean pigs early in infected herds. Save older sows to raise replacement gilts. Avoid stress conditions; enteritis, anemia, pneumonia, and parasites, which will make the effects of rhinitis more severe.	Chlortetracycline 100 g/ton Sulfamethazine 100 g/ton Penicillin 50 g/ton Chlortetracycline 100 g/ton Sulfathiazole 100 g/ton Penicillin 50 g/ton Tylosin 100 g/ton Sulfamethazine 100 g/ton	7 days 7 days 5 days

Disease	Management/Prevention	Drugs	Withdrawal
Inclusion body rhinitis (IBR) *Virus, may be observed in conjunction with Bordetella bronchiseptica rhinitis*	Keep cats and other carrier animals out of the farrowing house, as they can be carriers of the bacteria Bordetella bronchiseptica. Bordetella bacterin Injected at 7 and 28 days of age. Consider only as an aid. Maintain good preventive disease practices as well as good nutritional level.	Use for a minimum of 5 weeks, preferably to at least 75 lb in weight. Many strains of bacteria are resistant to sulfa drugs. To control secondary pneumonias it may be necessary to use these products to market weight. Antibiotics may be injected for treatment of individuals showing respiratory problems. (See Pneumonia, Baby pigs.)	
	The effects of the disease may be quite severe in very young pigs. Keeping older sows may be of value.	None	
Arthritis (pyogenic): *Bacteria* *Streptococci sp* *Corynebacterium sp* *Staphylococci sp*	Clip needle teeth in first few hours, ear notch and dock pigs in a clean and sanitary manner. Avoid rough floors. Mechanical abrasions of the feet and knees occur in first few hours of life. Disinfection of navels is important, but other sources of infection are the ears, knees, and tail in modern swine units. The use of epoxy paints to improve the floor surface may be helpful; avoid excessively smooth floors.	Oxytetracycline[2] Penicillin[2] Tylosin[2]	18–22 days 5 days 4 days
Lameness: *Navel infection* *Tail docking*	(See above) Use a sanitary method to reduce infection and control hemorrhage.	Injectable antibiotics (See above)	

307

Disease / Cause	Prevention[5]	Treatment[5]	Withdrawal
Foot and leg abrasions Other injuries	Chicken debeakers are useful for this purpose as they cauterize the tail stump.		
Bacterial enteritis: Bacteria E. coli most common Erratic diet sow's milk and creep feed Pigs immune system at low point	Avoid chilling and drafts. Keep pens dry. Consider using creep feeds with lower protein levels that have additional lysine and other fortification added. Use nitrafurazone or sulfas in the drinking water at weaning. Carbadox in the feed may be of value. See note concerning the use of carbadox under Weaning Pigs and Finishing Hogs (Necrotic enteritis).	Nitrafurazone or tetracyclines in pig's drinking water.[2]	5 days 4 days

Disease / Cause	Prevention[5]	Treatment[5]	Withdrawal
Colibacillosis (post weaning diarrhea) Feeder pig enteritis Nonspecific bacterial enteritis: Bacterial Usually E. coli	Avoid stresses, feed changes. Medicate feed and/or water for 5–7 days during stress periods	(See Necrotic enteritis) Correct anemia if present. Use injectable iron and feeds with additional iron and copper. Normal electrolytes may be of value in the water. Additional fortification with B vitamins in the diet may be helpful at this time.	
Edema disease (enterotoxemia): Bacteria E. coli Stress such as weaning, shipping, feed changes	Avoid stresses. Use feeds with higher fiber content during this period.	Starvation for 24 hours. Nitrafurazone or Tetracyclines in pig's drinking water.[2]	5 days 4 days

308

Condition / Cause	Prevention / Control	Treatment	Withdrawal time
Parakeratosis: *Zinc deficiency* *High calcium* *Rations or other mineral imbalances*	50 ppm of zinc added to the ration.	150 ppm of zinc added to the ration. Check the amount of calcium in the ration.	
Hemorrhagic syndrome (bleeding disease) *Anti-vitamin K factors? Mycotoxins Moldy feeds Unknown causes*	Menadione sodium bisulfite 2 g/ton of feed	Increased levels of menadione sodium bisulfite in feed and/or water.	
Jowl abscess (cervical abscesses): *Bacteria* *Streptococci sp most common Many others also associated with abscess formation*	Vaccination at 10–15 weeks of age[1,2] Chlortetracycline 50-100 g/ton to reduce incidence	Surgically drain abscesses. (limited value on a herd basis) Penicillin[2]—conduct sensitivity tests of bacteria present to determine correct antibiotic.[4]	None established 5 days
Erysipelas: *Bacteria* *Erysipelothrix insidiosa*	Erysipelas vaccine[1,3] (avirulent) Erysipelas bacterin[3] Oral erysipelas vaccine	Penicillin[2] Antiswine erysipelas serum[2]	5 days
Necrotic enteritis Necro bacterial enteritis *Bacteria* *Salmonella sp* *May be present as a systemic disease with little or no diarrhea present. Contaminated feed sources. Carrier animals. Isolate new animals for 3–4 weeks before mixing with other swine*	Bacitracin 50–100 g/ton of feed Chlortetracycline 50–100 g/ton of feed Furazolidone 150 g/ton of feed or Furazolidone 200 g/ton of feed, 2 wks 150 g/ton of feed, 3 wks	Bacitracin Not less than 100 g/ton of feed Carbadox* 50 g/ton Not to be fed to swine over 75 lb Chlortetracycline 100–200 g/ton feed Furazolidone 300 g/ton of feed Feed for 10–14 days	None established 70 days None established 5 days 5 days

Disease / Cause	Prevention[5]	Treatment[5]	Withdrawal
	100 g/ton of feed, 5 weeks	Neomycin sulfate 70–140 g/ton of feed	30 days
		Nitrafurazone 500 g/ton of feed 5-7 days	5 days
		Water-soluble form[2]	5 days
	Oxytetracycline 50 g/ton of feed	Oxytetracycline 100 g/ton of feed	None established
		Penicillin-streptomycin combinations Maximum 90 g/ton of feed in combination.	None established
		Sulfathiazole in drinking water.[2]	10 days
Hemorrhagic dysentery Vibrionic dysentery (bloody scours) *Vibrio coli* *Large spirochete* *Possibly other* *unknown causes*	Isolate new animals. Avoid contaminated trucks and equipment.	Carbadox 50g/ton. Not to be fed to swine over 75 lb.	70 days
	Arsanilic acid or sodium arsanilate 0.005–0.01% 45–90 g/ton of feed	Arsanilic acid or	5 days
		Sodium arsanilate 0.025–0.04% for 5–6 days 230–360 g/ton of feed	5 days
		Sodium arsanilate[2] Water-soluble for drinking water.	5 days
		3 Nitro-4 hydroxy phenyl arsonic acid[2] 0.02% feed for 5–6 days	5 days
	Furazolidone 150 g/ton of feed or Furazolidone 200 g/ton—2 weeks	Furazolidone 300 g/ton Feed for 10–14 days	5 days

Disease	Prevention/Control	Treatment	Withdrawal
	150 g/ton—3 weeks	Lincomycin hydrochloride 100g/ton for 3 weeks, then 40 g/ton	6 days
	100 g/ton—5 weeks	Neomycin sulfate 70–140 g/ton of feed	30 days
	Lincomycin hydrochloride 40 g/ton	Nitrafurazone—water-soluble	5 days
	Oxytetracycline 50 g/ton of feed	Oxytetracycline 100 g/ton	None established
	Tylosin 100 g/ton of feed for 3 weeks, then 40 g/ton of feed to market weight	Tylosin 100 g/ton of feed for 2–6 weeks after treating with tylosin in drinking water for 3–10 days[2]	None established
			2 days
	Virginiamycin Aid in the control, in swine up to 120 lb, 25 g/ton	Virginiamycin Treatment and control 100 g/ton 2 weeks followed by 50 g/ton	None established
		Treatment in nonbreeding swine over 120 lb, 100 g/ton for 2 weeks	None established
Pneumonias: *Secondary to atrophic rhinitis*	(See Atrophic rhinitis, Baby pigs)		
Secondary to influenza	Early treatment. Avoid drafts.	Individual injected[2] Oxytetracycline	22 days
Pastuerella sp.	Problem herds can use Pasteurella[3] bacterins.	Penicillin	5 days
Mycoplasma (VPP, SEP)	Avoid bringing in new animals; isolate all additions to the herd.	Herd[2] Chlortetracycline	1–2 days
	Reduce migration of ascarids (roundworms), makes the pneumonia more severe.	Oxytetracycline	1–2 days
		Sulfamethazine	7 days
		Sulfathiazole	10 days
		Other sulfa drugs	Dependent upon the drugs used
		Expectorant drugs	

Disease / Cause	Prevention[5]	Treatment[5]	Withdrawal
		All of the above drugs for herd use are to be used in the drinking water.	
		Tylosin plus sulfamethazine 100/100 (g/ton) in feed	5 days
Atrophic rhinitis: (See Baby pigs)	Avoid stresses. Enteritis, pneumonia, parasites all make rhinitis more severe. Sulfamethazine or sulfathiazole in the feed of small pigs, use for at least 5 weeks, preferably to 75 lb in weight. (Many strains of Bordetella are resistant to sulfonamide therapy).	Sulfathiazole or sulfamethazine in drinking water.	10 days 7 days
Arthritis: Bacteria Mycoplasma hyosynoviae (granularum)		Tylosin[2] Lincocin[2] Early treatment essential.	4 days 2 days
Erysipelas		Penicillin[2] Antiswine erysipelas serum[2]	5 days
Tail biting: Tail biting Injuries Crowding Dietary deficiencies Lack of enough feeders and waterers Lack of bedding (bare concrete floors) Weather changes Manure pit gases Unknown causes	Remove tails on baby pigs. Well-fortified rations. Avoid crowding.	Individual[2] Penicillin Oxytetracycline Early treatment is essential. Herd Organic iodides[2] Magnesium oxide in feed. Hay, paper sacks, tires, bowling balls, to give hogs something to reduce boredom. If closely confined, move pigs to a larger pen or outdoors.	5 days 22 days None established None established

Anemia:
  Nutritional
    (iron deficiencies)
  Eperythrozoonosis
    (blood parasite)
  Moldy grains
    (blood loss from hemorrhages)
  Gastric ulcers
    (blood loss)
  Vitamin K
    deficiency or interferences with absorption and utilization
  Postweaning diarrhea
    (secondary effect)

Acute hemorrhages as from ulcers and the effects of mold are seldom observed early enough to justify treatment. Other anemias are corrected by adding iron and copper to the diet. Injected iron is used in conjunction with other postweaning diarrhea treatments.

---

*(At this time carbadox has not been cleared for use in combinations with sulfa drugs. If you need sulfa drugs to aid in controlling rhinitis and pneumonia, consult your veterinarian for proper application of these products in your herd.)

Source: Dr. Vaylord D. Ladwig, Departments of Clinical Medicine and Continuing Education, College of Veterinary Medicine, University of Illinois, Urbana, Ill. Reprinted with permission from John B. Herrick, Feedstuffs. (Minneapolis, Minn.: Miller Publishing Company, Ref. Issue, Vol. 49, No. 30), 1977.

[1] Available through your veterinarian.

[2] Follow your veterinarian and the manufacturers' instructions.

[3] Slaughter not permitted for at least 21 days after biological products have been injected.

[4] Ideally the choice of antibiotics should be based on antibiotic sensitivity tests. Consult your veterinarian for details.

[5] Most of the drugs listed should be considered as aids in prevention and treatment of the disease. Combinations of several of these drugs are permitted. See Feed Additive Compendium for any recent changes.

This disease guide is a compilation in chart form of the more common disease and parasite conditions observed in swine. This information is generally available from many sources. Proper application of preventive measures are best programmed by a veterinarian as he establishes a herd health program for a given production unit. Due to the differences in management, facilities, and a host of other factors, no one herd health program can encompass all of the needs of all producers.

The necessity for the prevention of diseases in swine herds is becoming increasingly important. With diseases such as pseudorabies (Aujesky's disease), the introduction of carrier animals into the herd can start a costly disease outbreak for the pork producer. It is also important that the health history of the animals to be added to a herd be known and proper testing procedures be employed before bringing the animals to the production unit. Additionally, a strict isolation procedure should be developed before any new animals are added to the main herd. The veterinarian is the key individual in helping the producer to make knowledgeable decisions on the addition of animals to a herd. Adoption of a "closed herd" philosophy, or as nearly closed as possible, is very important in today's production enterprises.

brought about by weather or infection, may cause a panting that is abnormally fast. If hogs are panting and hanging around wet areas or lying in the mud constantly, this could be an indication of elevated body temperature. In hot weather, hogs need to have a sprinkler system or some other method of cooling off. For temperature elevations due to disease, the cause must be found and corrected.

The skin of a hog should be monitored for signs of numerous disorders. Hair loss or lesions in the skin are indications of vitamin or mineral deficiencies but more commonly are due to lice or mange infestations. Icterus (yellowing) of the skin is indicative of parasitic infection (eperythrozoonosis). Excessive oil on the skin indicates "greasy pig disease." Sensitivity to sunlight could be an indication of phenothiazine toxicity, moldy feed, or a reaction to some pasture legumes. Mineral deficiencies such as zinc show up as a thickening and infection of the skin (parakeratosis). Pellagra, swine pox, erysipelas, and hog cholera all show up as conditions affecting the skin as a part of their infective nature. Table 16-1 gives a swine disease guide in chart form.

RESPIRATORY DISEASES

General Respiratory Abnormalities

Respiratory disorders are a very common problem for the pig. Numerous disease organisms, anemia, parasite migration, and environmental conditions work together to cause respiratory problems. In addition to providing for the exchange of oxygen and carbon dioxide, the lung is an important source of heat reduction for the pig. Since swine do not have "sweat glands," their heat losses must occur through the lungs. Therefore, during hot weather, their respiratory rate may be 4 to 6 times as rapid as under normal situations. A normal respiratory rate is approximately 20 to 30 per minute. Signs of respiratory problems include coughing, sneezing, labored breathing, and panting. "Thumps" is a severe sign of respiratory disease; it may result from chronic pneumonia or severe anemia in young pigs.

Epistaxis (Nosebleed)

Nosebleed may occur due to a minor injury such as bumping the feeders with the snout. Some type of trauma is the most common cause of epistaxis, but generally this is not a condition to be worried about. However, nosebleed can be a sign of severe atrophic rhinitis and parasitic infections. If bleeding continues, further checks should be made for disease.

Atrophic Rhinitis (Infectious Rhinitis)

New entries into the herd are the primary reasons for atrophic rhinitis (AR) outbreaks. This is not a disease that causes many deaths, but it does create a tremendous economic loss because of irritation to the nose, inability to eat, and a generally deteriorated physical condition. Its greatest effect is the predisposition to secondary lung infections brought about by the reduction of the normal filtering activity of the nasal bones. The snout is affected by decreased growth of the small, thin bones that make up the nasal cavity (turbinate bones). The turbinates are reduced in size and are misshaped by this disease. Failure of normal turbinate growth causes a mishapen snout and severe pain. When severe degeneration occurs on both sides, the nose is shorter than the lower jaw. When one side of the turbinates is affected, the nose turns to the affected side.

Signs. AR develops first in young pigs about 3 weeks of age or less and becomes more chronic as the pig grows older. There is sneezing, coughing, blowing, and snorting. The tear ducts may also be plugged up, creating tear discharges or dirty rings under the eyes. The nose will occasionally appear bloody on the surface.

Cause. Numerous conditions probably contribute to the severity of AR, but the bacterium *Bordetella bronchiseptica* appears to be the primary infecting agent. This bacterium is found in most of the pig herds in the United States. It is very difficult to control because it is not exclusively an infecting agent of pigs. It can be carried by any mammal. The farm cat is the most common nonswine carrier beccause of its habit of sleeping under the heat lamp with new litters. Some strains of *Bordetella* are very mild, producing little or no lesion formation. Other strains are capable of severe lesion production. Dust and other irritants may also contribute to the severity of the attack. Researchers are not completely sure of all of the factors contributing to the condition, but *B. bronchiseptica* is considered the major initiative cause of atrophic rhinitis in the United States. Three things must occur for severe lesions to develop:

1. Infection with a pathogenic organism.
2. Infection by 1 to 3 weeks of life.
3. Persistence of the flu bug for 3 to 5 weeks in the pig's nose.

Animals infected later may carry the flu bug but may not have severe nose damage.

Prevention. Prevention is based on reduction of exposure and increased removal of flu organisms from the nose during early life. Established herds can remain free of the disease only by keeping a closed herd, raising their own replacements, using artificial insemination, or buying only SPF hogs.

It is recommended that all animals be purchased from one source that is free of *B. bronchiseptica* and that the owner provide adequate ventilation in swine houses and good care for nursing pigs because any other disease (scours, etc.) can make an atrophic rhinitis outbreak worse.

The Veterinary Research Institute of Iowa State recommends the following procedure to keep rhinitis out of an unaffected herd.

1. No exposure to other pigs.
2. Use of only *Bordetella*-checked boars.
3. Control of cat and rodent population.
4. Testing of each new crop of pigs for *Bordetella*.

A culture preparation made from infected pigs is 90% accurate in diagnosing the presence of *Bordetella*. Three negative cultures by a veterinarian over a 3-week period would allow the animal to be reasonably classified free of *B. bronchiseptica*. This test is most effective in testing on a herd basis or where animals are maintained separately until test results are returned.

Treatment. Sulfathiazole is used in the water and sulfamethazine is added to the feed continuously for 5 weeks as a treatment. Sows should be treated before farrowing to reduce the organisms transferred from the sow to her newborn litter. These sulfa drugs were effective in the early days of rhinitis outbreaks, but now it appears that more resistant strains have developed, and even this treatment is meeting with less than desired results.

There is a rhinitis bacterin containing killed *Bordetella* organisms that is now available. It is given during the first week the pig is born, and again at 28 days after birth to provide protection against the disease. Sows are injected with the same preparation 4 and 2 weeks prior to farrowing, and boars are injected twice annually to provide similar protection.

Tuberculosis

The incidence of tuberculosis is not as great in swine as it is in cattle. TB historically occurred in hogs when they were pastured with cattle; they picked up the disease from the bovines. Since the bovine TB eradication program began, however, the major cases have been of avian (poultry) origin. The main losses occur from condemnation of the hog carcass at the time of slaughter.

Signs. There are few or no outward signs. Occasionally, the joints of the hog will be stiff, indicating an involvement of the limbs by the organism. The major diagnostic signs are lesions in the intestinal lymph nodes and in the head lymph nodes.

Cause. The cause is a mycobacterium organism. Although swine are subject to infection by three types of mycobacteria, the most common one is the avian mycobacterium. For this reason it is recommended that swine not have contact with chickens, wild birds, or their droppings.

If you have poultry over a year old on your farm, chances are good that tuberculosis is present in them and represents a potential hazard to the hogs. For this reason old chicken houses should not be used as swine buildings, nor should chickens be allowed to run in the same area with swine. The TB organisms are very resistant to environmental conditions and may exist for years on infected premises.

Prevention. Prevention of tuberculosis in cattle is the main way in which the cycle has been broken. Because of an extremely effective tuberculosis test program in the United States, the disease has almost been eradicated. An ongoing program of testing cattle for TB protects humans and hogs from a spreading of the organism. However, the increase of avian-strain organisms indicates the importance of reducing exposure of swine to birds and their droppings.

Treatment. There are no effective treatments for swine.

Swine Influenza (Swine Flu)

Signs. The fall and spring with the sudden onset of cold damp weather bring about conditions favoring swine influenza development. It is a highly contagious, fast-moving outbreak that affects virtually every hog in the herd. There is a painful deep cough accompanied by rapid breathing and reluctance to move around. Temperatures may range as high as 107°F. Hogs will lie prostrate on the ground, refuse feed, and have a mucous discharge from the eyes and nose. There is a 1% to 4% mortality rate due primarily to secondary bacterial infections brought on by the initial viral infection. The outbreak usually lasts 3 to 7 days. The hogs that live recover quickly. Principal loss is economic, resulting from loss of weight and deteriorated physical condition.

Cause. The cause is a combination of the influenza virus and stress brought on by inclement weather in the fall and spring. Internal parasites may also precipitate an outbreak of swine influenza through lung migration and by reducing an animal's resistance to rapid virus replication. Ascarid migration also increases the severity of bacterial infections that accompany swine influenza.

Prevention. Protection from the weather and adequate health, sanitation, and nutrition factors are the chief remedies. Vaccines have been injected experimentally but have not proven economically practical. Once an animal recovers, he has strong immunity to swine influenza. Recovered swine act as inapparent carriers of the influenza virus and transmit it to susceptible pigs. Therefore in most swine herds the seed of infection is already present.

Treatment. Penicillin and sulfa drugs may be used once an outbreak occurs, to prevent death from secondary bacterial invasions.

Viral Pig Pneumonia (VPP, Mycoplasma Pneumonia)

Viral pig pneumonia actually is misnamed because the condition is not caused by a virus, but rather by a bacterium—*Mycoplasma hypopneumoniae.*

Signs. The most common sign is a dry, rasping, persistent, nonproductive cough, which is most noticeable when pigs are quiet. During the first 2 to 3 days of infection, young pigs 3 to 10 weeks of age may have mild diarrhea accompanied by this cough, but the diarrhea is very mild and short-lived and generally goes unnoticed by the producer. Slow growth and unthriftiness of litters are the major results of the disease.

Generally a simple *M. hypopneumoniae* infection is quite mild, but secondary *Pasteurella*, *Corynebacterium*, and *Hemophilias* may cause severe disease losses.

Cause. *Mycoplasma hypopneumoniae* is the cause.

Prevention. Pigs should be stocked from a known VPP-free source. The organism does not penetrate the placenta; so one source of pigs free of the disease is SPF pigs. These pigs are not immune to the attack of VPP but are free of the disease when introduced to your farm. Surveys indicate most swine are infected with the VPP organism during their lifetime. Stress of moving, mixing, and sorting; sudden weather changes; damp pens; effects of atrophic rhinitis; ascarid migrations; and influenza attacks are all intensifying agents. Stressful chores should be divided whenever possible.

Treatment. There is currently no specific treatment for *M. hypopneumoniae*, but the secondary bacterial infection can be treated. *Pasteurella* is the main bacteria in the secondary infection, and research has shown that *Pasteurella* bacterin can be used at 6 to 8 weeks of age to provide some relief. Tetracycline is a broad-spectrum antibiotic that is often used. Tylosin (Elanco) is effective when injected. Other products are Lincomycin (Upjohn), an injectable product, and Tiamultin (Squibb), a feed additive product that has been researched in both the United States and Australia with encouraging response.

Pasteurellosis (Swine Plague, Hemorrhagic Septicemia, Pneumonia)

Pasteurellosis is related to VPP and may be confused with it or may even occur in combination with VPP on occasions.

Signs. Coughing, 105°F to 106°F temperature, depression, very labored breathing, and occasionally "sitting dog" position are characteristic signs. Hogs have such difficulty and pain when breathing that they assume a position reclining on their posteriors (sitting dog) to get more relief while they breathe. This condition lasts 5 to 8 days and is accompanied by relatively high death losses unless proper treatment is instituted. Some pigs that live do not eat well or gain well after suffering the original signs. In the very acute septicemic form, the organism is carried in the bloodstream, affecting the whole body, and normally death will occur within 24 to 36 hours. Small hemorrhages (petechiae) occur throughout the body in this form and are a common observation on post-mortem examination. These animals may die with only a few or no outward signs.

Cause. A bacterium—*P. multocida*—is the primary organism that causes the disease, although other bacteria combined with parasite migration and dust problems contribute to the severity of an outbreak.

Prevention. There is a *Pasteurella* bacterin available in areas where the condition is endemic. Strict sanitation, avoidance of temperature variations and of cold damp quarters, and control of parasites and dust are keys to prevention.

Treatment. Even after hogs get over this disease, they still have sufficient lung damage to make them "poor doers," and it is questionable whether it is economically feasible to keep some of these survivors.

However, treatment may save most infected pigs. Treatment must include extensive, very high levels of medication for at least 5 to 6 days before going to a lower level of medication. Results must be monitored before deciding to reduce the level of treatment. This is where a veterinarian would be very helpful.

Sulfamethazine at the dosage of 1.5 gm/lb of body weight is recommended for the first 3 days. The second 3 days, dosage may be reduced to 1 gm/lb. Treatment may be lowered further after this, on a small group, to determine if the disease has been arrested or whether treatment should continue.

Fresh water, and dry, warm, well-ventilated buildings are essential during convalescence. High humidity and cold dampness contribute to a higher death rate.

REPRODUCTIVE AND GENETIC DISEASES

SMEDI

A group of viruses cause a complicated disorder that has been given the name *SMEDI*, based on the number of problems this term represents: stillbirth, mummification, embryonic death, and infertility.

The two key points in understanding this syndrome are to recognize (1) that the disease is caused by a group of viruses rather than by one specific virus and (2) that abortion is not a part of the signs. This disorder is very difficult to diagnose. When SMEDI is suspected, blood from stillborn pigs and complete mummies should be obtained for diagnostic tests. Paired serum samples from the sow taken before breeding and after the disorder occurs may help in diagnosis. However, whatever specific virus is the cause, prevention will be the same.

Signs. Any one or all of the following signs are characteristic of SMEDI. (Appearances will be extremely variable depending on stage of gestation when sows are affected.)

1. Very small litters (2 to 3 pigs).

2. Many mummified fetuses carried to full term.

3. Pigs that appear normal, but are born weak and die soon afterwards.

4. If the infection occurs before fetal bones begin to develop (less than 35 days after conception), sows may have appeared to have conceived in a

normal breeding pattern but return to heat in 28 to 45 days. If the infection occurs after the bones of the fetus have begun to develop (more than 35 days after conception), the sow appears to be having a normal pregnancy, but most or all pigs will be born mummies; or she may nest, produce milk, and show signs of farrowing but suddenly loose all these signs.

5. If the infection occurs in late gestation, the sow has stillborn pigs that look normal but are born dead. Most sows eventually return to heat.

6. Surviving pigs show weakened conditions and higher susceptibility to disease. The theory is that this is caused by a slow movement of the virus between each developing fetus in the uterus. The weak pigs are suspected to be the last infected; the virus is carried over and lesions have developed after birth, but have not caused death.

Cause. A group of at least eight enteroviruses and other viruses have been identified in the syndrome. These viruses do not affect other species with the same result.

Prevention. After the initial attack, sows develop an immunity to the specific agent involved and return to normal production. New outbreaks only involve replacements brought into the herd or new viruses that are introduced by new stock.

Pennsylvania State University recommends the following preventive measures:

1. Co-mingle sows and gilts for one month prior to the breeding season. One month is considered sufficient time to create immunity in gilts prior to pregnancy.

2. Isolate recently purchased animals that could introduce a virus to which other sows have not developed an immunity.

3. Keep affected sows if they return to heat and cycle normally. This would indicate an immunity to at least one type of virus. They are a better risk than replacing with sows or gilts with an unknown immunity.

Treatment. There is no vaccine available and no known treatment. The preventive measures to develop immunity are the best recourse. In addition to the above recommendations, fresh manure from new animals should be transferred to nonpregnant herdmates by fence contact, pen rotation, or direct feeding 30 days before breeding starts.

Myoclonus Congenita of Baby Pigs ("Jittery Pig," "Dancing Pig," "St. Vitus Dance")

Signs. At birth or shortly thereafter pigs develop tremors, occasional weakness in the hind limbs, and difficulty in nursing. The tremors usually disappear when lying down. The signs are aggravated by excitement and may persist for hours or months. The average recovery is at 5 to 6 weeks of age. Some pigs are poor "doers," however, even after recovery.

Cause. Exact causes are unknown, but viral infection of piglets before birth is one possible cause. Pseudorabies virus and other viruses have been implicated as causative agents. Hereditary "shaker" pigs have been reported in Britain but not in the United States. Boars may be carriers of the virus, but this has not been corroborated to date.

Prevention. Immunity should follow the initial outbreak. Therefore both boars and sows from that mating should be used again.

Treatment. There is no treatment for the precipitating condition, but pigs often develop hypoglycemia (low blood sugar) as a secondary condition because of inability to nurse. Administer 3 to 5 cc of a sterile 50% glucose solution intraperitoneally plus 1 teaspoon of Karo syrup several times per day until strength is recovered.

Thick Forelegs

Signs. Signs are enlarged forelegs (below the elbows) on pigs at birth. About 25% of the litter is affected. The piglets have difficulty walking and nursing and develop hypoglycemia.

Cause. The cause is an inherited factor passed on by the boar and sow.

Prevention. Avoid matings that have produced the condition before.

Treatment. There is no treatment for the precipitating condition, but pigs often develop hypoglycemia (low blood sugar) as a secondary condition. Moderate to severe involvement is considered lethal. This condition should not be confused with the thickening of the forelimbs seen with neonatal streptococcus (navel ill).

Brucellosis

Signs. Abortion is the key sign. It can occur at any stage of gestation but normally happens at 2 to 3 months or later. Retained placenta, temporary sterility due to inflammation of the uterus, lowered conception rate, pigs born weak, inflammation of the mammary gland, and arthritis are additional signs.

Males infected with brucellosis have signs of orchitis (swelling of the testes) and lameness.

Cause. A bacterium causes the disease. Swine are most often infected with *Brucella suis*, but are also occasionally infected with *Brucella melitinisis* and the bovine variety, *Brucella abortus*.

This bacterium is very resistant and hard to kill with any disinfectant unless protective organic material is removed. It remains in the soil, water, or aborted fetus for up to 60 days under natural conditions. Direct exposure to sunlight greatly accelerates *Brucella* death. Similarly dye, cresylic acid compounds, and sodium orthophenylphenate will kill the organism provided the area is well scrubbed with soap and water prior to disinfection.

Prevention. There is no vaccine to prevent the disease in swine. Herds should be tested annually, and reactors eliminated in order to control the disease. Buy replacement animals from brucellosis-validated herds or animals that have had a negative brucellosis test. Isolate breeding herds from feeder pigs, community boars, and other species of livestock. Brucellosis from goats and cattle may also infect contacted hogs, but the efficiency of transfer is not great.

Treatment. There is no treatment for brucellosis. Infected animals should be slaughtered.

Leptospirosis

Signs. The main signs are abortion, small weak pigs at farrowing, or a high incidence of stillbirths. The only other signs, in adult hogs, are a mild rise in temperature and a short loss of appetite. In some herds that have been exposed to the disease for the first time there is an abortion "storm." In other herds the disease spreads slowly, causing abortions that occur over a span of a month or more. Frequency of abortions will then diminish as immunity develops. Most abortions occur 2 to 4 weeks before parturition. Aborted fetuses have generally been dead several days before abortion.

Cause. There are five strains of the leptospirosis organism that swine are currently considered susceptible to—*Leptospira pomona, grippotyphosa, canicola, icterohemorragiae, and hardjo.* None of these seem to produce significant clinical signs of disease in adults other than abortion, stillbirths, etc. All five strains have an affinity for the placenta, liver, and particularly the kidney of infected swine. Contamination to feed, water, and pasture is through the urine of affected animals. Cattle, rats, raccoons, and other wildlife are also carriers of the organism and serve to spread the disease. The active organism is carried in the urine and excreted for up to 6 months in swine after clinical recovery. The reason for abortion is that the organism attacks the placenta (sac) and produces placental necrosis (a killing of the tissue), which kills the developing pigs.

Prevention. Several programs can be incorporated into the management system to help prevent the disease. The most common preventive measure is vaccination, which should be done 2 to 3 weeks prior to breeding but can be used at any stage, even during pregnancy. If the disease is suspected in the herd, blood samples should be taken, and a serological examination should be conducted to determine what types of organisms are involved. Then use the vaccine or bacterin that is specific in its control of the particular organism. All five serotypes have been isolated from swine-producing areas. Therefore, a good general recommendation would include vaccination with a five-serotype bacterin.

Control the rodent population on the farm, and keep dogs and other animals away from the swine herd since they are potential carriers.

Any new animal brought onto the premises should be isolated and tested for lepto prior to admission to the herd. Routine antibiotic treatment and vaccination of new additions have also been recommended.

Treatment. Streptomycin is usually the preferred drug. Two injections given 24 hours apart rid the animal of the disease and stop the carrier effect as well. The dose is 25 mg/kg or 12 mg/lb of body weight. Other antibiotics may be used such as oxytetracycline or chlortetracycline at 400 to 500 gm/ton for 4 weeks to stop the shedding of the leptospiral organisms from infected swine.

MMA (Metritis-Mastitis-Agalactia Syndrome)

MMA has become an increasing problem with the trend toward a large number of sows farrowing in confinement and with few vacant breaks between the farrowing groups.

Signs. Metritis means an infection of the uterus; mastitis involves an infection in the mammary gland; and agalactia means little or no production of milk. These are the major signs of MMA. The condition normally occurs in sows 1 to 3 days after farrowing, although it can occur at any time up until the baby pigs are weaned. Normally, the first sign is a hungry baby pig because of a lack of milk production in the affected sow. Vaginal discharge has been described as a consistent finding with agalactia; however, clinical observation indicates that the vaginal discharge has no value as a predictor of MMA or of a metritis in the affected sow. The sow will have a mild rise in temperature of 1 to 3 degrees above normal, she will go off feed, and she may develop a hot and painful udder with little or no milk production. Some sows have a yellowish white discharge from the vagina. Baby pigs nursing affected sows will become dehydrated due to a lack of liquid consumption. The baby pigs also often develop a diarrhea at this stage. Although the disease affects the sows primarily, the biggest problem is with a 50 to 100% loss in poorly nursed baby pigs. Even baby pigs that do make it are often runts and do not do very well.

Cause. Although exact causes are not known, research has indicated that a number of factors could be involved. Suspected are bacteria, fungi, viruses, and possibly hormone imbalances. There is evidence that milk production is a heritable trait that can be selected for. There is also some indication that nutrition is involved because overfat sows are more susceptible to the problem than others. This overfat condition may cause farrowing problems, exhaustion, and increased stress, thereby lowering the resistance of the sows to infection. The main infectious agent involved in MMA problems is probably *E. coli* and its endotoxins. *E. coli* may enter the mammary glands directly through the teats or indirectly by absorption of endotoxin from the gut, which then causes reduced milk production. Metritis is the least consistent finding with less than one-quarter of the affected animals having metritis. Agalactia without mastitis or metritis has been observed. It is due to inadequate mammary development caused by hormonal imbalances. Poor underlines and inadequate spacing of nipples may contribute to milking problems due to crowding of some glands by others. Pigs on the crowded glands will generally starve out by 1 to 2 weeks after birth.

Prevention and Treatment. Since so little is known about the actual causative factors of the disease, prevention and treatment are combined. The best preventive measure is strict sanitation, especially in the farrowing units.

Use of antibiotics in the feed prior to farrowing has been recommended as a treatment and preventive measure, but observation indicates that this is successful only part of the time. Nutritionally, animals on deficient vitamin E and/or selenium diets have had milking problems; therefore supplementation of the gestation and lactation ration with 20,000 I.U. of vitamin E and 0.1 ppm selenium is recommended.

Individual cases may be treated with injected antibiotics, uterine infusions, antiinflammatory drugs, vitamins, and hormones to induce milk letdown, depending on the causative factor.

The milk flow is the major problem because the little pigs starve so quickly. Adequate milk flow must be reestablished immediately. Milk under the influence of mastitis is alkaline and of questionable value to the nursing pigs; usually they will be reluctant to nurse or consume enough of this milk. However, if the nursing pigs will consume the milk present, some will survive, and normal milk quality and flow may be reestablished in 3 to 4 days. If the baby pigs can get colostrum in the first day, they can be shifted to another sow, but the colostrum consumption is a must before this is done. If you do not have a nurse sow, milk replacer can be used after colostrum consumption, by feeding it at body temperature (102° F) to pigs from a shallow pan. Young pigs usually will adapt to the pan and should be allowed all the milk they will consume in about 10 minutes. They should be fed 8 to 9 times daily for the first through fourth days, and 5 to 6 times daily for the fifth through seventh days. Thereafter, a gradual substitution of commercial pig starter can be implemented. Substitution must be gradual to avoid any abrupt change in diet and consequent problems such as diarrhea. These pigs must be kept in a very warm, dry place, which is cleaned often. Success with pigs will be variable.

SYSTEMIC DISEASES, VIRAL AND BACTERIAL DISEASES

Swine Pox

Signs. Swine pox is a skin disease characterized by small scabs that are brown and dry and are scattered all over the body. There is slight temperature elevation, but the swine do not appear to be very sick. There is a lot of itching and scratching, the disease running its course on individual hogs in about 2 weeks. Since it spreads so rapidly, various stages of swine pox will be seen throughout the herd, making the total effect of the disease much more extensive than the 2 weeks it takes to affect a single hog.

Cause. The cause is a virus spread by mosquitoes and lice.

Prevention. This is a self-limiting disease and will cure itself if left alone; however, spraying for lice and controlling these carriers will reduce the disease and subsequent loss in performance and economics.

Treatment. There is no recommended treatment because of the self-limiting nature of the disease. All animals in the herd should be treated for lice and mange immediately. However, you should be aware of the potential of secondary bacterial invasions, in which case antibiotics would be recommended.

325
SYSTEMIC
DISEASES
VIRAL AND
BACTERIAL
DISEASES

Ringworm

Signs. Signs include dry, crusty lesions, variable in size with some about the size of a 50¢ piece. Red discoloration occurs in the center of the lesion, and the outer edges of the lesion are crusted and matted with dead skin. Ringworm occurs most often in winter and in heavy crowding situations. The lesions start most often around the ears and neck and may spread over the entire body.

Cause. The cause is a fungus, usually *Microsporum nanum*.

Prevention. Since this is a disease brought about by heavy crowding and dark, damp housing, prevention naturally should be aimed at proper sanitation and housing measures. Because ringworm is spread by direct contact, infected swine should be isolated. Adequate A and E vitamins may also play a role in preventing ringworm. This organism may affect man; so care must be taken when handling infected pigs.

Treatment. Infected animals should be scrubbed and the lesions treated with tincture of iodine twice weekly for 2 to 3 weeks.

In severe cases, when a specific fungus is known, a specific fungicide such as griseofulvin or tinactin may be recommended. Generally this disease is self-limiting, and expensive treatment is not required.

Photosensitization

Signs. The appearance of sunburn (red, burned, or peeling skin) may be considered sensitivity to sunlight. The skin may blister on occasions; white hogs are much more susceptible than darker pigmented animals. In multicolored hogs, the white portions of the skin will be much more affected than the dark areas.

Cause. The cause is a sensitivity to sunlight brought about by a reaction to phenothiazine, or to some plants such as alfalfa, red clover, and rape, or to some types of oats.

Prevention and Treatment. You should avoid contamination of feeds by phenothiazine or by other compounds that cause the sensitivity. This is not always practical; so on the first signs of photosensitization, the hogs should be moved to a shady area and kept there until the condition passes. Some white hogs will sunburn due to intense sunlight without being influenced by any of the causative agents mentioned. This condition should not be confused with plain old-fashioned sunburn. Photosensitization is much more painful and serious.

Exudative Epidermitis ("Greasy Pig Disease," Pustular Dermatitis)

Signs. Exudative epidermitis affects young pigs, usually 3 to 55 days of age, and is a skin-irritating disease, producing greasy pigs with a foul odor. Signs include skin eruptions over the entire body, sudden onset and short duration, a loss of body fluids, dehydration, and death. Excessive secretion of the oil glands of the skin, sloughing off of the upper layers (exfoliation), and a serum secretion from the skin (exudation) are characteristic. Normally, there is no itch.

The disease develops in four distinct stages. First, a dry dandruff appears about the joints and flanks; second, reddish spots develop; third, blisters appear on the snout and feet; and finally, there is a rapid spread of lesions over the whole body, creating the greasy appearance with strong odor and subsequent dehydration due to the exudation of body fluids. Mortality rates are low. If animals do recover from acute symptoms, they may be affected permanently by the disease.

Cause. The exact cause is unknown, but a generalized staphylococcus infection is seen in all infected pigs.

Prevention. Cleanliness and sanitation are the best preventive measures. Some infections start following infection of a wound. Therefore, needle teeth should be properly clipped. The condition most often shows up under unsanitary situations.

Treatment. Treatment consists of large doses of antibiotics to individual pigs. Severely affected pigs may be bathed in an iodine solution; however, this bath treatment is generally not economical.

Listeriosis

Signs. This is a systemic (whole body) disease characterized by stiffness, posterior paralysis, trembling, incoordination, easy excitability, and occasionally diarrhea. However, a majority of *Listeria* infections probably cause no clinical signs.

Cause. The cause is a Gram-positive bacterium, *Listeria monocytogenes*, which can live in the soil for up to 200 days but is easily killed by the most common disinfectants and by pasteurization.

Prevention. There is no vaccine available. Control of rodents, separating of swine from cattle and sheep, proper sanitation, and isolation of affected swine are recommended as preventive measures.

Treatment. This organism appears to be slightly resistant to penicillin; so this drug should not be used as a treatment. Other antibiotics, however, can be of help in combating the disease. Sulfonamides have proven very beneficial in treatment.

The public health aspects of this disease are important to note. Listeriosis is contagious to humans and may be passed on in the form of meningoencephalitis (a disease of the membranes surrounding the brain). It can also cause ear infections and pneumonia in humans, and is responsible for death by abortion.

Aujeszky's Disease (Pseudorabies, False Rabies, "Mad Itch")

Signs. Aujeszky's disease affects young pigs more than older animals. Baby pigs that have no maternal antibodies develop high temperatures, convulsions, and paralysis, and usually die. In pigs less than 2 weeks old, death losses approach 100%. After 3 weeks, young pigs develop some resistance, and losses are considerably reduced.

In the adult swine, signs may be mild to nonexistent, or they may include abortion, stillbirths, infertility, mummified fetuses, mild respiratory signs, and lack of appetite. Death is rare for adults and generally occurs as a result of secondary pneumonia. Recovered hogs serve as a silent reservoir to carry the disease to cattle, dogs, cats, and wildlife.

The main effect is on pregnant and nursing swine. Depending on the stage of gestation, pregnant sows may have stillborns and weak pigs (late gestation), mummification (midgestation), and embryonic death and infertility (early gestation). Abortion may occur at any stage but is most prevalent during the last trimester of pregnancy. Piglets may develop signs as early as 12 hours after farrowing, but generally the first signs are seen at 5 to 7 days of life. Various central nervous signs may be seen, although in some cases sudden death without signs is reported. Severity of clinical signs is controlled by timing and quantity of exposure, strain of virus, age of pigs affected, and presence of protective antibodies. Pigs suckling immune sows may become infected but will show few or no clinical signs and minimal death losses. These pigs, however, are potential sources of infection for their lifetime.

Cause. The cause is a herpes virus. Since pseudorabies can occur in adult swine with few clinical signs and can persist in their system for long periods, these swine serve as the natural reservoir for the disease.

Swine can transmit pseudorabies by aerosol contact, by contaminated feed and water, and by biting cattle, dogs, cats, and sheep. It causes a fatal encephalomyelitis (inflammation of the nervous system) with signs of severe itching and self-mutilation—hence the name "mad itch." The disease also affects wildlife in a similar fashion and may be spread to other farms by movement of affected wildlife.

Prevention. A modified live virus vaccine (PR-Vac, by Norden Labs) has been released for use only on swine. Vaccination produces blood-test

327
SYSTEMIC
DISEASES
VIRAL AND
BACTERIAL
DISEASES

reactions identical to those of naturally infected swine. Vaccinated swine are protected from the effects of the disease for about 6 months, although they may become infected with a field strain virus and become carriers. Vaccines are restricted to use by veterinarians. Most states limit vaccination to infected or high-risk herds.

Since the major effects are on pregnant and lactating animals, vaccination of breeding animals before each breeding is recommended where applicable. This semiannual vaccination will protect both sow and litter during nursing. In herds where sows were not vaccinated or when persistent problems in "growing buildings" make growing-pig vaccination necessary, pigs can be vaccinated at 3 days of age if nursing nonimmune sows and at 3 to 8 weeks if the sows have immunity and are providing antibodies in her colostrum.

Whatever the circumstances, a decision to use the vaccine should be made after close consultation with your veterinarian and with an understanding of possible effects from vaccinating.

An important step in any future control and eradication program would be the establishment of procedures for identification and cleaning up of infected herds. Procedures would probably involve testing and removal of infected animals with negative periodic retests of herds before animals could be shipped. Although no cases of pseudorabies have been reported in man, reports of humans carrying the virus to new locations have been reported. Therefore, care should be taken to wash boots, equipment, and clothing before entering another farm. As an added protection, rubber gloves should be worn when posting (performing an autopsy) an animal or in cleaning up an outbreak area.

Treatment. Other than eradication, no treatment is known to be effective. Secondary infections in adult animals can be suppressed by the use of injectable antibiotics.

Meningitis

Meningitis is an infection or inflammation of the meninges (tissues that surround the brain and spinal cord). It is a sign of disease but not a disease by itself.

Signs. Clinical signs include elevated temperature, excitement, shaking of the head with a dazed expression, often walking in circles, depression, muscle spasms, convulsions, and death. Pigs will often walk into a corner and be so dazed they can't get out. These signs generally occur in very young pigs.

Cause. The cause could be a variety of viral and bacterial invasions. Very often, it is a whole body infection (septicemia) with some organism brought to the brain by the bloodstream. The disorder can originate from almost any infectious process such as a navel ill, castration, pneumonia, mastitis, pseudorabies, or listerioses; or from a noninfectious condition like water deprivation (salt poisoning).

Prevention. Use maximum sanitary measures in routine operations such as castrating, vaccinating, and so forth, by disinfecting all surgical instruments and using antiseptic procedures; dip navels in tincture of iodine at birth and insure adequate water is present at all times.

Treatment. High levels of antibiotics and, in some cases, steriods may be used to reduce the inflammation of the brain. Prevention is the key because once the infection starts, it is difficult to reverse.

329
SYSTEMIC
DISEASES
VIRAL AND
BACTERIAL
DISEASES

Tetanus

Signs. Clinical signs include mild depression, heavy salivation, little appetite, muscle rigidity ("sawhorse" appearance), muscle spasms set off by a slight noise or excitement, arched back, head drawn back, and death by asphyxiation due to paralysis of respiratory muscles.

Cause. The cause is a bacterium, *Clostridium tetani*, which is primarily a soil-borne organism. It survives well in many environments.

Prevention. Avoid sharp objects such as nails that cause deep puncture wounds. Strict sanitation must be observed with all surgical procedures.

Treatment. Pigs are not usually treated because of the expense involved and the poor recovery rate. If pigs should be treated, it is recommended that they be kept clean, quiet, with fresh water, and sedated. Antitoxins are available and are recommended to be used at 4 to 5 times the manufacturer's recommended dosage.

Malignant Edema

Signs. The chief clinical sign is a swelling around the area of a wound caused by gaseous air bubbles (edema) under the skin. With your fingers, press the swollen area and you can feel the gaseous accumulation under the skin. Body temperature will normally be elevated. If the disease goes the systemic route, there will be depression followed by the development of general toxicity and then death.

Cause. The cause is the bacterium *Clostridium septicum*. This organism gains entrance through cuts and scratches. The infection may also result due to unsanitary assistance with difficult births, vaccinations, castrations, navel infections, surgical procedures, or even parasitic wounds in the intestinal tract. This organism is also soil-borne and tends to build up in the environment following heavy use of an area.

Prevention. Strict sanitation and disinfection procedures during any surgical procedures should be followed to prevent occurrence of the infection.

Treatment. Massive doses of tetracycline and penicillin both systematically and around the wound have been useful.

Erysipelas (Diamond Skin Disease)

Signs. Clinical signs vary considerably because of the three forms: acute, subacute, and chronic.

In the acute form, some pigs may die very suddenly. Others may develop a high temperature, lack of appetite, appear physically sick, develop sore muscles or tender feet, have an arched back, and walk in a shuffling gait, often squealing because of pain in the feet and joints. Affected pigs may remain lying down or may protest loudly when they are forced up. About the third day of the disorder, red diamond-shaped or square patches may appear on the skin. Although these diamond-shaped areas rarely occur today, this is considered a diagnostic clinical sign of hogs infected with erysipelas.

Subacute forms produce milder signs with fewer deaths. This form is much more common in modern swine production than the acute form. Many pigs may show only reluctance to move and reddish skin discoloration of the ears, tail, jowl, and legs.

In the chronic form, the aftereffects are the main problem. There is a persistent arthritis and swelling of joints, and the tips of the tail or ears may blacken and fall off. In some instances, the heart valves are damaged due to the infection, impeding normal blood flow and bringing on cardiac failure.

Although the acute form would appear to be the most dangerous type, probably more economic loss is caused from the subacute and chronic forms because of developing lameness and arthritis, a condition that is very difficult to reverse once started.

Cause. A bacterium, *Erysiplothrix insidiosa*, is the cause. This organism is very difficult to control because it lives in a wide range of hosts including rats, birds, and insects, and can survive for extended periods of time (over 50 days) in alkaline soil. Recovered swine may also act as a major reservoir of infection in a herd.

Prevention. Vaccines are available and give immunity for about 6 months following use. Vaccination can be performed at any time during the gestation period but is recommended to be given initially 3 to 4 weeks before breeding gilts. The vaccines should be reinjected 3 to 4 weeks before farrowing in order to increase immunity in the baby pigs via colostrum milk. Revaccinate sows at each farrowing to maintain protection for the litter.

In herds where there is a real problem, young pigs can be vaccinated at 1 to 2 weeks and revaccinated at 6 to 8 weeks of age. Some lameness may occasionally be seen in pigs after vaccination, the theory being that the pigs were already in contact with the organism and the vaccine actually prompted the development of arthritis. Since erysipelas is carried by rats, predators, and flies, dead pigs should be disposed of properly by deep burial and lime covering or they should be cremated.

Isolate new stock 30 days before placing them with the rest of the herd; vaccinate all new herd additions while in isolation; and have a well-managed external parasite control program.

331
SYSTEMIC
DISEASES,
VIRAL AND
BACTERIAL
DISEASES

Treatment. If erysipelas is suspected, the antibiotics of choice are penicillin or chlortetracycline. If the disorder is in the later stages of development, arthritis may set in even with successful treatment.

A swine erysipelas antiserum is also available that can be given at the onset of an acute infection for immediate blocking effects.

Hog Cholera

Signs. Although not an explosive disease, hog cholera is a devasting problem with swine. Several stages may be present in a herd due to the often slow chronic spread, which requires 6 to 20 days to fully develop.

The first warning is several hogs dying with no clinical signs observed. The reason for this is that some swine are more susceptible than herdmates to the cholera virus, and they die very quickly. The strain and dose of virus, the presence of other diseases, and environmental factors play a part in determining the spread through a herd. After the initial unexplained deaths, the major signs are lack of appetite, elevated temperatures (104°F to 109°F), involvement of the central nervous system, depression, diarrhea, dehydration, weight loss, and a high death rate. Conjunctivitis (severe inflammation of the eyelids) in which the eyelids may be glued together due to exudates is common.

In the chronic form, pigs may recover but are susceptible to pneumonia, have intermittent diarrhea, and remain "poor doers."

Cause. The cause is a virus that is specific for swine. It is a contagious disease usually transmitted directly from pig to pig, although blood-sucking insects can transmit it. It is very often passed in uncooked garbage, and for this reason it is illegal to feed raw, uncooked garbage in the United States.

Prevention. Hog cholera virus has been the target of a massive and successful eradication effort by the swine industry. The original vaccine is no longer used in the United States because it was learned that the vaccine itself could cause the disease. When the USDA (U.S. Department of Agriculture) announced the withdrawal of the vaccine, some farmers stockpiled it in deep freezes and used it even though the regulation forbade its use. Since then, outbreaks that have occurred in the United States have been largely traced back to the use of the original vaccine, which was used to prevent the very disease that it caused, or to the importation of the virus in live swine or uncooked swine food products fed to hogs as garbage.

The best prevention is to avoid exposure by observing 30-day isolation of new swine, maintaining strict quarantine of the premises, and cooking all garbage fed to hogs.

Treatment. There is no present treatment. The disease is under U.S. government control by means of federal quarantine and slaughter.

Streptococcal Infection (Swine Abscess, Cervical Strangles)

Signs. The chief clinical sign is a cervical or jowl abscess with swelling of the lower jaw. There are several forms of this disorder. In the systemic form, the signs may also include diarrhea, anemia, depression, and icterus (yellowing of the membranes and skin) in addition to the abscess and swelling. The infection is usually seen in pigs weighing less than 100 lb.

Abscess formation may be due to arthritis, navel infection, or some forms of encephalitis. The abscesses are signs of a systemic disease that localizes in a particular area of the body.

In the more commonly seen form, a cervical or jowl abscess ("boil") occurs in which there is a swelling in the lower part of the jaw and occasionally drainage of pus from the abscess.

Cause. A streptococcus bacterium infects a localized area and the lymph nodes draining that area, resulting in the abscess formation.

Prevention. The infection is spread by contamination of equipment and waterers with pus, and by direct contact with infected sows during or after the farrowing process (navel infection). New animals should be isolated for 30 days and should be treated with long-acting penicillin before introduction into the herd. Infected swine should be quarantined until marketed. A vaccine is available, but the protection has been less than satisfactory.

Treatment. Broad-spectrum antibiotics, local drainage, and iodine packs are recommended. The disease may be eliminated from a herd by feeding 200 gm/ton chlortetracycline for 30 days to all animals in the herd followed by 10 gm/ton until hogs are sent to market.

PSS—PSE Syndrome

The initials PSS and PSE are used to describe this disease because of a complicated series of conditions that it represents. The initials actually stand for "porcine stress syndrome" and "pale, soft, exudative pork." These are all very important economical factors in the swine industry, creating a loss of value in the swine carcasses due to shrinkage and lower grades and a loss of sales because of the sudden death of afflicted animals during movement.

Signs. Each time pigs are moved, they may undergo an unexplained death loss up to 10%. These losses may occur at market time, breeding time, during farrowing and lactation, when swine are moved to grower units, and during hot periods of weather. The condition is related to stressful situations that occur during all these periods.

Cause. The cause is a hereditary problem predisposing animals to be susceptible to stress.

Prevention. Exercising and preconditioning hogs for adaptibility to stress may be of help, but since the syndrome is a genetic defect, such efforts will not correct or totally prevent the condition. Some selection techniques are used in order to select boars that are not likely to have the hereditary condition. There is a close correlation between nervousness, muscle tremors, and tail twitching in boars and this hereditary condition. Boars should not be selected that have a constant tail and ear twitching or develop red patches on the skin when excited. The carcass quality scores of littermates of boars should be checked for any exudative indications or lack of firmness and color in slaughter cutout data. A low score may suggest the possibility of high involvement of the boar in the PSS-PSE complex. Gilts may also be selected using the same criteria. The blood levels of creating phosphokinase (CPK), a blood enzyme, following excitement can be used as an indication of an animal's stress susceptibility. This test can be done easily and quickly with a commercially available test kit.

333
SYSTEMIC
DISEASES
VIRAL AND
BACTERIAL
DISEASES

If the condition has been noted in the past and genetic improvement has not been made, excitement should be held to the minimum as a short-term preventive measure until boars that are not stress prone can be introduced and can begin producing in a herd.

Vesicular Exanthena (VES)

Signs. An incubation period of 1 to 3 days is normal before the signs develop; these include an elevation of temperature (105°F to 106°F), followed by the development of small vesicles (blisters) on the snout, teats, udder, and feet (usually between the toes). These blisters last 1 to 2 weeks, and recovery is usually uncomplicated; but secondary infections of the blister drains may cause swelling of the mouth and feet areas, creating temporary lameness and reduced feed intake. Gestating sows may abort; lactating sows may go dry. Feeder swine may be severely stunted in growth.

Cause. A virus is the cause.

Prevention. The disease has been eradicated from the United States at present through quarantine and slaughter. Recent isolation of a virus in California sea lions similar to the VES virus opens the possibility that feeding of raw marine wastes may have been responsible for the original VES outbreaks. To date confirmed outbreaks have only been reported in the United States. However, because of its similarity to foot and mouth disease and other vesicular diseases, the signs may have been overlooked in other countries. Infected animals should be sold to slaughterers. There is no problem with the meat being consumed by humans in this case. The infected premises should be thoroughly cleaned and disinfected with a 2% sodium hydroxide solution before restocking the herd.

Treatment. There is no known treatment.

Gut Edema (Enterotoxemia)

Gut edema is characterized by sudden onset with the fastest gaining pigs most often affected. A change in ration and/or environment, weaning of the litter, castration, or other stressful conditions generally precede an outbreak. The primary cause is an endotoxin produced from *E. coli* and the changes in blood vessels that it produces. In times of stress or when rations are changed, there may be an explosive increase in the *E. coli* population with a concurrent increase in toxins and other bacterial byproducts.

Signs. Signs include central nervous system disorders in young pigs usually under 2 to 4 months of age. You usually find one or two of the best pigs in the herd dead unexpectedly. If you happen to observe these pigs before they die, the signs would be posterior weakness, convulsions, and puffiness of the upper eyelids.

Cause. Hemolytic *E. coli* growing in the gut produces endotoxins that are absorbed, causing changes in blood vessels that allow fluid to escape into the surrounding tissues (edema).

Prevention. Reduce stress by gradual changes in feed, in housing, and in working schedules. Addition of 5 to 10% ground oats to a starter or grower may help the transition to new feed. Oats can slowly be withdrawn over a 10 to 14 day period.

Treatment. Take pigs off all feed for 12 to 24 hours. Using 5 to 10% ground oats in the ration, gradually bring the ration back up to a full feed in about a week. Ground hay may be used to supplement the ration until full feed is reached. Feeding high levels of antibiotics during this period may be helpful but has been inconsistent in results.

Arthritis

In 1971 in the inspection of some 85 million hogs at slaughter, there were 20,000 hogs condemned, and 800,000 were retained for inspection and removal of infected parts before the carcasses were allowed to enter the meat market. This disease takes a heavy economic toll.

Signs. Lameness of one or more legs with puffiness and swelling are characteristic signs. The shoulder, hock, and stifle joints are most susceptible because of their structure and weight-bearing requirements.

There are two types of arthritis; an infective (the most prevalent type) and a noninfective variety.

Cause. In the noninfective type, a variety of conformation faults in feet and legs accentuate the condition because of undue stress on certain joint surfaces. Straight-legged, sickle or cow-hocked, buck-kneed pigs, and pigs that stand high on their toes are more prone to this type of arthritis.

The infective type of arthritis results from secondary infections caused by erysipelas, mycoplasma, streptococcal infection, and/or tail biting. Organisms gain entrance through the bloodstream and are filtered out by the small blood vessels in the joint. Once in the joint, the bacteria are protected from the body's defenses by a relatively poor blood supply to the area and inability for most antibiotics to reach therapeutic levels in the joint.

Prevention and Treatment. The noninfective type may be controlled now by close selection of breeding stock for good feet and leg conformation and by avoiding slick or very rough flooring that might cause injuries.

In the infective type, antibiotics such as tylosin (Tylan), lincomycin, and penicillin may be of help depending on the causative agent. Lincomycin has an added advantage of being able to achieve relatively high concentrations of drug in bone and cartilaginous tissues, which are major components of the joints. Lincomycin withdrawal time should be strictly observed to conform to federal regulations.

DIGESTIVE DISORDERS

Enteric Infections

Signs. Clinical signs include diarrhea, an increase in body temperature, and lack of appetite.

Cause. Ration changes and/or stress create conditions conducive to an increase in normal gut organism populations. Parasites may also contribute to the initial infection or may intensify an existing infection. Infectious agents causing diarrhea include *E. coli*, TGE, *Treponema hyodysenteriae, Salmonella sp., Clostridium perfringens* type C, and other minor bacterial and viral infections.

Prevention. Avoid stress and provide good parasite control. Vaccinate or control specific diseases with medication as required.

Treatment. Oral administration with stomach coatings like kaolin, pectin, or fiber (ground oats) to give soothing effects in the gut are recommended. When specific diseases occur, specific treatments must be applied quickly and correctly.

TGE (Transmissible Gastroenteritis)

TGE is an infectious, transmittable disease causing a high death rate in pigs less than 10 to 14 days of age. It affects older swine also, but it is seldom fatal in adult animals. Surviving animals may shed TGE virus for up to 40 days in manure and up to 120 days from the respiratory tract following recovery.

Signs. The disease spreads very quickly, producing poor appetite, vomiting, scours, and weight loss. Lactating sows stop giving milk, and there are high death losses in pigs under 2 weeks of age.

In young pigs, vomiting and diarrhea are constant. Whitish, yellowish, or greenish fecal material is passed through the digestive system. Ingested milk often appears in the manure unchanged. There is rapid dehydration and weight loss, with a high mortality rate in young pigs.

An enzootic or chronic form of TGE has been recognized as becoming increasingly important. Chronic TGE is characterized as a high-morbidity, low-mortality disease, usually affecting weanling pigs 3 to 7 days after entry into a nursery or feeder pigs following movement. The disease can occur at any time of the year, and the major losses are due to poor performance and production of some runt pigs upon recovery from the initial outbreak.

Cause. The cause is a corona virus usually passed through manure and the respiratory tract of infected swine.

Prevention. Sows should be vaccinated twice, 6 weeks and 2 weeks prior to farrowing. In serious outbreaks, a 2-month idle period or intensive sanitation procedures for farrowing and nursery facilities will allow the organism to die out. TGE virus is able to survive for long periods in frozen or cold, moist conditions. It is susceptible to drying, high temperatures and direct sunlight. This is one reason why TGE was originally considered to be a seasonal disease of the winter months.

Feeding infected material to pregnant sows to allow development of immunities has been successful for some producers. Sows should not be exposed to TGE within one month of farrowing.

Immunity to TGE virus and to other enteric problems is passed from the immune sow in two ways to the suckling pig. First, colostral immunity is absorbed by each piglet during the first 12 to 24 hours after farrowing. Second, a specific type of antibody is secreted into the milk each time the piglet drinks. This antibody travels to the gut, neutralizing the organism it is to fight. This protein is not destroyed by the stomach acids and is slowly "metered out" of the stomach into the intestine until the next feeding time. This "lactogenic" antibody is more effective in protecting the pig from TGE, rotavirus, and *E. coli* during the early stages of life than is colostral immunity.

A TGE vaccine is now available, and is considered to be the most effective method of prevention. Approved TGE vaccine given intramuscularly stimulates colostral immunity; whereas oral infection (feeding infected material) stimulates both colostral and lactogenic antibody production, giving a better protection. Currently efforts are under way to develop a TGE vaccine that will produce solid immunity but not produce clinical disease.

Prevention of enzootic TGE must rely on strict sanitation and disinfection, all-in and all-out nursery design (farrow house scheduling in which sows and pigs are moved in and out as groups so proper sanitation and disinfection procedures can be used to prevent TGE spread from one group to the next) or periodic breaks in the nursery, and possibly vaccination of pigs while they are suckling the sow. Vaccination offers the best future hope, but today sanitation and building design are the keys to success.

Treatment. There is no effective treatment. Avoid outside exposure during farrowing time.

Colibacillosis (Baby Pig Scours)

Estimates of 10% are not unusual for the number of pig deaths brought about by this disease. Infection rates may be as high as 50% of all the pigs born in the United States.

Signs. Clinical signs are usually seen in the farrowing pen during the first week of life. Baby pigs develop a profuse yellow diarrhea, dehydration, staggers, trembling, and go off feed and die. This disease can be confused with TGE; so it is important to get an accurate diagnosis, so that the proper measures can be taken.

Cause. *Escherichia coli* is the causative organism, usually combined with a stress factor such as chilling.

Prevention. Oral vaccines made from *E. coli* cultures can be fed to sows for three days 3 to 4 weeks prior to farrowing, resulting in antibody production in colostrum and milk (lactogenic effect) to protect pigs. These live cultures are made from isolation on individual farms. As many as four *E. coli* types may be needed to insure complete control. There are also injectable vaccines (bacterins) available. The vaccine is injected twice (at 4 weeks and 2 weeks) prior to farrowing, and once at farrowing time.

Strict sanitation of farrowing houses and washing of sows prior to entry are most important because *E. coli* is present in the sow's manure and on the muck attached to her skin. Keep baby pigs warm and dry to promote resistance. Chilled pigs, weak pigs, and pigs not nursing or on sows without milk are generally the first to break out with the infection. It is important to remember that *E. coli* populations build up over time, causing earlier outbreaks and with more severity as time passes. Therefore, production breaks and good sanitation must be practiced. Use of medications to "sterilize" the sow's gut prior to farrowing have been suggested, but the results are not always beneficial. The herdsman should also go first to the farrowing house, then to chores with the other animals on the farm, in order to prevent the spread of disease organisms. This is a good management procedure for all diseases.

Treatment. Neomycin, furazolidone, polymycin, streptomycin, and tetracycline have been effective, but the number one treatment is prevention through strict sanitation.

Swine Dysentery (Bloody Scours)

In the opinion of many veterinarians, the most important intestinal disease of weaned pigs is swine dysentery. It is a contagious disease and can result in severe economic loss to pork producers. Swine dysentery was first described in 1921 by American workers. It has been a problem ever since.

Signs. Bloody scours commonly affects pigs after weaning, usually 10 to 16 weeks of age; but unweaned animals as well as adults are susceptible. Reduced appetite is often the first noticeable sign, accompanied by soft, off-colored bowel movements, which have been described as appearing like "wet cement" or milky coffee.

The stool becomes streaked with blood as the disease progresses and usually contains undigested food as well as mucus from the intestinal wall. The blood increases progressively because of shredding of the intestinal mucosa. For this reason the term *bloody scours* is often used.

The rear of affected pigs becomes wet and stained, and pigs take on a characteristic gaunt appearance. Although the death rate is not particularly high, some sudden losses can occur early in the outbreaks.

Cause. Early researchers thought that swine dysentery was caused by *Vibrio coli*, a bacterium. However, although the exact triggering mechanism is still in dispute, it is now accepted that a large spirochete, *Treponema hyodysenteriae*, is the causative agent with several normal gut bacteria acting as intensifying agents.

Studies of outbreaks suggest that in the majority of cases carrier pigs are the most likely source of infection. These pigs show no signs of the disease, having developed an immunity, but spread it to others that have not been previously exposed. There is also speculation that the organism is carried commonly by many hogs, but that the disease does not become active until some stress-producing change in the pigs' environment occurs, precipitating the development. Birds, dogs, man, and equipment have been identified as mechanical carriers. The spirochete can survive in lagoons or manure pits for unknown but significant lengths of time.

Prevention. The first step towards effective control is to obtain an accurate diagnosis. Swine dysentery can easily be confused with other causes of bloody scours such as salmonellosis, whipworms, and even gastric ulcers.

The second step in controlling the disease is a good sanitation program. The severity of the problem is directly proportional to the level of manure contamination in hog facilities. Clean, dry floors and uncontaminated feed and water will reduce losses. Steam-cleaning to remove organic matter and chemical disinfection of facilities at routine intervals will greatly reduce this disease. Environmental stress factors such as overcrowding, chilling, and poor ventilation should be eliminated. With proper sanitation and attention to a comfortable environment the condition will be less likely to occur.

Treatment. Organic arsenic preparations have been used for many years and are thought to have considerable value in some cases today. The preferred method of drug delivery is via the drinking water rather than in the feed. After the initial outbreak is controlled, medicated feed can be used to hold the disease in check until the pigs are marketed.

Tylosin has proved beneficial in injectable form but does not work in feed or water at currently approved levels. However, individual pigs that show extreme weakness may be injected with Tylosin. Drugs to be mixed with feed are available, such as Mecadox, Virginianycin, and Lincomix.

Salmonellosis

Signs. Young weanling pigs, found dead with no previous signs of illness, is characteristic of salmonellosis. Older pigs are affected and may show high fever, depression, and weakness. Quite often a reddened area shows up on the skin of the ears, inner thighs, armpits, and abdominal walls. There is generalized congestion and hemorrhaging of the lymph glands. These signs characterize the acute form. Definite diagnosis can only be made by isolation of the organism and identification of typical lesion formation.

In the chronic form, the signs are a profuse scouring, which may be confused with swine dysentery. After scours begin, a progressive loss of flesh follows. Pigs may survive for weeks and recover, but are usually stunted, have a rough haircoat, and remain unthrifty. High fever is not usually present, although pneumonia often accompanies an outbreak of salmonellosis.

Cause. Two bacterial organisms, *S. cholerasuis* and *S. typhisuis*, are most commonly associated with outbreaks. These organisms are widely distributed in nature and are often found in normal healthy swine. If hogs are severely stressed, the organisms may develop to the point that scours and other signs are triggered.

Prevention. The organisms causing salmonellosis are present in most hog barns, lots, and facilities, and must be controlled through proper cleaning and sanitation. Management in providing a comfortable environment free from serious stress is the key to prevention. No vaccines are available for salmonellosis prevention.

Treatment. Furazolidone (NF 180) and Mecadox are used widely with good results. Antibiotic treatment must be accompanied by strong sanitation and environmental controls.

POISONS

Nitrate (Nitrite) Poisoning

Nitrate consumption causes gastroenteritis, but swine are only poisoned by the nitrites that are formed in the gut from the nitrates. Nitrite poisoning causes respiratory distress. The amount of oxygen in the bloodstream is reduced, resulting in oxygen starvation to the tissues.

Conditions conducive to nitrate problems or nitrite poisoning are consumption of not thoroughly boiled whey in which potassium nitrate has been added in the cheese-making process, butcher-shop scraps containing sodium nitrite, water wells that have an accumulation of nitrates, and drainage that comes out of some silo materials. Levels of 100 ppm nitrates in water are considered safe for all ages of swine. Baby pigs and newly weaned pigs are most susceptible to nitrate problems. Resistance develops with age.

In the case of nitrates, the direct causative action is on the gastrointestinal tract. Absorption of pure nitrite causes the formation of methemoglobin, developing anemic anoxia (a lack of oxygen-carrying capacity in the blood).

Signs. Nitrite poisoning causes difficult breathing, muscular tremors, weakness, staggering gaits, bluish discoloration of normally pink membranes (cyanosis), rapid weak pulse, and subnormal temperature. Severe convulsions can terminate in death.

Treatment. Methylene blue can be injected intravenously in a 1% solution at the rate of 1 to 2 mg/kg of body weight. You may have to repeat this injection at intervals if the toxic dose has been very high.

Mycotoxicoses

Toxin-producing molds that occur when feed gets spoiled due to high-moisture content in storage, accidental wetting, or the ergot condition (fungus disease) of some types of grasses cause mycotoxicoses.

Signs. The most common poisoning in swine is the toxin produced from feeding moldy corn silage or grain. A common mold is *Fusarium sp.*, which produces the estrogenic syndrome. The signs are swelling of the vulva, irregular heat cycles, reduction of the sex drive, rectal and vaginal prolapses, and abortions.

Prevention. Avoid feeding moldy grain particularly to baby pigs and gestating or lactating females. If moldy feeds must be used, they should be fed to a few individuals and the results observed before feeding to the entire herd.

Salt Poisoning

Salt poisoning, more correctly termed *water deprivation toxicity*, is most common in swine. It occurs under field conditions when there are inadequate water supplies. When fresh water is available in adequate quantities, swine can endure salt content of feeds up to 10% salt. However, reduction or cessation of water intake for a period may bring on toxicity with near normal (0.5%) salt feed levels. Hot weather, dietary regime, water restriction, and dehydration of the pig all play a part in salt poisoning. The more severe the water restriction and increased dietary salt level, the more rapidly and severely signs develop.

Signs. This disorder affects the central nervous system within 1 to 5 days of water restriction. There is often mental derrangement, weakness, muscular tremors, blindness, and constipation; affected pigs may fall over and die within 2 to 48 hours of clinical onset. There are epileptic-type convulsions in severe cases, always accompanied by twitching of the snout, progressing through the muscles of the face, neck, forelegs, trunk, and finally to the hind limbs. The pig may move backward rapidly and assume a sitting dog position or fall over backward. Each convulsion lasts about 1 minute and in typical cases ends with profuse salivation, complete exhaustion, and collapse. Mortality will range from 0 to 100%, but generally few animals (less than 10%) die and some severely affected swine make spontaneous recovery.

Treatment.   Remove all feed. Give small amounts of fresh water to the least affected animals. Repeat at regular intervals. Do not offer free-choice water immediately as this could make the problem more severe. Severely affected animals should be kept in clean, spacious quarters with a minimum of noise or stress. Swine should not be forced to drink water. Drenching should be avoided because of the potential for aspiration pneumonia.

METABOLIC DISEASES

Hypoglycemia ("Baby Pig Disease," "Three-Day Pig Disease")

Hypoglycemia means low blood sugar. This condition is due to inadequate food intake and may develop in 24 to 36 hours after birth. Stress also plays a significant part, particularly cold stress during the first 10 days of life. Baby pigs don't have the ability to produce glucose as do adults and therefore must depend on daily intake from milk. If milk intake is inadequate or if demands are too high because of environmental conditions, hypoglycemia develops. Death losses may be very high during the first few days of life.

Hypoglycemia is a significant disease of suckling pigs, although in many cases it is secondary to other problems.

Signs.   Pigs newly born show signs of shivering, erection of hair, squealing, weakness, a rolling of the eyeballs, and coma. Without treatment, death usually occurs within 36 hours.

Cause.   The most common causes are agalactia (a lack of milk production) in the sow, inadequate functional teats for litter size, and diarrhea in baby pigs. Inherited weakness (in splay legs) and exposure to cold may be contributing causes and will aggravate the condition.

Prevention.   Prevention can be achieved by selection of breeding stock for mild temperament and high-milking qualities and by the provision of supplemental heat for pigs farrowed during the colder parts of the year. Controlling litter size (by redistribution of piglets) also help reduce starve-out pigs in individual litters.

Treatment.   Provide a warm environment through heat lamps and supplemental feeding, and if signs are severe, use an intramuscular injection of 5% glucose solution given every 4 to 6 hours. A satisfactory supplement is evaporated milk diluted with $\frac{1}{2}$ tsp. water.

Parakeratosis

Parakeratosis is a nutritional deficiency disease characterized by thickening and cracking of the skin. It frequently affects young pigs between the ages of 6 and 16 weeks, reaching a level of 60% in some herds.

Signs. This disease is characterized by the formation of horny crusts, cracks, and fissures. Brown spots first appear on the abdomen, pastern, fetlock, hock, and tail; these spots become progressively more abundant until the entire body may be affected. The crusts are dry and are usually easily removed. This problem may be confused with severe mange infections. Secondary infections may set in on occasions, confusing the disease with exudative dermatitis ("greasy pig disease").

Cause. The cause is metabolic disturbance resulting in either a deficiency of zinc or an imbalance between the zinc and calcium dietary levels. The condition is most prevalent in pigs on diets consisting primarily of vegetable proteins and excess calcium supplements.

Prevention. Feed rations should have zinc and calcium properly balanced. The calcium level should be maintained between .65% and .75%, with the addition of .4 lb of zinc sulfate or zinc carbonate (40 to 70 ppm as Zn.) per ton of feed.

Agalactia

Agalactia is a total stoppage or lack of milk production. This condition may be caused by a variety of problems including mastitis, metritis, high environmental temperatures, infectious diseases causing high body temperatures, constipation, and absorption of *E. coli* endotoxins from the gut, difficult farrowings, hereditary factors and hormonal imbalances.

Signs. Signs will vary, depending on the cause. Generally agalactia is noticed within the first 3 to 5 days after farrowing. The piglets are hungry, attempting to nurse, but are unable to receive adequate quantities of milk. In some hereditary and hormonal problems, mammary tissue does not adequately develop prior to farrowing. Agalactia can be caused at any time during lactation when a sow becomes ill and runs a high fever.

Cause. Agalactia is considered a multifaceted problem with environmental, genetic, dietary, and disease components. One or more problems may occur simultaneously, and together create a more severe outbreak than one problem alone.

Prevention. Select for good milking gilts by saving only gilts from good milking sows. Insure maximum sow comfort during farrowing and following farrowing. Maintain sows in good flesh but do not overfatten during gestation. Feeding of bulk in early lactation can be beneficial in reducing constipation problems. Where mastitis is a problem, strict sanitation and farrowing stalls that are clean and dry will help solve the problem.

Treatment. Treatment consists of periodic injections of oxytocin, use of injectable antibiotics, warm compresses on the udder, and provision of palatable laxative rations at farrowing. The primary treatment should be to relieve the underlying problem causing the agalactia.

Anemia

Anemia is a sign of inadequate red blood cell or hemoglobin production and has been a more common occurrence since moving hog operations from outdoors to concrete or slatted floor operations. Iron deficiency is the major cause of anemia. Pigs are born with minimal iron stores, and sow's milk supplies only one-seventh to one-tenth of the pigs' daily iron requirement. In older pigs and sows, infectious diseases like eperythrozoonosis (a blood parasite) may cause anemia, even with adequate iron in the diet.

Signs. Anemia is a condition primarily of rapidly growing baby pigs. The affected pigs are listless and droopy-eared; they have a rough haircoat and a pale color to membrane of the eyes and mouth. Signs generally start about 10 days after farrowing and become severe by 2 to 3 weeks in unsupplemented litters. In the advanced stages, breathing becomes very labored and produces the characteristic abdominal breathing. The heart enlarges and pumps more forcefully and rapidly than normal in an attempt to compensate for the reduced blood capacity. When a severely affected pig is handled, this increased heart action may sound like "thumping" against the chest wall. Baby pigs have their resistance to disease lowered because of this condition and become susceptible to respiratory and intestinal disease organisms, creating major death loss.

Cause. Pigs are born with minimal levels of iron in their bodies and can't satisfy their iron requirements for growth by milk alone. Under natural conditions, after the first few days the piglets would be able to root around in the soil, picking up sufficient iron to enable required hemoglobin production. However, since most hog operations have now moved away from dirt, this problem has become more common.

Prevention. Inject each baby pig (at 1 to 3 days of age) with an iron dextran solution in the muscle of the neck. This injection should be repeated at $3\frac{1}{2}$ weeks if the pigs are not on creep feed by this time. You should watch out for leaks at the time of injection to make sure no material is lost from the puncture nor accumulated under the skin without being absorbed. All air should be removed from the syringe and needle before injection. Slide the skin backward and insert needle; give 1 to $1\frac{1}{2}$ cc; then let go of the skin and withdraw the needle. Leakage is minimized by these procedures.

There are two types of injectable iron solutions, a highly viscous and a nonviscous iron dextran solution. Difference between products is minimal. Available data support the more slowly absorbed iron dextran as more effective. Viscosity of product should have little effect on IM iron absorption. The iron dextran is readily absorbed by the pig following the injection.

A variety of other iron products are also on the market. There are iron supplemental blocks that may be offered free-choice, and crystals that can be sprinkled on the floor. Sod may be taken from a hog manure-free pasture and thrown into the pens to correct iron deficiency. In cases where pigs are reared on slatted floors made of iron, the oxidation of these floors may release enough iron for the pigs to nibble on, providing the needed iron to prevent anemia. Another development is an acid-iron chelate fed to the sow just prior to farrowing, which supposedly provides the needed iron in the sow's milk to the baby pigs. However, researchers found the baby pigs got most of their iron from the sow's droppings, not from the milk. Most authorities still agree that injectable iron is needed and is cheap insurance even if not needed.

Iron absorption from the gut is controlled by an unknown but very sensitive system. During times of deficiency, considerable absorption takes place. When iron stores are adequate, most iron passes through the gut unabsorbed. Coupled with the absorptive mechanism is a very sophisticated iron recovery system in the body. Very little iron is lost even during times of disease, but significant iron losses can occur from bleeding wounds or blood losses in the intestines.

Adult swine may be affected by diseases that cause destruction of red blood cells, including epirythrozoonosis, leptospirosis, and lice and mange infestations. When these disorders are corrected, hemoglobin will rise to normal levels. Accepted normal hemoglobin levels are as follows:

Newborn	8–11 gm/100 ml
Weanling	9–12 gm/100 ml
Growers	10–13 gm/100 ml
Sows	11–14 gm/100 ml

Research indicates that levels above 9 gm/100 ml are adequate to support function in all ages of swine.

Treatment. Injection of iron dextran is the preferred treatment once the condition arises. If pigs are severely affected and are comatose, a calcium gluconate or dextrose solution should be given to provide an extra boost of energy.

PARASITES

Internal Parasites

Heavy losses to swine producers occur every year from internal parasites. The major species of worms are roundworms (*Ascaris*), nodular worms (*Oesophagostomum*), whipworms (*Trichuris*), lungworms (*Metastrongylus*), threadworms (*Strongylus*), and kidney worms (*Stephanurus*).

Threadworms and kidney worms are much greater problems in the south than elsewhere in the states. They are rarely seen in the Corn Belt states. However, the roundworms, lungworms, whipworms, and nodular worms are common throughout the United States.

345
PARASITES

Damages from diseases and unthriftiness resulting from internal parasites come to an estimated $100 million per year. Management of the internal parasite problem should be aimed at breaking the cycle to control most parasites.

In general, the effect of internal parasites on hogs is a loss in weight or condition and if severe enough, diarrhea and/or respiratory difficulties. External signs are not as pronounced as in some other species. Swine are much more susceptible to internal parasites because of their habit of rooting in soils that may be heavily ladened with infective parasite eggs.

As with any animal, the signs of internal infestation must be determined by visual or microscopic examination of the feces. In the case of swine, there are few internal parasites, except when present in heavy concentrations, that exhibit external signs. Therefore, it is very important to use a preventive program of routine worming in a management program. The key to internal parasite control is breaking the cycle of exposure. The sows are the most logical place to accomplish this because of their smaller numbers and natural immunity that develops over time.

Diagnosis of swine parasitism is important. Fresh fecal samples can be used for examination for eggs of roundworms, nodular worms, whipworms, and lungworms. Threadworm eggs can also be found in excrement and kidney-worm eggs are found in the urine of infected animals. Other species of parasites' eggs are routinely found only when a post-mortem examination or condemnation of carcasses is made. Use of anthelmentics (deworming agents), well-drained lots, pasture rotation, and good cleanup procedures will help control parasites. Success of your program should be verified by fecal examination by a veterinarian at least twice yearly.

Hot lye solutions, saponated solutions of cresol, sodium orthophenylphenate, organic iodide or iodophores, and fumigation with formaldehyde gas are satisfactory disinfectants. Whether preceded by mechanical cleaning and/or the use of a steam cleaner or a detergent solution, the important consideration is the thorough cleaning of the facility to remove all the manure from contact with the animals.

Sows should be washed with a mild soap solution and rinsed with a mild antiseptic solution just before going into the farrowing house. The udder and feet should be given special cleansing attention. These procedures will keep down the spread of internal parasites by removing their eggs and will reduce the exposure of baby pigs to infective eggs.

Four chemicals, among the many products, are commonly used to control internal parasites—piperazine, dichlorvos, tramisol, and banminth. The newer parasite control products kill the adult worms, and the pig partially digests them before they are passed in the excrement. This is true of all the wormers listed in Table 16-2 except piperazine. Therefore, do not judge effectiveness based on the number of roundworms seen after worming.

Piperazine in the feed or water is used to worm pigs at 7 to 8 weeks of age. Repeat treatment again in another 3 to 4 weeks or as often as necessary.

With all products, frequency of worming is influenced by rate of reinfectivity. Pigs in high-exposure areas will need additional wormings. Worming the sow with piperazine 1 to 2 weeks before entering the farrowing house will help protect the baby pigs from roundworms.

Piperazine is a relatively inexpensive product, but it also has the limitation of being very narrow in its scope of activity (see Table 16-2). Dichlorvos (Atgard) is effective against the immature stage of the large roundworms as well as being effective against whipworms and nodular worms. It is available only in feed mixes. Tramisol is effective against lungworms, as well as the large roundworms and nodular worms, and is available in both feed and water formulations.

Banminth is used in the feed to control large roundworms and nodular worms. It is similar to piperazine in its range of activity; but when fed continuously, it stops migration of ascarid larvae in the liver and lungs. This is particularly important for young pigs held in high-exposure areas such as dirt lots or pastures that have had pigs on them for extended periods. Hygromycin B is useful in controlling whipworms, nodular worms, and roundworms. It is used in the feed. Thiabendazole paste is recommended for use against threadworms in baby pigs.

Internal parasites, especially ascarids (roundworms), are controlled by manure removal (sanitation) and by proper timing and selection of wormers. Control through prevention is stressed because damage due to the migration of immature worms (larvae) occurs to the liver and lungs before the parasites arrive at the intestines where most medication is effective. For pigs in confinement, thorough and frequent cleaning of buildings and floors and the use of drugs are the best means of control.

Routine worming is recommended if autopsy or fecal examination reveals adult worms or worm eggs. Administer all preparations according to the directions of your local veterinarian.

Table 16-2. Percent Removal of Common Swine Parasites

Anthelmentic[a]	Ascaris (Roundworms)	Oesophagostomum sp. (Nodular worms)	Trichuris sp. (Whipworms)	Metastrongylus sp. (Lungworms)	Strongylus sp. (Threadworms)
Dichlorvos (Atgard)	99–100%	95–100%	90–100%	0	60–80%
Hygromycin B (Hygromix)	95–100%	95–100%	85–100%	0	0
Levamisole (Tramisol)	99–100%	80–100%	60–80%	90–100%	80–95%
Piperazine	75–100%	50%	0	0	0
Pyrantel (Banminth)	96–100%	99–100%	0	0	0
Thiabendazole (Thibenzole)	0	0	0	0	100%

Source: Iowa State University.

[a]Several trials reveal that efficiency in feed may approach 100%.

Table 16-2 lists most of the anthelmentics (dewormers) commonly on the market today. The percent removal of the various swine parasites is indicated. In order to properly use these products, information about each life cycle must be understood.

Roundworms. Roundworms are the most common internal parasite found in swine. Signs of infestation include unthriftiness, weight loss, and respiratory problems. There is also a yellowing of the skin and pigments around the eyes from a jaundiced condition (icterus) caused by blockage of the bile ducts. Economic damage comes from decreased feed efficiency, lower growth rates, and condemnation of livers and carcasses due to the presence of icterus.

The small intestine is the site of activity for the large roundworm. Eggs are picked up in the pasture by grazing hogs, and these eggs burrow through the wall of the small intestine, migrating to the liver, lungs, and to the throat area in 9 to 10 days. This causes the main clinical signs of coughing, wheezing, and difficult breathing. The larvae are then coughed up and reswallowed to migrate back to the small intestine where they develop into adults. Adults do not attach to the wall of the intestine but swim upstream against the flow of digesting material to maintain their position. This adult stage lasts for 2 to $2\frac{1}{2}$ months. Eggs are laid in the small intestine and are passed out onto the pasture. One female may lay as many as 250,000 eggs per day; so it is easy to see how an infestation can develop into major proportions. Migrating larvae also predispose the animal to bacterial pneumonia, increase the severity of mycoplasmal pneumonia by irritating the lungs, and increase the intensity of swine influenza when both the virus and larvae are present in the lungs.

Thorny-Headed Worms. Signs of infestation are nonspecific. Determination is by microscopic fecal matter examination or on post-mortem.

The thorny-headed worm is a large, flatlike parasite that has a strong attaching point on the tail that fastens itself to the wall of the small intestine. This causes a severe drain on the animal as well as internal lesions, which allow secondary infections to develop.

There are several beetles that serve as an intermediate carrier for the thorny-headed worm. The larval stage occurs in the grub of the beetle, which is eaten by hogs.

There is no effective chemical wormer for this parasite. The only recommended control is to avoid contamination. For this reason a rotation system and a rest period for large lots or pastures are a must.

Intestinal Threadworms (Strongylus). In a light infestation, there are no clinical signs. In heavy concentrations, signs will include diarrhea, anemia, and weight loss. Infestation is quite common in the southern United States.

The intestinal threadworm has several larval stages. One is free-living and may become parasitic at anytime. The larvae enter the pig by ingestion or through penetration of the skin. They affect the heart, creating a fatal condition. There is also research that indicates that the larval stage can be transmitted from the sow to the baby pigs while in the uterus and through the colostrum (first milk). These internal parasites are extremely dangerous to baby pigs if the mother is a carrier. A yellowish diarrhea and death in young nursing pigs are observed. Up to 75% of affected pigs may die before 2 weeks of age if treatment is not adequate.

Thiabendazole is recommended for both young and adults.

Nodular Worms (*Oesophagostomum*). In heavy infestations of nodular worms, the signs are digestive disturbances, weight loss, and loss of appetite. In light infestations, no signs are present.

The nodular worms develop in the large intestine, producing larvae, which are excreted directly to the ground where they are then consumed by the hog and develop again in the large intestine. The cycle is short and direct. The nodular worm is especially destructive to the large intestine wall because of its habit of burrowing into the wall, creating abscesses. These abscesses reduce food absorptive potential, and if they rupture into the body cavity, can cause infection and death.

Whipworms. Signs of whipworm infestations are bloody diarrhea and unthriftiness. Mild cases may show few signs if any.

Whipworms attack the cecum and large intestine mainly, creating a severe internal irritation and lesions, which allow secondary infections to develop. A heavy whipworm infection may intensify a swine dysentery outbreak.

See Table 16-2 for treatment.

Lungworms. Lungworms lodge in the small branches of the lungs. This results in inflammation and production of an exudate that blocks the air from these small passages, making a portion of the lung nonfunctional. Adult lungworms use this exudate as a source of food.

Adult lungworms produce eggs that are coughed up and swallowed by the pig. These eggs are passed out to the pasture where they are eaten by earthworms. Infective larvae develop in the earthworm. When the earthworm is eaten by pigs, the larvae are released in the small intestine and migrate back to the lungs.

This migration through the lung tissue causes a major portion of the damage due to lungworm infestation. The damage may also open the way for serious respiratory problems caused by secondary infections. This is the major potential danger with lungworms, even though they are not as common as other intestinal parasites.

Swine Kidney Worms. The adults of a swine kidney worm, as the name implies, are found in the kidneys. The eggs are passed in the urine and hatch shortly thereafter, reaching an infective stage in about 3 to 5 days. The eggs are ingested and migrate through extensive areas of the liver, finally entering the abdominal cavity. After some wandering, the larvae migrate permanently to the kidney. The kidney worm rather than the larva is the destructive form. In warmer climates of the South, the kidney worm is the second most important parasite of swine, exceeded in potential damage only by the roundworm.

The principal economic losses result at inspection time through condemnation of affected livers and kidneys and surrounding muscle tissue.

Currently there is no known treatment for kidney worms once the parasites gain a foothold.

A control program is based on the fact that initial infection may take 10 months to develop. Pastures are disinfected by natural sun and drying conditions 18 to 36 months after egg contamination is stopped. This is done by using only first litter gilts as breeding stock and disposing of them as soon as their pigs are weaned. Older boars should also be removed and replaced with clean boars. In this way, new eggs are not added to the pasture by the young breeding boars. A longer period may be required to eradicate the kidney worm from shaded feed lots because of reduced sunlight.

Stomach Worms. There are three types of stomach worms that affect swine. The thin worm (red worm) and two thick stomach worms; all three have the potential to cause economic loss. Stomach worms are a common internal parasite in swine and are widespread throughout virtually every state in the union and country in the world.

The thin stomach worm is generally not observed in the northern United States because of its inability to survive the severe winter conditions. Signs of infestation of stomach worms include a reduced appetite and/or diarrhea; however, high populations are required before these signs are observed. The only real way to diagnose their presence is by a fecal egg count or observation of adults on post-mortem. Hog manure can be analyzed by your veterinarian under a microscope to determine the presence of stomach worms.

An intermediate host, the coprophagus beetle, is a carrier of the thick stomach worm larval stage and serves as a source of reinfestation since hogs commonly eat these beetles. The thin stomach worm has a direct life cycle from egg back into swine by ingestion of the eggs. No intermediate host is required.

Treatment with Thiabendazole, Atgard, or Tramisol is effective in removing the adult worms. However, the stomach worm is seldom justifiably treated. Only with very heavy concentrations is treatment recommended. Prevention is by good sanitation.

Trichinosis. The swine trichina worm is found throughout the world in the pig and other carnivorous mammals including man. The highest infection rate is associated with the feeding of uncooked garbage to swine. There have been estimates that as many as 50 million Americans live with trichina larvae in their muscles. In swine there are seldom any observable signs except after slaughter where cysts can be seen within the muscles of the pigs.

These cysts contain the live larvae, which may be passed onto man or other animals by ingestion of improperly cooked pork products. This is the reason most housewives are aware that pork should always be thoroughly cooked. By raising the temperature to 137°F at the innermost point, the trichina larva are killed, and the parasite is not able to be transferred to another host. Occasionally improperly prepared or uncooked pork containing trichina is consumed. Depending on the amount of meat eaten and the level of trichina larvae, some human symptoms may occur. Rarely, following severe exposure, death may occur. The potential for infection reminds us to properly prepare pork and wild animal meats to kill any trichina present.

External Parasites

Louse and mange control is a part of good swine management. Heavy infestation can lower feed efficiency, stop growth, weaken animals, cause discomfort, and make swine susceptible to other ailments.

Lice are large and easily seen, especially on white hogs. A simple visual check can detect their presence. They are relatively easy to control. Chemical treatments are constantly being changed and regulated by the government; so check for current farm chemical registration with farm dealers, veterinarians, or local extension agents.

Mange mites are very small and are not as easily detected as lice. Mites burrow into the skin, making them more difficult to control. Scruffy, scabby skin and constant rubbing are signs of mite infestation, commonly known as *mange*. Most veterinarians are equipped to make an accurate diagnosis based on microscopic examination of skin scrapings from the inside of the ear or other affected areas.

Mange and lice are highly contagious and will spread throughout the herd if not contained quickly. Both lice and mange mites are host-specific (swine lice infect only swine, human lice infect only humans, etc.) and cannot live separate from swine for more than several days under ideal conditions. Transfer of lice and mange mites occurs readily from sows to suckling pigs. The small pigs are particularly susceptible to the adverse effects of the pests. The life cycle of lice and mange mites takes approximately 10 to 25 days. Current insecticides are not able to kill the eggs prior to hatching. For this reason several sprayings 10 to 14 days apart are advised. Repeat control procedures should be done as needed. Control of louse and mange infestations is best accomplished in the breeding herd.

A variety of insecticides are approved for use in swine. Some are toxic to suckling stocks under 30 days of age. Therefore suckling pigs should not be treated with these products, nor should sows within a week of farrowing be sprayed with these products. Replacement and new herd additions should be treated two times, 10 to 14 days apart, before being allowed into the herd.

Read and follow insecticide directions carefully. Failure to follow these rules may result in toxicity for the pigs and for the person doing the application, or may result in illegal tissue residues that could cause carcass condemnation.

17

Reproduction in Swine

The reproductive system of the male and female in swine is covered in Figures 17-1 and 17-2. The function of the male is quite similar to that of other species. Sperm is produced in the testicle of the male. Seminal fluids are produced by the secondary sex glands represented by the prostate, Cowper's, and seminal vesicles glands. The major difference between swine physiology and other species is that the swine male produces a much larger volume of seminal fluid, but this semen has not lent itself to the usual methods of storage and preservation through freezing. This has made artificial insemination a much more difficult practice than in other species, but with recent advances in frozen semen techniques, artificial insemination has become more practical for swine.

CHARACTERISTICS OF SWINE REPRODUCTION

The female reproductive system is essentially the same as in other species as far as the production of eggs and fertilization is concerned. However, the swine ovaries produce many more eggs, generally in excess of 15 to 20 with each ovulation. About 90% are fertilized by the male, so that it can be readily seen that the chief advantage of swine over other species is in the production of large litters rather than just one or two offspring. The major difference after fertilization is in the development of the sac (placenta), which in other species such as cattle allows for individual fetus envelopment and has attachments to the uterus called *cotyledons* or "buttons." The sow, on the other hand, does not have cotyledons but rather a zonary attachment of numerous points scattered all over the surface of the sac. Shedding of the sac (afterbirth) is important for normal health and should occur within a few hours after birth to prevent internal decomposition and possible infection. The afterbirth should be removed and burned. There is some evidence to

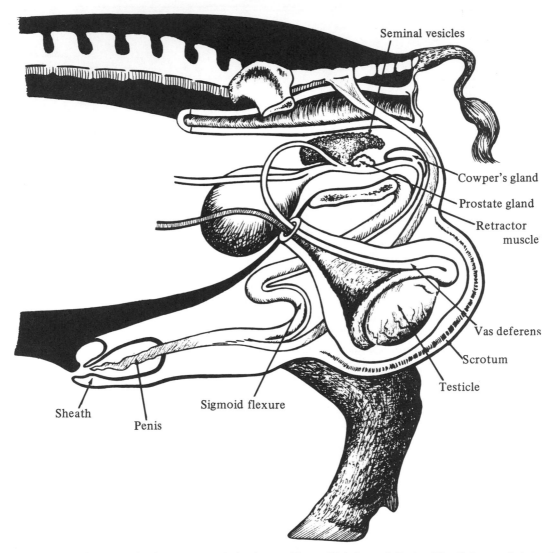

Figure 17-1. The reproductive system of the boar. (From Blakely and Bade, *The Science of Animal Husbandry*. Reston, Va.: Reston Publishing Company, Inc., 1976)

indicate that allowing a sow to eat the afterbirth leads to the vice of eating her own offspring.

Table 17-1 illustrates in short form the reproductive characteristics of a hog. Hogs reach sexual maturity (puberty) quickly, making it possible to produce a generation every 12 months. Because of this short generation interval and long-term profitability, hogs have often been referred to as "mortgage lifters." The female reaches sexual maturity at 5 to 8 months of age, normally weighing 150 to 250 lb. The male reaches puberty at 5 to 8 months, normally weighing 175 to 250 lb.

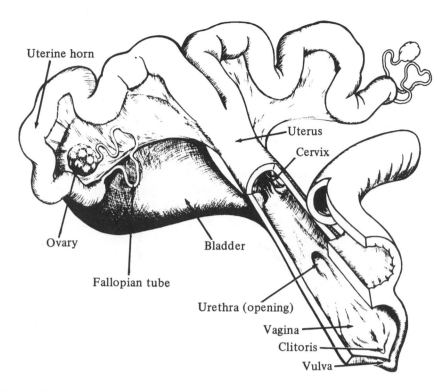

Figure 17-2. The reproductive system of the sow. (Blakely and Bade, *The Science of Animal Husbandry. Reston, Va.: Reston Publishing Co, Inc.*, 1976)

Table 17-1.   Reproductive Characteristics of Hogs

Gestation period	114 days (range 109–120)
Interval between heat periods	21 days (range 18–24)
Heat occurs after weaning pigs	5 days (range 2–10)
Length of heat period	2–3 days (range 1–5)
Best time to breed in heat period	1st and 2nd day
Number of services per sow	2 at 12 to 20 hr intervals
Gilts:	
Age to breed	8 months
Weight to breed	250–300 lb
Boars:	
Age at puberty	5–6 months
Minimum age to breed	7 months

ESTRUS

Estrus (heat) occurs in young gilts at about 5 to 8 months of age. Although this may be delayed to 9 to 12 months in confinement operations, sexual stimulation from contact with a nearby boar and increased space can be helpful to induce puberty. If the gilt is not bred, this estrous cycle will be repeated every 21 days. A gilt will vary in length of time that she stays in heat, ranging from 2 to 3 days. Sows may be in heat for 24 to 36 hours longer than gilts. Usually gilts are not bred until the third heat period or about 8 months of age. According to research, delaying breeding until the third heat results in one to two more pigs being born per litter. The gilt sheds most of her ova (eggs) the second day of the heat period. This is the maximum point of fertilization and therefore the best time period to breed her. If hand mating, the gilt should be bred twice, approximately 12 and 24 hours after the onset of heat for maximum conception and litter size.

Signs of estrus can usually be observed well before the sow actually comes into heat. Swelling and reddening of the vulva may begin 2 to 6 days before actual estrus. The sow becomes restless, frequently sniffs at the genitals of others, and utters typical grunts. Mounting of other sows may begin the day before actual receptivity to a boar.

Sows will accept a boar during a period of about 56 hours. Ovulation occurs about 40 to 42 hours after standing heat begins. As shown in Figure 17-3, the period of peak fertility begins some 14 hours after the onset of heat and generally corresponds to the period when a sow will stand to pressure applied to the haunches. However, only about 80% of the sows and half of the gilts will respond to haunch pressure in the absence of a boar.

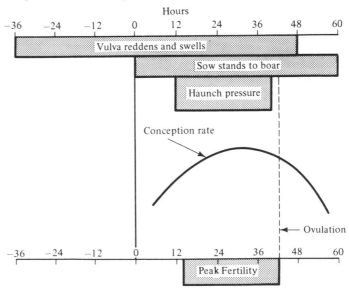

17-3. Optimum breeding time during standing heat.

In practice, best conception is usually obtained by breeding about 20 hours after the sow will stand to the boar, followed by a second mating 12 to 18 hours later. If only one mating is made, wait until about 30 hours after the sow first enters standing heat.

GESTATION

The gestation period for swine is, on the average, 114 days, enabling swine to be produced from litter to litter in one year's time. This has been the chief advantage to this species, and combined with the factors of high fertility and ease of handling, has made them extremely popular with small farmers who have to rely on maximum production with minimum amounts of feed. Swine are very efficient converters of grain to meat, as compared to other species, and no doubt will be around the farm as long as there are farm enterprises.

The nutrition of swine is extremely important because of the production of multiple fetuses. Flushing (increasing the total feed 10 days prior to breeding) in gilts is practiced to increase the number of ova (eggs) shed. Nutrition is important in order to get the maximum potential from breeding, and it is equally important for embryonic survival. The first 30 to 35 days of the gestation period are critical from the standpoint of the mother and the embryos that she carries.

PREGNANCY AND FERTILITY TESTING

Pregnancy testing in sows in the past was mostly a matter of observation of a lack of heat cycles. Now ultrasonic devices are available that determine pregnancy. Some models also measure back-fat thickness and estimate loin-eye depth. A variety of types and models exist, but their capabilities of detecting pregnancy are all very similar. The machines are most effective in measuring pregnancy from the 30th to 75th day of gestation. The device has a probe that looks something like a doctor's stethoscope; this is placed on the flank right above the udder line. It sends out and receives ultrasonic waves, which bounce back off the different tissues at different rates (much like a sonar works). These incoming results are analyzed, and indicator lights or a screen gives the results. This reading will tell if the sow is pregnant. Under old methods, a sow would have to be kept about 90 days before this determination could be made. Using the ultrasonic device, 60 days of feed could theoretically be saved, making the cost of the machine quite attractive. If you determine that about 20% of your stock was kept for replacement, 60 days off that 20% could amount to a sizable savings. There are several inexpensive ultrasonic scanners on the market, and as they become more widely used, the price will no doubt drop to even more attractive levels. These machines are very reliable and useful as a management tool, primarily in preventing and maintaining an open sow in a group of gestating sows.

Table 17-2. Recommended Breeding Load per Boar

| AGE OF BOAR | NUMBER OF SERVICES | | NUMBER OF FEMALES PEN MATING |
	(daily)	(weekly)	(21-day period)
Young (7–9 months)	–	2	–
Young (9–12 months)	1	7	8–10
Mature boar	2	10	10–15

Many producers will find such a tool useful, particularly if their operation is large enough to justify the purchase of such a unit, or if they can share a unit with a neighbor.

Fertility testing through semen evaluation is highly recommended and can be done by your local veterinarian. The boar can be tried on several sexually mature market gilts to determine his willingness and ability to breed. In this way, feet and leg and natural sex drive can be observed. Boar soundness is strongly related to his general health, usefulness, and fertility. Even though a semen evaluation proves the boar fertile, steps should be taken in very hot weather to provide the necessary cooling and shade needed for top performance, because semen quality can be reduced for 4 to 10 weeks following high environmental temperatures.

The recommended breeding load per boar is given in Table 17-2.

PARTURITION (BIRTH)

The time of farrowing, or parturition, is noted in several ways: the most common of which is the keeping of accurate records so that a herdsman knows within 3 or 4 days of when a sow is likely to farrow. As parturition nears, a gilt or sow will begin to rearrange her bedding, become restless, have slightly swollen external genitals and enlarged teats, and will noticeably be producing milk within 12 to 48 hours prior to birth. Most herdsmen will move a sow to a farrowing house 3 to 5 days prior to birth in order to acclimate her to her new surroundings. The prospective mother is normally cleaned thoroughly with soap and warm water in order to remove any worm eggs and manure from her udder or other parts of the body, and is placed in a previously sanitized farrowing stall. The farrowing stall has guard rails and other protective equipment to prevent the newly born pigs from being accidentally crushed. Also having the necessary equipment in the farrowing house makes for an easier operation should any difficulties arise. There are a number of chores that must be done even under the modern system, and equipment should be readily available.

Gestation ranges from 112 to 117 days, averaging 114 days. At farrowing time, the litter size will average about 11 piglets (the range is 1 to 15). The duration of labor may be as short as 30 minutes or as long as 10 hours, with the average being about $2\frac{1}{2}$ hours. The interval between piglets can be as short as 1 minute or as long as 4 hours, but the normal expected delivery time between piglets is 15 minutes. Approximately 50 to 75% of the pigs will be born head first, and 24 to 25% will be born in a posterior presentation. The afterbirth should be passed within 30 minutes to $2\frac{1}{2}$ hours after the last piglet. If it is longer than this, steps should be taken to assure that no infection develops. Although the incidence of difficult birth is generally less than 1% of all farrowings, it is always a good idea for the herdsman to be on hand at farrowing time.

Once farrowing begins, it should be completed within 2 to 6 hours. No assistance should be given unless it is obvious that difficulties are developing. Any departure from the normal birth averages previously described should be regarded with suspicion. Although nothing may be wrong, you should be ready to act in the event you are needed. Some of the signs of difficult birth are prolonged gestation, foul discharge from the vulva, a failure to start the birth process, straining, premature cessation of labor, prolonged labor, distress or exhaustion during labor, and hysteria.

Prolonged gestation is when any sow carries its litter over the normal 114-day period. She should be checked twice daily if this is the case, and any signs of vaginal discharge should be taken as a positive indication of impending problems.

A foul discharge at the vulva indicates decaying afterbirth and the good possibility of death of some or all of the piglets. A veterinarian should be called without delay in this case because it is generally beyond the scope of the average farmer.

When birth is obviously near, but no birth process has started, this could be an indication of a condition known as *uterine inertia* or lack of contraction of the womb.

If the sow is straining but no piglets are being delivered, there may be a malpresentation (a pig coming in the wrong position).

Premature cessation of labor sometimes occurs when piglets are still left in the sow. This is another form of uterine inertia and can be recognized by a very small number of piglets being expelled. Examination of the vaginal tract should be made to determine if other piglets are still in the birth canal. After this determination has been made, oxytocin injections may be given to create uterine contractions and continuation of the birth process.

Distress or exhaustion during labor is a serious sign of birth difficulties. If the sow is gasping, hot to the touch, or the skin is obviously discolored because of heat prostration, adequate ventilation should be given and the sow sponged with water. Oxytocin injections and veterinary help are generally necessary in these situations.

Hysteria is a rare condition in sows but is sometimes seen in gilts. Affected gilts become so excited at the time of birth that the process is completely inhibited. Sedation is normally helpful. Animals that must be sedated to farrow should be sold at weaning and none of their offspring kept for replacement stock.

The types of difficult birth may be divided into either faults in the piglet or faults in the sow. In the case of piglets, the normal presentation is either nose first or hind feet first. Any departure from these two presentations spells trouble. The two main types of malpresentation are if a pig is coming bottom first without the feet leading the way, or if two or more pigs are in the birth canal in the same spot. A lesser problem is oversized pigs; this occurs chiefly in cases of small litters or fat accumulation in the pelvis decreasing the size of the birth canal.

The main faults in the sow are uterine inertia, obstruction of the birth canal, and a condition known as *deviation of the uterus*. This latter situation normally occurs with deep-bodied sows and involves an "S" curve in the reproductive tract. The S-curve slows down the birth process much as an S-curve slows traffic on the freeway. Fortunately, when the first piglet is born, the S-curve usually straightens out, and the others are usually born without difficulty.

If birth problems are obvious, it should be within the capability of most hog farmers to carry out an internal examination of the sow. However, you should not be too proud to call a veterinarian in the event a situation occurs that is beyond your ability to master. This is a case of judgment every time the situation occurs. In the event you decide to do an internal examination, it can be an effective tool readily available to aid the sow in the case of minor difficulties such as malpresentations. This palpation is performed by introducing the hand and forearm into the birth canal. This is much easier to do if the sow is on her side; so if she is lying on her belly, she should be rubbed on the udder to encourage her to roll to one side. If the sow is on her left side, use the left hand; if on her right side, use the right hand. The back of the farrowing crate should always be removed to prevent injury should a sudden move occur. The hands should be thoroughly washed, the fingernails clipped short, and a mild disinfectant used on the hands, arms, and the area of the sow's vulva.

The hand is formed in a cone shape with the thumb and forefingers forming a point. This cone is gently inserted through the vulva into the birth canal. Be careful not to introduce foreign material such as bedding into the canal. Although gilts may show resentment at this treatment, older sows usually show little objection.

After passing into the canal, the first point of reference for the layman is the front of the bony pelvis, which can be felt below and at the side of the hand as it passes along the birth canal. This is usually an easy passage in sows but may be difficult or impossible in gilts.

As the hand explores the canal, the fingers should gently feel the wall of the canal for signs of tearing, lack of lubrication, or damage.

Any obstruction in the canal should be a piglet. You should be able to feel either the snout or the hind legs depending upon the type of presentation. Do not put your fingers into a piglet's mouth because it is quite capable of biting even before it is born. Make sure that the piglet's feet are not stuck against the walls, and then gently ease it back by pulling on the snout if a head-first presentation, or on the back legs otherwise. The amount of force needed to do this is about the same as pulling a cork from an average bottle.

The normal birth process may resume at this point, and further assistance may not be necessary. Resist the temptation to feel too often, and let nature take its course as much as possible. When no more piglets can be felt, the hand may be allowed to rest in the uterus for a while to assess the state of contractions. If contractions are occurring, as should usually be the case, they can be felt as pressure on the arm by the walls of the uterus every few minutes.

After feeling for obstructions and determining that the reproductive tract is functioning without obstruction, it may be necessary to use a pituitary extract such as POP (Purified Oxytocin Principal), more commonly referred to as *oxytocin*, in order to induce uterine contractions. The dose is 1 to 2 cc, intramuscularly or subcutaneously, if contractions are not present or if there is more than 30 minutes between pigs. This dosage may be repeated every 20 to 30 minutes as needed. Where strong uterine contractions are present in the internal exploration there is no need to use these drugs. The skilled farmer should be quite capable of this internal exploration to relieve any uncomplicated malpresentations or minor obstructions, and if he has access to oxytocin, he may be able to help in case uterine inertia is a problem. These drugs should never be used without first doing the internal exploratory examination.

As a result of your preliminary examinations, you must make a decision as to whether to cope with the situation yourself or call your veterinarian. Specific examples of when a veterinarian is needed are when you have damage to the birth canal, you are unable to withdraw a piglet, there is heavy loss of blood, the vagina and/or rectum develops a prolapse, or when stillbirths occur. In these cases it is necessary to make a quick decision and call the veterinarian before you have allowed so much time to lapse that he is unable to be of any help.

After the pigs have been expelled or delivered, you should examine them, and if breathing normally, dry them off, especially if it is chilly weather, and place them near the heat lamps. A check should be made of the nose and mouth to be sure no mucus is obstructing the air passages.

If the newly delivered pig is not breathing, grasp the head between your thumb and index finger with the pig's back lying in your palm. Bring the pig over your head and then slowly, in a large arch, bring it down between your legs. Two or three gentle swings should stimulate normal respiration. Once the pig is breathing, remove any mucus from the nose and dry and place the pig under a heat lamp. Another method for pigs that are not breathing is to fit the larger end of a small plastic funnel over the snout. Gentle breaths are blown into the small end, helping to fill the piglet's lungs and initiate respirations.

The needle teeth should be clipped (Figure 17-4), and nursing should be supervised to assure that all pigs get colostrum (first milk) during the first few hours after birth.

Shortly after farrowing (2 to 7 days), the sow will return to heat. This is a sterile heat and should be ignored even though the temptation may be to breed her again. This false heat is the last one the sow will produce until she weans the pigs that she is now nursing. Three to 5 days after weaning, the sow

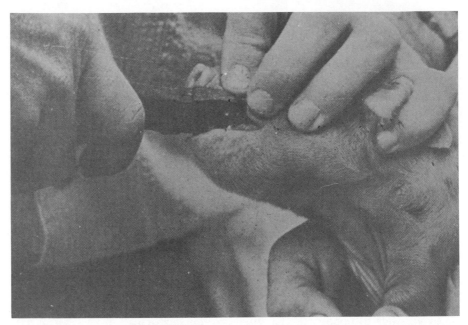

Figure 17-4. Needle teeth are clipped to prevent nursing discomfort to the sow. (*Photo courtesy of H. D. Wallace, University of Florida*)

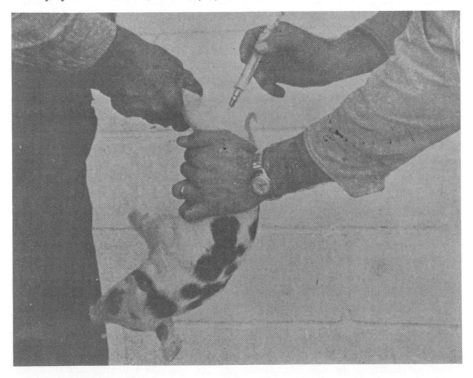

Figure 17-5. Injectable iron dextran compounds are easily administered to baby pigs. (*Photo courtesy of H. D. Wallace, University of Florida*)

normally will return to heat and will breed at this time. Early weaning is practiced by some swinemen in order to produce another litter in a shorter period of time. There is no economic advantage to early weaning before 20 days of lactation. Another practice that has received some attention is removing the pigs for several nights in a row, producing a heat period in the sow that quite often results in a new litter being started before the current one is weaned. This is not normally recommended unless it is desirable to try to get one sow into sequence with others.

At 3 to 5 days of age, baby pigs should be treated for anemia with capsules, solutions, or injections. The most common method today is an intramuscular injection of 100 to 150 mg of iron dextran per pig (Figure 17-5).

CARE OF THE BOAR

The main precaution in handling the boar is to be sure not to overwork him during the breeding season. A young boar should be bred to no more than 7 to 10 sows per three-week period. A mature boar may service as many as 10 sows per week. It is extremely important, also, to make sure that the boars are well fed and "flushed" 10 days prior to the breeding season just as are the females. This high level of nutrition for the male should continue throughout the breeding season, and during the off season it should be reduced to keep the boar in a lean, trim condition. This will improve or maintain a high level of fertility throughout the year.

SPF PIGS

In recent years, there has appeared a technique to produce swine that are free of certain pathogenic organisms that cause the greatest amount of economic loss in the swine industry. It was determined that if a farm could be sanitized or in some manner cleaned up to be free of certain disease-causing organisms, that swine could be reared in this environment completely free of those diseases.

This program was developed through the use of Caesarean operations on sows by trained veterinarians and complete isolation of the pigs from the sows. In this way the cycle of certain diseases from sow to litter was broken. The only way this is possible is to take the piglets from the mother in a sterile environment—the placenta (sac). All natural-born animals living today have been exposed in one way or another to some pathogens. They have been affected by these pathogens but have developed an immunity to them; otherwise they would have succumbed. Therefore, pigs that are taken by Caesarean operation may be considered unexposed to certain diseases. If placed in a clean environment, they would be free of these diseases as long as the sanitary measures are maintained. The development of this type of program through veterinary science is referred to as *SPF* (specific pathogen free) pigs. These pigs are free of atrophic rhinitis, brucellosis, mycoplasma pneumonia, swine dysentery, lice, and mange, the most crippling of the diseases that affect the swine industry. These diseases aren't generally fatal, but they take such a heavy toll in reduced feed efficiency and lowered gains that they are worth controlling or eradicating.

SPF hogs are no guarantee against MMA, *E. coli* scours, gut edema, SMEDI viruses, enterotoxemia, pseudorabies, internal parasites, bacterial pneumonia, or TGE.

The closed herd concept is the key to making the SPF program work. There are two types of SPF hogs currently on the market: primary and secondary. Primary SPF hogs are those that are delivered by Caesarean operation in a laboratory. Pigs are raised for 4 to 6 weeks under laboratory conditions, then moved to a farm where lots and buildings have been thoroughly cleaned, disinfected, and left idle for at least 6 weeks. The secondary SPF pigs are those that are raised from this primary stock by mating and natural farrowing. Because of the time and expense involved in producing primary herds, the secondary concept has become very popular.

To maintain an SPF herd of primary or secondary nature, the producer has to be accredited by state and national associations before he can advertise as a producer of SPF pigs. In order to do that, he has to send at least 10 hogs from each farrowing through a slaughter check. Noses and lungs are checked by a veterinarian for atrophic rhinitis and mycoplasma pneumonia. If diagnosis confirms either of these diseases, the producer loses his SPF accreditation.

Precautions must continuously be taken by any person or animal entering the premises where SPF hogs are kept. Generally, very strict measures are provided for visitors or the introduction of new animals onto the premises. Any visitor must step into a vat of disinfectant or be sprayed in some way in order to protect the clean environment.

Once swine leave this area and go to market or go to other operations, they may become exposed to pathogens, but are guaranteed not to carry them. The reason for the development of SPF pigs is simply to produce a line of hogs that will be good producers, fast growers, and efficient converters of feedstuffs, due to the fact that they are free of the normal disorders and discomforts caused by the diseases mentioned above.

The public often mistakenly refers to SPF hogs as "disease-free." This is incorrect; they are free of only a few "specific" diseases.

ARTIFICIAL INSEMINATION IN SWINE

In recent years, interest has surfaced concerning the use of artificial insemination techniques in swine. Frozen semen is now available on a commercial basis in Iowa and perhaps other states, indicating growing improvement in technology. Artificial insemination can't yet be considered routine or necessarily economical, but it is on the increase. The swine industry is at about the same point where the dairy industry was approximately 25 years ago.

Advantages to using artificial insemination in swine are:

1. Use of genetically superior sires. One ejaculation from a boar may be used to breed 10 to 20 females. On this basis, a boar could serve an average of 16 to 24 females per week or 830 to 1250 females per year.

2. Disease control. Boars from other herds can be used without violating closed herd principles. Semen is especially known to be an unlikely transmitter of organisms that cause atrophic rhinitis, erysipelas, TGE, leptospirosis, and mycoplasma pneumonia. However, where fresh semen is used, care must be taken that the herdsman does not bring disease back on his clothing or boots. Another positive benefit is that transmission of internal and external parasites can be eliminated. The most obvious advantage is to the herdsman who wants to maintain a completely closed herd yet introduce new bloodlines on occasion. Addition of antibiotics to the semen is an additional precaution in holding down disease transmission.

3. An entire group of sows may be bred to a single boar at the same time using the postweaning estrus for breeding.

The disadvantages to AI are:

1. Boar training is needed for semen collection.

2. Semen dilution and evaluation are time-consuming and difficult.

3. Heat detection requires extreme patience.

4. A minimum of equipment is required. A thermos bottle or an insulated semen-collecting bottle is usually the collecting receptacle (Figure 17-6). However, a plastic bottle with a 1 in. foam rubber washer around it can be used. There are two types of insemination catheters (Figure 17-7): a bovine type, which is disposable, and the rubber spirette, which is reusable. The technique for using the spirette is easy and simple. Tapered threads on the ends of the spirette are used to actually screw into the cervix after the tube has been inserted in the vaginal tract. The technique is actually easier to learn than artificial insemination in cattle.

5. When using frozen semen, a liquid nitrogen tank must be rented or purchased. Frozen semen at approximately $4 to $16 per tube are commercially available. Two inseminations are normally required to insure conception. Swine AI can be a very useful tool for those who are willing to put forth the high managerial effort needed. Although some word-of-mouth stories indicate that conception is low and litters are smaller in AI, research has not proven this to be the case. Conception rates of current users run as high as 87% on the first insemination. However, some people have poor results. This is partly due to technique and partly to inability of some humans to accurately predict the optimum insemination time.

In spite of the current problems encountered with AI, it will continue to grow because of the ability to genetically improve a closed herd without risking the threat of major disease outbreaks.

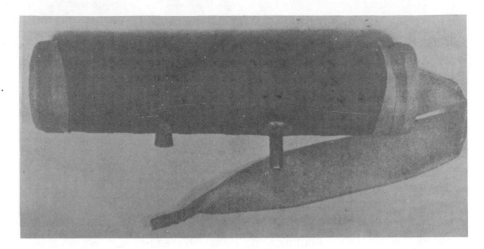

Figure 17-6. The artificial vagina shown above is one method of collecting semen from boars for use in artificial insemination. (*Photo courtesy of H. D. Wallace, University of Florida*)

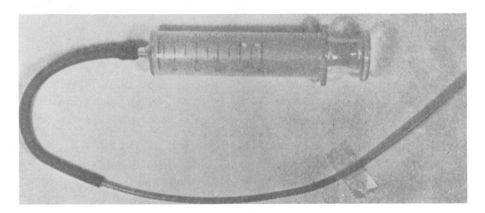

Figure 17-7. A 50 cc glass syringe attached to a rubber tube and a plastic tube is one method used for depositing semen in the uterus of the sow. (*Photo courtesy of H. D. Wallace, University of Florida*)

18

Swine Herd Management

SOWS

A blood test should be made each year for brucellosis. Any reactors should be marketed immediately.

Vaccination Program

Erysipelas. Erysipelas is known to exist widely in nature. There is a good vaccination program for it. Some areas of the United States vaccinate for erysipelas as a routine procedure. Check with your local veterinarian for recommendations in your area.

The erysipelas bacterin gives good immunity when given in two administrations subcutaneously at 2- to 4-week intervals. About 3 weeks is required to obtain maximum protection. Gilts are normally given this vaccine at 2 to 3 months of age with two administrations protecting them up to 6 months. They are revaccinated when added to the breeding herd. Sows are then vaccinated 3 weeks prior to farrowing, giving them maximum protection at farrowing and also protecting the pigs because of a transfer of the immunity through the sow.

Leptospirosis. Five strains of leptospirosis are available in commercial vaccines. A local veterinarian's recommendations should be followed. Results of blood tests of the herd and types of lepto found in the area will determine what vaccine strains to use. If vaccination is necessary, it will need to be repeated each season before breeding because immunity lasts only about 6 months.

SMEDI. Cross-exposure of boars and gilts and co-mingling sows with gilts and boars 30 days before breeding will generally spread available viruses

Table 18-1. Common Parasites—Internal

Parasites/Cause	Prevention	Treatment	Withdrawal
Ascarids Large roundworms: *Ascaris suum*	Worm the sow prior to breeding and/or 2 weeks prior to farrowing. Wash sow thoroughly before farrowing. Raise pig in cleaned buildings or new hog pastures. Avoid old lots.	Sow Dichlorovos 7–10 days prior to breeding and/or 2 weeks prior to farrowing. Piperazine in feed or water, same schedule as for Dichlorovos.	None established None established
		Pig Dichlorovos mixed in feed at 4–12 weeks of age.	None established
		Piperazine compounds in feed or water 6 weeks of age or older.	None established
		Levamisole hydrochloride in feed or water at weaning.	3 days
	Pigs Hygromycin B 12 g/ton of feed Thiabendazole 0.005–0.1% (45.4–908 g/ton) in feed (administer continuously, feed containing 0.05–0.1% for 2 weeks followed by feed containing 0.005–0.02% Thiabendazole for 8–14		2 days 30 days

Parasite	Prevention / Control	Treatment	Withdrawal
weeks). Pyrantel tartrate 96 g/ton (0.0106%) 21–28-day feeding.		Pyrantel tartrate 800 g/ton (0.0881%)	1 day
Lungworms: *Metastrongylus sp.*	Raise pigs in confinement. Avoid ingestion of earthworms.	Levamisole hydrochloride in feed or water at weaning.	3 days
Whipworms: *Trichuris sp.*	General swine sanitation.		None established
	Hygromycin B 12 g/ton	Dichlorovos in feed as needed. Have your veterinarian check for the presence of parasites. Hygromycin in feed. (an aid in treatment)	2 days
Nodular worm: *Oesophogostomum sp.*:	Hygromycin B 12 g/ton of feed Pyrantel tartrate 96 g/ton (0.0106%) 21–28-day feeding.	Hygromycin B in feed. Dichlorovos in feed. Phenothiazine in feed. Piperazine in feed or water. Levamisole hydrochloride in feed or water. Pyrantel tartrate 800 g/ton (0.0881%).	2 days / None established / None established / None established / 3 days / 1 day
Strongyloides *strongyloides ransomi*:	Strict sanitation in the farrowing house. Maintain sows and gilts in clean dry pastures during gestation. Thiabendazole in feed at a level of 0.05–0.1% has been reported to be of value.	Thiabendazole Baby pigs 1–8 weeks of age 200 mg to each 5–7 lb of body weight. Repeat in 5–7 days if necessary.	30 days / 30 days

Source: *Feedstuffs* (Minneapolis, Minn.: Miller Publishing Company, 1977); reprinted with permission.

and stimulate immunity to SMEDI. Avoid exposure of pregnant animals to new herd additions during this co-mingling.

Pneumonia and Enteric Diseases. Mixed bacterins are often used to protect sows against pneumonia and enteric (intestinal) organisms. This may be done 4 to 6 weeks prior to farrowing. Generally a second injection at 2 to 3 weeks before farrowing is required for maximum colostral immunity.

TGE (Transmissible Gastroenteritis). A vaccine is available for use where TGE is a problem. It should be used at 6 weeks prior to farrowing and repeated at 2 weeks prior to farrowing.

E. coli Scours. Sows can be exposed to manure from the farrowing house 2 to 3 weeks prior to farrowing. Bacterins also are available and may be helpful. Feeding of live milk cultures of pathogenic *E. coli* has also proved effective in reducing *E. coli* scours during the first 2 weeks of life.

Clostridial Enteritis. A clostridium bacterin-toxoid is on the market to be used at 6 weeks and 2 weeks prior to farrowing to protect baby pigs from enteric (intestinal) disorders through the colostrum of the sow. Clostridial antitoxin can be given to each pig at birth to increase immunity, but this is used only in cases where clostridium-type diarrhea is known to be a problem.

Deworming and Parasite Control

Internal. The most damaging internal parasites of swine are round-worms, nodular worms, and whipworms. These parasites are almost always present in any swine operation, and lungworms and strongyles may be present as well. For this reason sows should be scrubbed down with a brush using mild soap and warm water to remove all mud and any worm eggs that may be attached to the mammary system to reduce infection of the newborn pigs. Treatment of these internal parasites and preventive measures are given in Table 18-1.

External. Lice and mange are always a threat to the effective operation of a swine farm and an extreme discomfort to the animal, resulting in economic loss. If it is obvious that external parasites exist, commercial sprays are also available. As a precautionary measure sprays are often routinely used as recommended in Table 18-2.

Breeding Season

Flushing. Flushing is generally not beneficial with sows. In the case of gilts, an increased level of feeding should begin 3 weeks prior to breeding but not be continued after conception because the higher energy flushing rations have been shown to increase embryo death, thereby negating the flush advantage in some cases. See Table 18-2 for specific recommendations for summer and winter variations. Sows, if thin, may need to have their ration increased 1 to 2 lb, 3 to 5 weeks prior to farrowing.

Table 18-2. Common Parasites—External

Parasite/Cause	Prevention	Treatment	Withdrawal
Mange: *Sarcoptes scabiei* *Demodox phylloides*	Dip or spray all new animals arriving at the farm. Routinely schedule spraying, at 2-week intervals, of animals and premises until control is achieved.	Toxaphene Malathion Lindane.	28 days None established None established
Lice: *Hermatophinus suis*	Dip or spray all animals arriving at the farm. Routinely schedule spraying, at 2-3 week intervals, of animals and premises until control is achieved.	Use above as a dip or spray. Toxaphene Malathion Coumaphos (Do not use on pigs before weaning.) Use above as a dip or spray. Crotoxyphos (Ciodrin) Fenthion (Tiguvon) Use above as a single application; pour on the back line.	 28 days None established 14 days None established 14 days

Caution: In the use of products for mange and louse control, follow manufacturers' instructions for proper mixing and application. Avoid medicated hog oils on pregnant animals as abortions may occur. It is not safe to spray small nursing pits.

Source: John B. Herrick, Feedstuffs (Minneapolis, Minn.: Miller Publishing Company, 1977; reprinted with permission.

When to Breed. Sows should be bred to coincide with the farrowing house schedule and be grouped according to age and/or weight to produce uniform pigs. A 48-day farrowing schedule is shown in Table 18-3, which illustrates one system of breeding sows to obtain the maximum use of farrowing facilities. Breeding of the sow, of course, will depend on the time of the year and in which farrowing schedule she is included. The 48-day farrowing schedule allows 35 days from farrowing to weaning with an adjusting period of 13 days to allow for disinfecting the premises, adjustment of the pigs, and moving in a new group of sows and allowing them time to get settled in the quarters. Similar 35-day schedules can be developed along the same lines with weaning at 28 days, allowing 3 days for a cleanup and 4 days for an adjustment period for the new sows.

Pregnancy Testing. Ultrasonic devices are on the market that are portable and highly efficient for testing sows any time between 30 and 75 days after conception. A probe is placed on the flank of the sow, sending out ultrasonic waves that bounce back to a sensing mechanism in the probe. If certain lights or lines are produced on a screen or if a buzzer goes off, the sow is pregnant; if not, she is open. These devices are very accurate and are becoming inexpensive enough to be within the reach of most serious swine farmers.

Farrowing

When to Farrow. The time to farrow will be dictated by space available in the farrowing house and the system selected by the individual. Table 18-3 gives examples of farrowing schedules. The normal time on most smaller farms is a farrowing in the spring and again in the fall. This theoretically provides for two litters per year, and it is not uncommon for above-average swine breeders to average 1.7 to 2.2 litters per year with a more intense farrowing schedule, although 1.5 to 1.8 litters is more likely.

Farrowing House Sanitation. You should allow for a break between sows being brought into the farrowing house to control the buildup of organisms. The farrowing house should be cleaned, disinfected, and fumigated thoroughly between each group of sows. Specific recommendations and products are given in Chapter 2, Sanitation.

Table 18-3. 48-Day Farrowing Schedule

Sow Group	Date Bred	Date moved to Farrowing House	Farrowing Date	Date Weaned
A	Jan. 1	Apr. 19	Apr. 24	May 29
	June 3	Sep. 20	Sep. 25	Oct. 30
B	Feb. 12	June 7	June 12	July 17
	July 22	Nov. 7	Nov. 12	Dec. 17
C	Apr. 7	July 25	July 30	Sep. 3
	Sep. 8	Dec. 27	Jan. 1	Feb. 3

Feet and Leg Problems on Concrete. Feet and leg problems are frequently associated with concrete feed lots. Some hogs are susceptible to a development of tenderness around the pasterns and soles of the hoof because of their leg conformation. Many hogs will develop lameness in the joints and will walk on their knees, and quite often they will become lame enough to refuse to walk. A short-term solution is to provide an area with a different type of surface so that the hogs may go to that area for a convalescent period on their own. Eventually conformation must be improved by using breeding animals that have remained sound under similar conditions.

Hogs also develop this same condition on slotted floors because of increased pressure applied to their feet and legs. The same corrective measures must be taken as above.

Tail-Biting and Ear-Biting. Tail-biting and ear-biting are apparently caused by overcrowding in feed-lot situations or in confinement operations and by the social stresses that occur, because this activity is seldom seen on open pasture or in a natural environment. The vast majority of confinement operators are now "docking" their hogs as a routine procedure to prevent tail-biting. Ear-biting or sucking of pen mates' ears still can be observed.

A solution is to provide sufficient space in confinement or feed-lot operations. Recommended space allowances are 4 to 5 sq ft per hog from weaning to 100 lb and 8 to 10 sq ft for hogs over 100 lb. This does not include feeder and alley space. Toys, tires, and bowling balls have also been used but without uniform success. The addition of EDDI and magnesium oxide to a ration has been beneficial in some situations. Generally, the smaller pigs in a pen are the biting ones. You should remove them to a pen of smaller pigs.

Pasture Management

Sanitation. Pasture management should always consist of proper rotation and a reasonable stocking rate. Manure should be spread as well as possible after grazing has been completed and the soil turned over deeply and thoroughly. If possible, rotations should be such that swine do not follow swine on a pasture in order to break the cycle of disease organisms that are specific in their nature of attack. For example, cattle should be grazed on a pasture one year, swine the second, with perhaps crops the third year before swine return in the rotation.

BOARS

Special Needs

Exercise. Exercise is extremely important to keep boars in prime shape for the breeding season. Feet and legs must receive sufficient exercise to meet the demands placed on them during the breeding season. If a boar is in total confinement, he should be released to an exercise area and encouraged to walk. This is not necessary for all boars because some boars are now being successfully held in gestation crates for life except when called upon to breed a sow.

Weight. Keep lean but well-fed. A fat hog is not the most aggressive nor the most fertile. Hogs that are lean, in trim shape, and free of parasites and major disease should be your goal.

Health. Health is as important as performance when buying a boar. Records should determine weight gain, feed efficiency, etc., but the health of the boar's herd should be investigated to determine what diseases he has been exposed to. A blood test for brucellosis and pseudorabies is also recommended.

Sanitation Procedures

Buying. Buy your boars 60 to 90 days early. Completely isolate them from the herd for 30 days and observe them for any disease or disorders. Inspect feet and legs. Look for signs of arthritis. Do a blood test for pseudorabies 21 to 30 days after the boar is home.

Worming. Deworm the boars 30 days prior to adding to the herd. Dichlorvos, levamisol, piperazine, and pyrantel are recommended dewormers used at levels suggested by the manufacturer or your veterinarian (see Table 18-1).

Spraying for lice. Spray the boars for lice and mange using an approved insecticide prior to adding to the herd (Table 18-2).

Fence Contact. Allow fence contact with gilts 30 days prior to actual breeding to transfer SMEDI immunity. Try the new boars on several sexually mature market gilts to determine the boars' ability and desire to mate.

Fertility Tests. Every prospective herd boar should be checked for infantile reproductive organs, penile abnormalities, or cryptorchidism (undescended testes). When in doubt about a boar's fertility, have his semen evaluated.

Vaccination Program

Buy from a validated brucellosis-free herd or have a blood test made. You might consider buying boars from an accredited SPF herd. Erysipelas vaccination is recommended in areas where it is known to be a problem. Leptospirosis vaccination is given 30 days prior to adding to the herd on the advice of your veterinarian.

Heat Stress

In the boar, sperm count goes down to one-fifth the normal level and does not return to normal until 8 to 10 weeks after a boar has been stressed by heat. As little as 90° F for 72 hours can create this heat stress. You may find it economical to house herd boars in air-conditioned breeding buildings or at least provide a sprinkler for boars and sows in order to get around this problem during the summer months. This makes it doubly important to try the boars on a few gilts and have a semen evaluation run by a veterinarian before you breed them.

REPLACEMENT GILTS

If at all possible, you should maintain a closed herd, raising your own replacements to assure that no unknown diseases are brought onto the hog farm. If this is not possible, extreme care and close observation will determine whether or not purchased hogs are free of problems. It is best to purchase from only one source if possible or to buy SPF hogs to maintain a herd with minimal disease levels. The same health program as for sows, Table 18-1, should be followed.

Avoid bloodlines that have shown genetic abnormalities such as inverted teats, less than 12 functional teats, hernia, poor milking ability, atresia ani (no anal opening), and nervous disposition.

Breeding Practices

When to Breed. Gilts are selected at 5 to 6 months of age and usually are ready for breeding at 7 to 9 months of age, weighing 250 to 300 lb. Moving to another pen and regrouping will help induce heat. Gilts should be selected for 12 to 14 well-developed teats and should be allowed two heat cycles before breeding to insure maximal litter size.

What to Breed. Purebred breeders will naturally select matings according to size, type, bone development, and other breed characteristics. Market hog producers will want to consider crossbreeding. The advantages of crossbreeding are well known, and approximately 90% of commercial sows are now crossbred. Crossbred pigs are stronger at birth and grow faster, thus producing heavier pigs at market time. Crossbred sows produce more pigs. Most crossbreeding is not a single cross of two purebred parents, but some type of crossing using crossbred sows. This is accomplished by using two breeds in a crisscross or backcross system or using more than two breeds in a rotation crossbreeding program. Figure 18-1 shows the process of rotating breeds without backcrossing to one of the original breeds, thus maintaining high levels of hybrid vigor.

3-breed rotation system

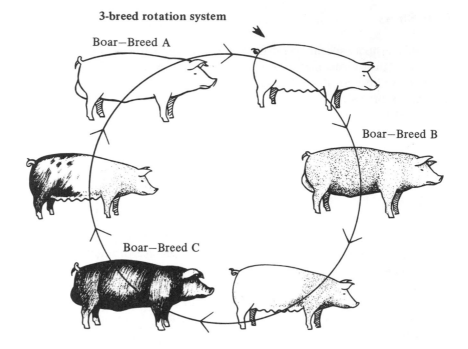

Figure 18-1. A rotational crossbreeding program for swine. (From Blakely and Bade, *The Science of Animal Husbandry*. Reston, Va.: Reston Publishing Company, Inc., 1976)

BABY PIGS

Management

1. Remove newborn pigs from membrane. Clean mucus from nose and mouth.

2. Place pigs under heat source in the brooder area. Pigs placed on chilled floors are subject to diarrhea and pneumonia. The temperature of the brooder should be kept at 90° F for the first week.

3. Help weak or chilled pigs to nurse to assure consumption of colostrum (first milk) soon after birth. Disease resistance in the form of antibodies comes from this milk. It is important that all pigs nurse within a few hours after they are born.

4. Transfer pigs from large litters to other sows to even up size of litters. Orphan pigs can be handled in a similar manner. Sows that farrow within 24 to 48 hours of each other can serve as foster mothers with few problems. Attempts to transfer pigs to a sow that has farrowed 3 to 4 days prior are seldom successful. Teats that are not continually nursed generally dry up in 24 to 48 hours. If it is necessary to try a delayed transfer, moving the oldest and largest pigs to the new foster mother may help.

5. Sever the navel cord at $1\frac{1}{2}$ in., not by cutting but by grasping it between the thumb and forefinger and pulling it apart. Use a 7% tincture of iodine solution to spray or dip the cord to prevent bacterial infections from entering the navel.

6. Clip "needle teeth" soon after birth to prevent injury to sow's udder. Cut the tip of the tooth off with a sharp pair of side-cutter pliers, taking care not to crush the teeth, injure gums, or leave jagged edges that could provide more damage than the original tooth.

7. Dock tails if close-confinement feeding operations have shown a problem with tail-biting. This is best done within the first 3 days after birth. Use a cutting-crushing instrument such as "side-cutters" or an emasculator. Sharp instruments are likely to cause more bleeding. Cut tail about $\frac{1}{2}$ inch from its base, taking care not to pull the skin as it will then draw back after cutting, exposing tissue and bone. Disinfect the stub with iodine.

8. Ear-notch pigs 24 to 36 hours after birth. Numerous notching identification procedures are used. Some simplification may dictate only notching large litters that show promise as replacement gilts or boars.

9. Prevent iron deficiency in pigs kept on artificial floors for 2 weeks after farrowing by injecting an iron-dextran compound (150 mg of iron) during the first 3 days after birth. Inject into the neck muscle and repeat 2 to 3 weeks later. Use a plastic disposable syringe and a new needle for each injection.

An alternate method for the small hog farmer is to place hog manure-free sod in each farrowing pen several times a week. Pigs get iron from the soil. Some herdsmen may prefer using iron pills, dusts, or liquids given at weekly intervals.

10. Castrate male pigs before 2 weeks of age to reduce shock and possibility of infection.

11. Feed antibiotics or growth-promoting drugs in the creep feed, when disease conditions dictate, until pigs reach 75 to 100 lb (or as directed by the manufacturer).

12. Provide clean, fresh drinking water for both sows and pigs.

Parasite and Scours Control

See Table 18-1 for parasite control measures.

If scours are a problem during the first 2 or 3 weeks, feed or use medicated water containing sulfas or antibiotics for 5 to 7 days during the stressful period.

Start pigs on feed at 7 to 10 days of age, so that they are eating feed with high levels of antibiotics in preparation for the stressful period occurring at 3 to 4 weeks of age.

The lowest point of protection in the pig's life is at 3 to 4 weeks after farrowing. Passive (colostral) immunity is greatly reduced, and active immunity produced by the pig has not begun to fully protect the pig. For this reason it is important that stresses (castration, movement, weaning, vaccination, and parasite control) be minimized.

Avoid social problems such as tail-biting, ear-biting, and fighting by sorting pigs according to size, and limit the number of pigs per pen. Open wounds can lead to bacterial invasion.

Vaccination

Generally, the only diseases to be vaccinated for as a routine measure are erysipelas and atrophic rhinitis. If the sow was vaccinated for erysipelas prior to farrowing (to protect the nursing pigs), the baby pigs should be vaccinated at 8 weeks or older, as better immunity is developed at this stage than if vaccinated younger. Vaccines are currently available from local veterinarians and appear to be effective when directions are followed exactly.

Feed Supplementation, Protein Requirements

If pigs are weaned before 3 weeks of age, they should be placed on a milk replacer and fed until approximately 12 lb in weight. The protein requirement at this age is very high, 18 to 20% crude protein.

If pigs are not weaned until 8 weeks of age, they should be creep fed with a full-fed complete ration containing 15 to 16% crude protein. Sow lactation feed makes an excellent feed for pigs when sows are lactating normally. After weaning, at about 40 lb, the protein requirement decreases to 14 to 16%, and pigs should be full-fed a complete ration until reaching market weight at approximately 220 lb. Table 18-2 gives a condensed version of requirements and specific feeding recommendations during a life-cycle feeding program.

SUMMARY OF HERD HEALTH-MANAGEMENT PROGRAM

The specifics of management have been covered for sows, gilts, and baby pigs. A complete hog management calendar might be more readily understandable if condensed into a herd management system, divided into four basic procedures: prebreeding, gestation, farrowing to weaning and growing, and finishing. The following information is from a farrow-to-finish management system recommended by Iowa State University.

This management calendar is not intended to be all-inclusive. To set up the program, it is recommended that you confer with your veterinarian and select those procedures most needed for your hogs. It may also be that your consultant will add one or more items to the system to fit your particular situation.

Prebreeding Management of Gilts

377
SUMMARY
OF HERD
HEALTH-
MANAGE-
MENT
PROGRAM

1. Select gilts from good milking dams at 220 and 240 lb with well-developed external genitalia, and 14 good, well-spaced nipples. Breed on the second or third heat cycle.

2. Vaccinate for leptospirosis (five-way) 2 to 4 weeks before breeding. Vaccinate for pseudorabies if recommended by your veterinarian.

3. Co-mingle with boars and older sows 30 days before breeding for SMEDI virus control.

4. Vaccinate for erysipelas 2 to 4 weeks before breeding.

5. Vaccinate with autogenous or mixed bacterins as needed at 3 to 4 weeks before breeding. Repeat 1 week before breeding.

6. Spray for lice and mange as needed.

7. Use broad-spectrum wormer as needed.

8. Add 200 gm of absorbable antibiotic (i.e., aureomycin or terramycin) to ration 1 week before breeding. Remove after breeding.

9. Flush (increase energy intake about 50%) during breeding period only. Restrict intake from day bred.

10. Double-mate during heat period.

Gestation

1. Limit feed to 4 to 5 lb daily during gestation.

2. Check pregnancy at 30 to 35 days after breeding.

3. Inject *Clostridium perfringens* bacterin-toxoid 5 to 6 weeks before farrowing. Repeat in 2 to 3 weeks.

4. Vaccinate for TGE 6 weeks before farrowing.

5. Feed *E. coli* milk cultures to sows for 3 to 4 days at 3 to 4 weeks before farrowing.

6. Repeat erysipelas vaccination at 2 to 4 weeks before farrowing.

7. Vaccinate with mixed or autogenous bacterin at 2 to 4 weeks before farrowing.

8. Start lactation ration 1 week before farrowing.

9. Wash sow before placing in farrowing area.

10. Worm with broad-spectrum wormer 3 to 7 days before putting in farrowing area.

11. Spray for lice and mange 4 to 6 weeks before farrowing. Repeat at 10- to 14-day intervals until control is achieved.

Farrowing—Lactation

1. Farrow in clean, disinfected, and fumigated (if practical) house.

2. Limit feed during farrowing period. Gradually increase lactation ration after first 3 days to full feed by 7 to 10 days.

3. Clip needle teeth and tails 1 to 3 days after birth. Disinfect or tie but do not clip navel cord at birth.

4. Inject 100 to 150 mg of iron per pig at 1 to 3 days after birth. Repeat in 14 to 21 days as needed.

5. Maintain farrowing house temperature at 65 to 70° F until the pigs are four weeks old.

6. Vaccinate pigs at 7 days with atrophic rhinitis bacterin. Repeat at 4 weeks of age.

7. Add 100 to 200 gm of antibiotics to a well-balanced creep ration.

8. Castrate boar pigs by weaning age.

9. Vaccinate pigs for erysipelas at 6 to 8 weeks.

10. Deworm pigs at 6 to 8 weeks with a broad-spectrum wormer. With high roundworm exposure, consider continuous feeding of wormer to stop roundworm migration.

11. Spray for lice and mange at 6 to 8 weeks. Repeat at 10- to 14-day intervals until control is achieved.

Rebreeding Sows

1. Vaccinate for lepto (5-way) at or before weaning.

2. Limit feed to maximum of 6 to 8 lb daily. Antibiotics may be added to ration during this period.

3. Put in small groups (ideal is one per pen) to reduce fighting and stress.

4. Place in fence contact with boar on day 4.

5. Double-mate during heat period.

Growing—Finishing

1. Observe twice daily for gaunt or "off-feed" pigs, lameness, or other signs of illness.

2. Provide adequate water and feeder space.

3. Spray for lice and mange.

4. Deworm with a broad-spectrum wormer about 30 days after original worming—when pigs are 6 to 8 weeks of age. Repeat if pigs are maintained in high-exposure conditions.

5

Horses

19

Nutrition of Horses

THE DIGESTIVE SYSTEM

The horse, although it eats hay and grass, is not a ruminant. Its digestive system is unique among domestic farm animals. The horse is not able to regurgitate and form a bolus as cattle can, and therefore, it does not ruminate nor digest roughage as efficiently as the ruminant. It lacks the large fermentation vat, or paunch, and the type and/or quantity of bacteria that do the work of digestion for cattle. Figure 19-1 shows the digestive system of the horse.

The key to understanding the nutritional aspects of horses is the cecum. This is the large storage area where the bulk of hay and grasses is stored when eaten by the horse. Most digestion and absorption occur in the stomach and small intestines, and little digestion takes place in the cecum. However, there are bacteria in the cecum that break down some roughage material and allow it to be absorbed into the system. Because the cecum is located beyond the stomach and small intestines, it is understandable that the horse's digestive efficiency is not nearly as good as in ruminants. This is evident in the droppings of horses, which are comparatively drier and bulkier because of the passage of undigested fiber.

Because the horse is less efficient in its forage conversion, it is often necessary to provide nutrients through concentrates (grains), to provide the necessary energy. If grain is not fed, horses tend to eat more forages to compensate for a lack of energy, increasing the size of the cecum, which shows up externally in the form of a large barrel. Some horses have a greater tendency to exhibit this characteristic than others, and this gave rise to the early term *hayburner*, because they were able to utilize large amounts of forage.

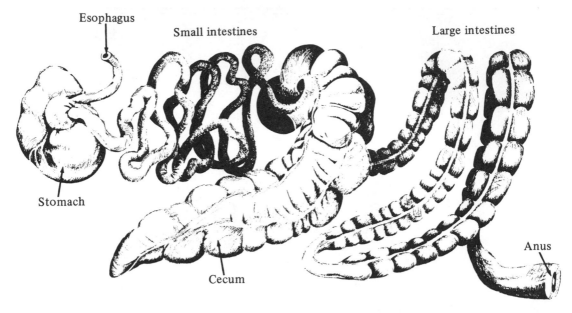

Figure 19-1. The horse's digestive system. Note the size of the cecum. (From Blakely and Bade, *The Science of Animal Husbandry*. Reston, Va.: Reston Publishing Company, Inc., 1976)

The key to feeding horses from a health and safety standpoint is relatively simple but often overlooked. Because of the unique character of its digestive system, the horse must receive a high-energy feed; and the feed must be relatively bulky, so that compaction does not occur in the digestive system, creating severe problems. For this reason oats have long been associated with the feeding of horses. The horse owner's admiration for oats is exceeded only by the horse's desire to consume them. The old song "Mares Eat Oats" hinted that there must be a reason for this happy arrangement. There is—a lack of digestive disorders. In the southern states, many horsemen have found that ground ear corn (corn and cob meal) makes a suitable substitute for oats. Either oats or ground ear corn, when used with common sense, is unexcelled in feeding horses without causing problems. Other safe mixtures are given in Table 19-1. Digestive disorders are probably the number one problem faced by any horse owner; these will be discussed later in this chapter.

NUTRITIONAL DEFICIENCIES AND SIGNS

Calcium and Phosphorus

The function of calcium and phosphorus in the horse is the same as that previously discussed for other species. Bone development is extremely important in horses, perhaps more so than in other animals because of the extreme pressures exerted on their feet and legs through work or recreation. A lack of either mineral may cause rickets in the young horse or osteomalacia in

Table 19-1. Some Example Grain Mixtures for Horses

| | \multicolumn{6}{c|}{MIXTURE NO.[a]} | | | | | |
| | 1 | 2 | 3 | 4 | 5 | 6 |
	%	%	%	%	%	%
Rolled oats	15.0	25.0	31.0	45.0	35.0	41.0
Cracked corn	15.5	20.5	29.5	25.5	25.0	35.0
Oat groats	15.0	—	—	—	—	—
Soybean meal	15.0	10.0	10.0	5.0	10.0	5.0
Linseed meal	10.0	10.0	5.0	5.0	10.0	—
Dr. skimmed milk	5.0	5.0	5.0	—	—	—
Dehy. alfalfa	5.0	10.0	10.0	10.0	5.0	—
Wheat bran	10.0	10.0	—	—	5.0	10.0
Molasses	7.0	7.0	7.0	7.0	7.0	7.0
Dical. phosphate	—	0.5	1.0	1.0	1.0	—
Gr. limestone	1.5	1.0	0.5	0.5	1.0	1.0
T.M.salt	1.0	1.0	1.0	1.0	1.0	1.0
Vitamin premix	+	+	+	+	+	+
	100.0	100.0	100.0	100.0	100.0	100.0
DE mcal/lb[b]	1.4	1.4	1.4	1.4	1.4	1.4
CP%[c]	20.2	17.8	15.9	13.2	16.1	11.9
DP%[d]	15.8	13.7	11.9	9.4	12.0	8.0
Ca%	0.82	0.81	0.72	0.65	0.79	0.46
P%	0.53	0.57	0.54	0.49	0.58	0.37

Source: Blakely and Bade, *The Science of Animal Husbandry*. Reston, Va.: Reston Publishing Company, Inc, 1977. Courtesy of Dr. John P. Baker, University of Kentucky.
[a]Type of ration: (1) milk replacer; (2) creep feed; (3) postweaning; (4) grower; (5) broodmare; (6) maintenance and working.
[b]DE = digestible energy
[c]CP = crude protein
[d]DP = digestible protein
Note: All grain mixtures are to be fed with grass or grass-legume hay.

mature mounts. Rickets is a deformation of the young, soft growing bones, whereas osteomalacia is a brittle development in mature horses causing leg problems, even broken bones. The calcium-phosphorus ratio in horses should be maintained at 1.1 part calcium to 1 part phosphorus to prevent the occurrence of these problems. The range up to 1.4 to 1 is acceptable. Horses require rations with .6% to .7% calcium and phosphorus. Bonemeal should be served as a source in feed mixtures or be given free-choice mixed with an iodized trace mineralized salt.

Salt

Salt is also extremely important in horses because they are one of the few domestic farm animals that sweat extensively. This sweating mechanism allows them to cool their systems, and in hard-working horses, salt can be, and often is, expelled from the body in very large quantities. If free-choice salt is not allowed, the feed ration should contain salt in quantities of .5% to 1% of the feed. A deficiency of salt leads to heat prostration, tiredness, and exhaustion.

Iodine

A deficiency of iodine can create goiter in the horse, although it is not a very common occurrence. Iodine is used by the thyroid gland to regulate body temperature. It is add to the trace mineralized salt mixture or in the ration as a precautionary measure. The more common form is to use an iodized salt mixture.

Iron and Copper

Owners of working horses have a tendency to worry about anemia (iron poor blood) and therefore give excessive iron injections. If parasite control and nutrition are adequate, most animals do not need iron injections. But if in doubt, blood tests are available through your veterinarian to determine if there is a need.

A deficiency of iron and/or copper can create the anemic conditions previously discussed in other species.

Zinc

There is some indication that zinc is utilized by horses for proper skin and hair maintenance, and recently there have been reports that added zinc to a ration appears to have some influence on the well-being of race horses. There are some breeders who feel that zinc added to the ration keeps their horses eating better, more alert, and running faster than the competition. However, this is purely speculation at this point. Any level of zinc added to a ration should be checked thoroughly with a competent nutritionist because of the possibility of creating an imbalance with other minerals. The safest way to provide zinc is in a trace mineralized salt as suggested in Table 19-2.

Manganese

A deficiency of manganese has not been proven to exist on a widespread basis under natural conditions, but it is known that manganese is required by the horse and is added in most rations for safety reasons. A trace mineralized salt mixture complete with levels recommended is given in Table 19-2 from the heart of horse country, Kentucky.

Fat-Soluble Vitamins

Good, clean, fertile pastures on fertile soils offer the best insurance against vitamin shortages. However, in the absence of green pastures, or when a horse is being stall-fed, it is important to provide as much green, leafy forages as soon as possible to prevent a deficiency of the fat-soluble vitamins: A, D, E, and K. The owner is cautioned, however, against feeding very large quantities of alfalfa hay because digestive problems can occur from a very rich, straight diet of legume hays.

Water-Soluble Vitamins

Water-soluble vitamins are not as necessary in the diet of a horse as for other species because of a sufficient amount of bacterial activity in the cecum, which produces a great number of B-complex vitamins; however, for safety's sake, thiamine, riboflavin, pantothenic acid, and vitamin B_{12} should be included in a horse's ration.

RATIONS

The average horseman doing recreation riding will do well to forget about all of the exotic sweet feeds that are on the market and stick to a relatively simple concentrate ration containing 95% oats and 5% oilseed meal (linseed, soybean). A bright, clean, leafy nonlegume hay is recommended for roughage. The grain portion, of course, is fed at a specified level to be explained at the end of this chapter. An alternate ration suggestion is a grain portion of half oats and half "sweet feed" (a commercial mixture of grains and molasses) and free-choice bright clean, leafy hay. There have been very few reports of digestive problems with horses fed totally or largely on oats and hay. Almost all of the digestive disorders come when man tries to improve on nature by mixing an exotic feed.

Each horse should be fed as an individual because some eat very rapidly and some are very slow eaters. It is extremely important to keep feed boxes free of moldy feed and to allow a horse about 30 minutes to clean up his feed. If he does not, it should be removed in order to prevent digestive disturbances. Hay is, of course, left. Horses should always be fed at the same time(s) each day, whether fed once, twice, or three times daily. Fast eaters may be slowed down (to prevent digestive disorders) by placing a few large round stones in the feedbox so that the horse has to eat around them to clean up the feed.

Rations should never be changed abruptly, and a week's time should be allowed when gradually switching to a new mixture.

Table 19-1 gives some example grain mixtures for horses that have been proven to be excellent, safe mixtures for the horse's digestive system when hand-fed at recommended levels. Tables 19-2 and 19-3 give the trace mineral-ized salt and vitamin premixes referred to in Table 19-1 for the horse owner who wishes to mix his own ration.

Feeding Hints

As previously stated, each horse should be fed according to his own particular condition. Some horses get too fat, others too thin, depending on what they do and what they eat. Although the horse owner or handler will

Table 19-2. Trace Mineralized Salt

| | TRACE MINERAL CONTENT | |
| | | AMOUNT PER LB OF |
MINERAL	T.M. SALT	GRAIN MIXTURE
Iodine	0.007%	318 mcg
Iron	0.80%	36 mg
Copper	0.16%	7 mg
Zinc	1.00%	45 mg
Manganese	0.40%	18 mg

Source: Blakely and Bade, *The Science of Animal Husbandry*. (Reston, Va.: Reston Publishing Company, Inc., 1976.) Courtesy of Dr. John P. Baker, University of Kentucky

Table 19-3. Vitamin Premix for Horses

| | | AMOUNT PER LB FEED | |
| | PER LB | WHEN PREMIX ADDED AT: | |
VITAMIN	PREMIX	5 LB/TON	1 LB/TON
Vitamin A	1,000,000 I.U.	2,500 I.U.	500 I.U
Vitamin D	100,000 I.U.	250 I.U.	50 I.U.
Vitamin E	5,000 I.U.	12.5 I.U.	2.5 I.U.
Thiamine	1.2 gm	3.0 mg	0.6 mg
Riboflavin	800 mg	2.0 mg	0.4 mg
Pantothenic acid	800 mg	2.0 mg	0.4 mg
Vitamin B$_{12}$	5 mg	12.5 mcg	2.5 mcg

Source: Blakely and Bade, *The Science of Animal Husbandry*. (Reston, Va.: Reston Publishing Company, Inc., 1976.) Courtesy of Dr. John P. Baker, University of Kentucky

modify diets according to individual body and flesh conditions, some helpful rules to serve as guidelines follow:

1. Horses doing light work (under 3 hours)—0.5% of body weight in concentrate (see the sample rations in Table 19-1), 1 to 1.25% hay.

2. Horses doing medium work (3–5 hours)—1% of body weight in concentrate, same amount of hay.

3. Horses doing hard work (over 5 hours)—1$\frac{1}{4}$% of body weight in concentrates, 1% in hay.

Breeding stallions should be fed as a horse doing hard work and should be exercised thoroughly prior to and during the breeding season.

4. Pregnant mares—0.75% to 1.5% of body weight in concentrate, 0.75% to 1.5% of body weight in hay.

5. The total combined consumption of concentrate and hay should be kept in the range of 2% to 2.5% of body weight.

6. Foals—The mare's milk will sustain adequate growth until about 6 weeks of age, when it is advisable to begin creep feeding. The foal should be consuming about .75% of its body weight in a good legume or grass hay and

an equal amount of concentrate creep feed. The concentrate mix should contain a minimum of 12% crude protein and at least 5% fiber. A standard ratio is 9 parts grain to 1 part oil meal. No more than one-half the grain mix should be corn, milo, or wheat combined with oats or barley because of the possibility of compaction due to the heavier concentrates. This same mix can be continued after weaning to about 1 year of age. Consumption by this time will have increased to 1% of body weight in concentrates and 1.5% in hay. A suitable mineral mixture should be supplied free-choice as for other horses.

Management Suggestions

1. Withhold half of the grain ration and increase hay on days that working horses are idle.

2. Use only dust-free and mold-free feeds.

3. Water before feeding. If horse is heated, avoid excessive watering.

4. Feed hay before grain.

5. Do not feed a tired horse his total allotted diet of grain at one time. Feed half the grain, then feed the rest 1 hour later.

6. Do not work a horse hard after feeding a full grain allotment.

7. Feed and water regularly and not less than twice daily.

8. Observe the condition of the horse and feed accordingly.

20

Diseases of Horses

HOW TO IDENTIFY A SICK HORSE

The general behavior of any horse under healthy conditions must be known before the handler can determine if the behavior is normal. Any act contrary to normal behavior should be viewed with suspicion as to the possibility of disease or disorder being the primary cause. An animal shows its feelings through its actions just as humans do. But how do you know something is wrong with an animal? You must first "suspect" some problem, and then draw conclusions based on evidence. The art of diagnosis is supplemented by conclusive tests and/or closer examination.

If a horse goes off feed, becomes wild-eyed, appears very sleepy for long periods of time, lies down excessively, or varies in its daily routine habits, the handler may suspect a problem.

Some ailments only occur during certain times of the year, and can be ruled out at other times even if similar signs occur.

Early detection of abnormal signs is extremely important in horses because early detection not only aids in a more rapid cure of the condition, but it also prevents a spread of the disease to other animals in the herd.

If, for instance, a horse lies down often, this could be a sign of illness. A horse usually stands even while sleeping. In the rare instances that it does lie down, the normal position is on one side. If a horse should be seen lying on its belly for long periods of time, this is a good clue that something is wrong. When you approach a horse that is lying down, it will invariably get up and move off or run away if it is healthy. If the horse does not offer to get up when you approach, this could be an early sign of trouble.

In the case of foot problems, the horse will naturally want to get the weight off of its feet. Close examination of feet, legs, and hooves by palpation of tender spots or by noting unnatural odors from the hoof area, may discover possible inflammation or infection.

When a horse sweats profusely, paws the dirt, rolls on the ground and groans, it is a probable sign of colic and attention should be given immediately.

The stance of a horse tells a lot about its health. The normal stance will be loose, with ears erect or forward. When the horse's head is down, its back arched, and its ears droopy, it is a sign of disease or disorder.

For instance, a horse suffering from early signs of tetanus will show a wide "sawhorse" stance and will have difficulty in moving sideways. The condition gets progressively worse as tetanus develops into the later stages. If sleeping sickness is suspected, the stance will be different, with most of the weight shifted to the hindquarters and the horse exhibiting a wobbly, uncertain gait.

The refusal of feed is frequently a sign of problems because the normal horse eats all the time. The refusal could simply be due to moldy feed or even a sudden change of feed, because a horse is a finicky eater, although once it gets accustomed to a feed, it quite often becomes a glutton. So, if the horse is on a standard ration and suddenly refuses it, the feed should be checked to determine quality. If the feed is okay, the handler may suspect disease or digestive upset.

A rapid loss of condition is a sure sign of difficulty in any animal. In the horse, internal parasites, digestive disturbances, or even a sore mouth, tongue, or bad teeth can be serious problems.

The skin of horses is a reflection of their internal health. It should be soft and pliable, and the haircoat, especially, should be bright, smooth, and shiny. Any variation from this normal skin and hair condition could indicate problems. Allergies are not uncommon in horses. A characteristic sign is small bumps that look like mosquito whelps on the skin. Patches of hair may be missing due to scratching. External parasites, a mineral deficiency, or internal organ malfunctions may all exhibit themselves outwardly through a change in skin and hair condition. The hair of chilled animal will stand on end.

Unexplained unpleasant odors from the mouth or body parts could also be an indication of a problem. Excessive salivation or dry mouth is a sign of many disorders.

If the eyes lose their moist appearance, it is an early indication of trouble. The pupil should become smaller when a light is shined into it. If it doesn't, this is a probable indication of a disorder somewhere. Both eyes should be checked for normal constriction of the pupils to rule out the possibility that there is simply a problem in one of the eyes. If the pupils do not constrict, then more extensive examinations can take place in putting the pieces of the puzzle together.

Other indications of illness or disorder are when droppings are no longer in round balls that break upon hitting the ground; or when there are bad odors and/or consistency changes in the droppings; or when there are mucous or parasite excretions.

Because of the common occurrence of feet and leg disorders, the legs should be observed frequently for swelling or an obvious difference in circumference of one leg compared to the other.

Temperatures above or below the normal (100 to 101°F) should be viewed as conclusive evidence that a problem exists. Temperatures should be taken with a thermometer placed in the rectum. Be sure that the thermometer is well lubricated and if available, use a thermometer designed for horses so that it's long enough to reach far enough into the rectum to get an accurate reading. Leave it in the rectum 2 to 3 minutes. The thermometer should be secured by a string and clamped to the tail to prevent losing it due to rectal muscle movement.

RESPIRATORY DISEASES

Colds, Upper Respiratory Infection (URI), Distemper

Signs. A thin, nasal discharge that gradually becomes thicker is the chief clinical sign.

Cause. The cause is generally thought to be a virus or bacteria.

Prevention. Avoid subjecting the horse to extremes in temperature and keep away from other horses that have obvious signs of colds.

Treatment. Isolate the horse. Consult a veterinarian if signs appear extreme. Keep it warm and administer antibiotics such as penicillin or streptomycin.

Coughs

Signs. The sign is a hacking cough much like that seen and heard in humans.

Cause. A cough could be brought on by a variety of conditions. A change in food or temperature, even an allergy to grass, could bring on the condition. It could also be brought about by a roundworm infestation causing a tickling sensation in the larynx.

Prevention. Keep the horse out of extreme variations in temperature. Provide it with shelter, constant quality of food, and a regular program of worming.

Treatment. A good home remedy is to keep the horse warm and give small doses of a common cough syrup placed on the back of the tongue two or three times a day. If the condition is determined to be caused by worms, a laxative diet should be established, the proper chemical treatment given, and be sure not to overexert the horse during the recooperative period. If the cough persists for more than 48 hours, seek professional help.

Whistling

Signs. The chief clinical sign is a high-pitched noise coming from the larynx of a horse when it is worked hard, particularly at the faster paces.

Cause. The disorder is thought to be caused by a rupture of one of the nerves of the larynx, resulting in paralysis of the vocal chord and a partial blocking of the larynx.

Prevention. This condition is thought to be hereditary, and very little can be done to prevent it. It does not normally occur in smaller breeds of horses.

Treatment. The veterinarian can perform a "tubing" operation in which a tube is inserted into the larynx, allowing free passage of air. Another operation allows for the removal of a membrane from the pouch directly behind the vocal chord.

Heaves (Broken Wind)

Signs. The chief sign is a persistent deep cough, which if not treated often turns into a more serious condition. The name is derived from the movement of the horse's flank, which can be seen to heave twice, rather than once, as normal, during exhalation. The extra muscle effort from the abdomen causes the secondary reaction in the flanks.

Cause. The cause is thought to be dusty food, especially just prior to excessive strain or work. Asking a horse to work excessively while it has a cough can also lead to this condition.

Prevention. Take care not to feed horses dusty feed or house them in an area where there is obvious air pollution.

Treatment. The condition is incurable, although it can be improved or alleviated by avoiding dust through the use of small amounts of water on the feed, or better yet, by the use of linseed oil in the feed about three times a week. The bedding should also be kept slightly damp in order to keep the dust particles down. Precaution should be taken not to use excessive moisture because this could lead to other respiratory ailments. Stable bedding should be shavings or peat so that the horse won't eat these materials and stir up more dust. Antihistamines in the feed offer aid in controlling this condition.

Strangles

Signs. Horses become very lazy in appearance, temperatures may rise to 105°F, generally there is nasal discharge, and the key sign is a swelling under the jaw, which eventually forms an abscess and usually bursts.

Cause. Strangles is a disease of the lymph gland, usually only affecting horses under 6 years of age. It is thought to be caused by a virus.

Prevention. There is little to be done in preventing the first case, but much to be done in preventing spread of the disease because it is highly contagious. Any horse contracting the disease should be isolated and all items that came into contact with it disinfected.

Treatment. Keep the horse warm, provide a laxative diet, and call your veterinarian. The course of the disease is usually about 6 weeks. Convalescence is normally very slow. The normal period for regaining strength and health is 2 to 3 months of gentle work. After that, horses can be gradually returned to their usual activities.

Roaring

Signs. The clinical sign is a deep rumbling noise made by the horse when exhaling, particularly when doing heavy work.

Cause. The cause is a paralysis of the soft palate of the mouth, or laryngeal paralysis.

Prevention. Avoid excessive working after an attack of strangles. This is the primary cause of the disease.

Treatment. The condition is very difficult to treat, but live firing (using a hot iron) of the soft palate has been used by some veterinarians and may be recommended for specific cases, although the practice is no longer in general use.

Equine Viral Rhinopneumonitis

Signs. Clinical signs include a fever that ranges between 102 and 107° F, cough, nasal discharge, either constipation or diarrhea, and a severe deformation of the nasal bones (rhinitis). There is also a very high rate of abortion, generally 1 to 4 months after the onset of the respiratory signs. If a mare carries her foal to full term, it is more often than not born weak, develops pneumonia, and dies shortly after birth.

Cause. The cause is an airborne virus that can also be carried in water. It can contaminate hay and feed as well as drinking water. The organism may be spread in a variety of ways, including man and dogs.

Prevention. Proper sanitation is of utmost importance. Adequate ventilation in the stables and isolation of infected patients are recommended. There is a vaccine for protection against the disease, but it does not confer permanent immunity. Horses must receive a regular inoculation schedule complete with booster shots for full protection.

Treatment. There is no effective treatment against the virus. The secondary infections created by the weakened condition can be treated through the use of antibiotics such as penicillin and streptomycin. Other supportive treatment is recommended such as rest, shelter, and proper temperature.

Pneumonia

Signs. The onset is usually sudden. A rapid rise in temperature and dullness are initial signs, with the highest fever occurring during the early part of the disease. There is an increased pulse and respiratory rate, a painful cough, and discharge of mucus from the nose.

Cause. A variety of agents such as viruses, bacteria, parasites, fungi, hot or cold air, dust, or even foreign matter can be the precipating factors in this disease. However, the most common causative agents are either a virus or bacteria, alone or in combination. The condition is most often brought on by exhaustion, sudden changes in the weather, or confinement in damp quarters.

Prevention. Dry, well-ventilated quarters and a minimum of stress with an adequate level of nutrition are considered supportive measures for prevention.

Treatment. Because pneumonia is contagious, sick animals should be isolated, provided with adequately ventilated quarters, and the temperature kept at a comfortable level. Blanketing is recommended for horses kept in unheated pens or stalls. Treatment with antibiotics, such as penicillin, streptomycin, or in combination, should be given at full dosage for at least 4 days or until the patient has been afebrile (body temperature returns to normal) for at least 24 hours. Be sure adequate water is available.

Influenza

Signs. The chief sign is an abrupt onset with a fever ranging from 102 to 106° F, lasting 1 to 6 days. There may be excessive discharge from the nostrils, tears discharged from the eyes, and nasal congestion. A cough appears often during the early stages, especially in working horses, but is slight or absent in nonworking horses. Foals may become quite ill and can even die. Uncomplicated cases in adults usually result in recovery within 7 to 10 days.

Cause. This is a virus infection of a specific nature that also attacks swine. It first appeared in the United States in 1963, but is now found in most countries throughout the world.

Prevention. Rigorous sanitation and isolation between groups that have outbreaks are the chief preventive steps. An immunity develops in those animals exposed to it, but the immunity gradually wears off after a year or two, and the infection may return again. However, the second time is usually not as severe as the first. Vaccination is effective in prevention.

Treatment. Treatment is seldom necessary except in very young foals; it is recommended that they receive antibiotics throughout the course of the disease. After 24 to 48 hours of normal temperature and normal respiration restoration, treatment can be discontinued.

REPRODUCTIVE PROBLEMS

Difficulties of reproduction in horses have always been a major concern for their owners.

Mares must have good housing, adequate nutrition, regular exercise, and proper parasite control in order to breed efficiently. Infectious diseases cause very few disorders in horses, but a combination of diseases and other factors have made a 50% foal crop quite ordinary in the average operation. Given adequate grass, breeding in the spring, exercise, care and attention to parasites, and other measures, the conception rate in captivity can approach a high efficiency. In the wild, conception rates may exceed 90% if breeding occurs during the spring. On specialized horse farms where strict sanitary measures are maximized and other problems minimized, a 60 to 80% foal crop may be expected.

Abortions

The main problem with reproductive diseases in horses are abortions, some of which are caused by bacterial and viral infections. The cause of about 40% of the abortions are never known; so antiseptic measures are extremely important both at breeding and at the time of foaling. A mare's genitals should be washed and scrubbed clean with disinfectant and her tail bandaged prior to breeding. The stallion's penis should also be cleaned in a similar manner, the reason for this is to prevent organisms from being introduced into the reproductive tract of the female, bringing contamination. Foals may be carried by the mare for several months before the abortion occurs.

About 20% of abortions are caused by a streptococcal organism that affects the fetus frequently in the early months of pregnancy, but that may affect it at any stage of gestation. There is no vaccine available for streptococcal abortion. Since it cannot be avoided, the main thrust of defense is through sanitary conditions. In cases where the foal may not be affected by the streptococcal organism, a difficult birth can predispose the mare to infection from the organism. A retained placenta (afterbirth, sac) can also create a condition conducive to streptococcal invasion.

Contagious equine abortion is caused by a bacterium called *Salmonella abortivo-equinus*. Although infrequently found now, this abortive organism may make its presence known about the fourth to eighth month. A good preventive measure for any abortion, but especially in this case because of its contagious nature, is to bury any dead fetus and the afterbirth deeply, or burn them. Stalls and equipment should be cleaned and disinfected immediately. Aborting mares should not be bred again until the reproductive tract is determined free of the infection.

There is no treatment for abortive conditions once they develop, but the problem may be controlled by eliminating reacting mares and stallions, and may be prevented by vaccination with a salmonella bacterin.

Other infectious diseases, in addition to those caused by the salmonella and streptococci organisms, may cause abortion; but since they account for less than 3% of the known abortions, they lack sufficient importance to cause concern.

395
SYSTEMIC
DISEASES,
VIRAL AND
BACTERIAL
DISEASES

Control procedures are necessary during outbreaks of infectious disease to stop the spread of disease and to assure prompt return to normal health. Restricting employees to specific quarantined areas and sterilization of equipment are necessary in a cleanup. A mare that aborts should be left in the stall or barn where the abortion occurred unless she can be moved to a more isolated spot without danger of contaminating other mares, especially pregnant mares in the herd. Bedding and the manure should be removed and burned. The lack of proper sanitation during both breeding and foaling does often allow entrance of an organism that can bring about an abortive disease. Therefore strict sanitation measures are a necessity for proper horse reproduction.

Equine viral rhinopneumonitis (EVR), a disease of the upper respiratory tract of the horse previously discussed in this chapter, is another virus that commonly causes abortion and affects horses of all ages.

Abortions also may be caused by certain drugs, deworming agents, poisonous plants, chemicals, and moldy or spoiled feed.

SYSTEMIC DISEASES, VIRAL AND BACTERIAL DISEASES

African Horse Sickness (Equine Plague)

African horse sickness is caused by an insect-borne virus and has a very high mortality rate. It has been of epidemic proportions in Africa since the early 1700s. Although the disease is not known to exist in the United States, it is mentioned here in order to inform foreign horse breeders who find this book useful.

Signs. The clinical signs involve an incubation period of less than 10 days in which a gnat is generally the insect vector spreading the virus. The disease may take either a pulmonary or a cardiac form. In either case the animal is not likely to recover. Temperatures will be high (105° F plus), but horses will continue to eat normally up until the last 24 to 36 hours before death.

In the pulmonary form there is a severe accumulation of fluid in the lungs blocking the respiratory passages. Horses with the cardiac form show an accumulation of the fluid around the head and neck. The cause of death in this case is generally from cardiac failure.

Cause. The cause is a virus with nine distinct forms. Gnats are the principal carrier. For this reason, among others, importation of horses into the United States from countries infected with this disease is very strictly regulated.

Prevention. One preventive method is the use of quarantine measures to isolate the virus to those countries of its origin.

There are also vaccines available for use in preventing the disease before an outbreak occurs. A nine-strain vaccine has been in use for the past 30 years that produces a satisfactory immunity. Horses from infected countries should be quarantined for 30 days in insect-free isolation. A negative virus test is required for release of the horse to United States owners.

Treatment. There is no known treatment.

Azoturia (Monday Morning Disease)

Signs. Azoturia is referred to as "Monday morning disease" because it most often occurs after a horse has been rested over the weekend while still consuming a customary heavy ration of grain.

It is most prevalent in hard-working, well-fed horses during cold weather. The attacks usually appear during the first hour of exercise, most often during the first 15 minutes. The animal begins to sweat and shows stiffness in the legs. This stiffness may occur in either the front or back and may affect one or all four legs, but it most often affects the hind legs. Affected mounts become stiff, try to extend the hind legs, and eventually assume a "sitting dog" position. Later, the horse lies down, and urination becomes difficult if not impossible. The urine, if it is still possible to be passed, is discolored red, brown, or almost black. The horse will remain down usually for 2 to 4 days, after which recovery is possible; in severe cases, death may occur. Those animals that do not go down or those that are affected only in the forelegs stand the greatest chance of recovering.

Cause. This is an unusual disorder caused by an accumulation of lactic acid in the tissues and blood. The cause of the buildup is a lack of exercise without a decrease in metabolism.

Prevention. Management is the key to prevention through restricting the diet of horses that are worked very hard if they are to be off this strict exercise program for even one day. The most often used method of prevention is to give a wet mash on Saturday night if the weekend is to be the off period and a very light feeding on Sunday. The normal resumption of heavy feeding can begin Monday at the regular work hour.

Treatment. If the horse is affected while you are riding, do not ride the horse further. If the attack is obviously severe, dismount and allow the animal to rest or walk slowly until a veterinarian can arrive. In the event it is a mild attack and only the front legs are involved, a laxative should be given, preferably 2 to 4 liters of mineral oil to act as a purgative. In more severe cases if a veterinarian is not available, tranquilizers may be used to aid in lessening the muscle tension. Keep the horse comfortable. Sedatives or antiinflammatory substances may be prescribed for pain.

Navel Ill

Signs. Newborn foals develop a high temperature, but there may be little involvement of the joints of the legs in contrast to the effect on cattle or hogs. Death can occur in this early stage within 1 to 3 days after onset if treatment is not commenced. In the case of foals 2 to 3 weeks or older, the course of the disease is less acute, and there is a greater tendency for stiffness to develop in the joints, tendon sheaths, and lymph nodes.

Cause. Numerous microorganisms can invade the umbilical cord of the foal to create an infection giving rise to navel disease. However, about five organisms normally are the cause, with the most common being streptococcus.

Prevention. Good management and strict sanitation practices are the key to prevention. Also, the umbilical cord should always be dipped in tincture of iodine as soon after birth as practical. The umbilical cord should not be cut unless it is absolutely necessary because this is often a point of entry for disease—when man uses an unsterile instrument such as a knife to cut the cord. In the fly season, a repellent should also be used to prevent infection due to fly problems. Animals that are properly treated at birth seldom require subsequent treatment.

Treatment. Treatment should commence immediately because there is imminent danger of death. Injectable penicillin-streptomycin mixtures are commonly used and are quite effective. The dosage should depend on the streptomycin requirement rather than the penicillin portion. A dose containing 1 to 2 grams of streptomycin should be given every 12 hours for at least 3 days or longer.

Poll Evil or Fistula Withers

Signs. The clinical signs are identical for both poll evil and fistula withers, even though the outbreak may be in two different places. A bursa (a saclike structure containing lubricating fluid to cut down on friction) is the normal site of the infection, which deteriorates into a running sore. A bursa is infected at the top of the poll in poll evil, or at some point on the shoulder in fistula withers. There is never any indication as to which of these points will be the point of attack.

Cause. It is known that some organisms attack the bursa of the horse, creating a running sore. It is thought that this is due to mechanical injury in some instances, but there is no evidence to indicate that this is always the case. It is also known that the brucellosis organism that causes abortion in cattle can be injected into horses and can cause the condition. Simultaneous outbreaks of brucellosis (Bang's) in cattle along with poll evil in horses have been quite commonly recorded. It is therefore thought that the main invading organism creating the condition in horses is *Brucella abortus*. There have been

397
SYSTEMIC
DISEASES,
VIRAL AND
BACTERIAL
DISEASES

instances in which horses have developed an infected bursa, and shortly thereafter cattle break out with brucellosis.

Prevention.   Strict sanitation and separation of horses and cattle are required in the event an outbreak of either brucellosis or poll evil occurs because of the contagious nature and the ability for the organism to infect both species.

Treatment.   The brucella vaccines have not proven effective for horses; therefore treatment is essentially a surgical proposition requiring the drainage of the infected bursa on horses and treatment with sulfa drugs following surgery. It is highly recommended that a veterinarian handle this treatment because of the contagious nature of the organism involved and because of the possibility of contamination to other species on neighboring farms and ranches.

Sleeping Sickness (Equine Encephalomyelitis)

Signs.   The signs of equine encephalomyelitis, commonly called *sleeping sickness*, include impaired vision, a drousy appearance, pendulous lower lip, a dazed look, fever, irregular gait, wandering around, a reduction of reflexes, incoordination, yawning, grinding of teeth, inability to swallow, inability to rise, paralysis, and death.

Cause.   There are a group of viruses that create sleeping sickness in a horse. The virus is carried by mosquitoes and birds. Common domestic birds such as chickens, quail, turkeys, pheasants, etc., act as hosts for the virus. The mosquito attacks the bird, which keeps the virus alive. The horse, in most cases, is a dead-end host. Mosquitoes may also transfer the disease from horse to horse. The disease is therefore common in areas with a large bird and mosquito population. Pasture horses rather than stable animals are most susceptible.

Prevention.   The disease is caused by an eastern or western-strain virus, either of which can be fatal; but the eastern variety has about 90% mortality rates, while the western is only 20 to 50% fatal. In most instances a bivalent vaccine is recommended that will cover both strains. Immunity lasts only for the current season. Vaccination is recommended annually to prevent the disease. Control of mosquitoes is the most worthwhile objective, but this is seldom possible.

Treatment.   There is no effective treatment for the condition other than supportive measures during mild cases of the less deadly western strain. Food, water, shade, and proper rest are recommended for those affected by the disease.

Swamp Fever (Equine Infectious Anemia, EIA)

Signs.   Swamp fever is characterized by an intermittent fever, depression, weakness, loss of appetite, loss of weight, and, as the name implies, anemia. Horses will develop high fever, sweat profusely, and often lie down and appear listless. The fever may be very high and continuous, or it may go away and return quite often. The attacks in some instances decrease in severity, and an animal appears to have recovered. The fact is that animals once affected with swamp fever never lose the virus from their bloodstream, and even though they appear healthy, they serve as a source of infection to others. Mortality rates range from 30 to 70%.

Some horses appear to recover but develop subsequent signs in a pattern that appears to reoccur about every week or two. This is a key sign of the disease.

Cause.   A virus that is transmitted by the blood of blood-sucking insects such as flies and mosquitoes transfers the virus strictly through mechanical means. The virus can also be mechanically transferred through the use of unsterilized instruments, particularly hypodermic needles.

Prevention.   Control of mosquitoes and flies in an area where outbreaks are known to occur and strict sanitary measures with hypodermic needles and other instruments are a necessity. Be sure that all new animals brought on a farm have had a Coggins test in the last 30 days. If you suspect EIA is a problem on a farm, your veterinarian can run a Coggins test on all animals.

Treatment.   There is no effective treatment. Infected animals should be separated from the herd and kept in isolation until they can be disposed of. Flies and mosquitoes must be controlled, and sterilized instruments should always be used if they could cause even a skin wound.

Tetanus

Signs.   Tetanus is an infection caused by bacteria that live in the soil and invade through a puncture or open wound to create a fatal condition unless quickly treated. Signs are usually not noticed until the disease has progressed. The horse shows stiffness in the joints, begins to move about in a shuffled stiff gait, and the third eyelid flickers across the eye. Coordination is restricted, and the jaws eventually lock.

Cause.   The cause is a bacterium that lives in the soil all around us. It theoretically enters the bloodstream and releases a toxin that causes the disease.

Prevention.   Immunization is the only sure way to prevent tetanus, and it is especially recommended in any area where tetanus has been known to occur. Two injections followed by an annual booster shot are often required to create immunity. If the disease has developed, a veterinarian must be called immediately. If a puncture wound occurs, or if an animal is suspected of coming down with tetanus, the veterinarian should be called to give an antitoxin serum.

Treatment.   The veterinarian must be called once signs develop or there is no hope of survival. Even then the chances are slim. The stable should be

399
SYSTEMIC
DISEASES,
VIRAL AND
BACTERIAL
DISEASES

kept darkened and absolutely quiet because of the animal's nervous reaction to noise during this time. Diet should be laxative, and plenty of water should be available.

Tying Up Syndrome (Myositis or Cording Up)

Signs. There is a rapid increase in respiration, dilation of the nostrils, profuse sweating, and a stiffness in gait. Coffee-colored urine excretions are seen in very severe and prolonged untreated cases. This disorder may be confused with azoturia; the chief difference in signs is that the tying up is not as severe in the incidence of stiffness as in azoturia. Many authorities think this tying up syndrome is simply a mild form of azoturia. However, the difference is that tying up occurs in horses that are being worked every day, regardless of the feeding program, whereas azoturia usually occurs when horses are rested for a day or more while continuing on a heavy grain diet.

The mortality rate in tying up is almost zero, whereas azoturia is much more dangerous. Horses will commonly come down with tying up syndrome and recover in an uneventful manner.

Cause. Tying up is a muscular disorder of unknown origin, probably metabolic in nature.

Prevention. There is no sure way to prevent this disorder. It affects all light horses and occurs during work or exercise only.

Treatment. Some work has concluded that vitamin E therapy has a place in treatment, but the only known recommended method of handling horses is to stable them, rub them dry, and if during the winter, apply a blanket. Veterinarians may use sedatives and tranquilizers to ease the pain.

Many new treatments are evolving from research in this area. Check with your veterinarian for the latest techniques.

GASTROINTESTINAL PROBLEMS IN HORSES

Equine Colic

The primary problem in all colic cases is distention of the stomach or intestines. This may be static distention, which is due to an accumulation of food material; or it may be a transient type of disturbance, where periodic distentions occur as a result of spasms and increased intestinal motility. The static type is often called physical colic because it requires physical treatment. For the functional, or transient type, the treatment is relief of both the spasm and intestinal movement.

There are several things that can produce blockage of the intestines (physical colic): bad teeth; lush, green feeds; obstructions due to foreign bodies; engorgement with grain; acute intestinal twists (strangulations);

and/or mesenteric arteritis (bloodworm infestations). All of these factors can produce distention, gas, and in some cases, fluid accumulation.

Transient colic is due to inflammation of the intestines from parasites, bacterial viruses, chemical poisons, or spasmodic pause of intestines due to excitement, cold water, thunderstorms, etc.

Clinical Signs of Colic. Depending on the cause of colic, the pain may be a very sudden onset that is continuous, or it may be a gradual onset and be intermittent. These animals are usually depressed and may have periods of profuse sweating. The pulse may be up to 80 to 100 beats per minute. Affected horses usually walk very stiffly and kick toward the stomach or abdomen. They may assume a "sitting dog" position. In advanced stages the mucous membranes around the mouth may be very red, later changing color to a bluish tint. There may not be a temperature increase, but usually it's up to 102 to 103°F. By putting your ear up against the abdomen or side of the horse you may hear a foaming or explosive gas noise. Respiration may be very shallow or very rapid. These animals usually will be up and down, acting nervously. One characteristic sign is to see the animal do complete continuous rolls on its back. If the animal is not rolling at the moment, you may suspect intermediate signs of colic by observing where the hairs are rubbed off the back and the head, an indication that it has been rolling.

Treatment. The most important thing is to try to judge the degree of severity. If it's a mild colic, walking will usually relieve it in an hour or so. In severe cases, it can be a life-threatening situation. These animals are in intense pain and need help and relief right away. Calling a veterinarian is recommended when the problem is first noticed. Walk and keep the animal up until the veterinarian can get there.

Cantharis Poison

Cantharis poison is caused by the Spanish beetle, which is common in the southwestern United States. These poisonous insects are often found in alfalfa hay. The horse eats the hay, and a toxic substance in the dead beetle causes severe irritation to the mouth and throughout the intestinal tract. The animal shows signs of colic, but the pain is not relieved by the normal methods of treatment of colic. There is no effective treatment. This condition is very common in colts that go along behind the mother and eat the tender leaves that have been shaken out of the hay. The beetles are usually in these leaves, and the colts can get a large dose of them.

Choking

It is very common for horses to choke on ears of corn, or apples, or any type of fruit. Many times the blockage will pass, through a motion of the esophagus, but if the choking persists for 3 or 4 hours, a veterinarian should be consulted.

Verminous Arteritis, Mesenteric Arteritis, Bloodworm Colic

Verminous arteritis is an inflammation of the arteries, causing an intestinal upset that is due to a blockage of one or more branches of the mesenteric artery by strongyle (worm) migration and the emboli that are formed there by the parasite. This blockage can sometimes rupture, and the horse can die. Other times the blockage will cause periodic bouts with a coliclike syndrome. The very best prevention is treatment by a systematic deworming program where the animals are started out young—when they are 4 to 6 months old—and are dewormed regularly three to five times a year throughout their entire life. As far as treatment for a condition that is already there, massive doses of thiabendazole have been effective along with other types of medication, but the problem should definitely be handled by a veterinarian.

Simple Diarrhea

Simple diarrhea is not as common in horses as it is in other species, but it can occur due to a number of conditions, including parasites, abrupt feed changes, too much milk, and several bacterial and viral diseases.

Treatment.   Kaolin/Pectin-type products are used as treatment. These products normally will take care of the problem. If anything stronger must be used, a veterinarian is suggested.

Colitis X

Colitis X is a disease that needs mentioning. It is also called *Ruidosa disease*. It is a serious inflammation of the large intestine.

Signs.   Clinical signs include sudden profuse diarrhea, a very depressed animal, elevated temperature (in later stages it will be subnormal), and a very rapid pulse. Horses with this condition usually stay on their feet until they die. The cause is unknown, but the disorder may be associated with a severe stress respiratory disease outburst 3 to 4 weeks before, such as extremely hard training or hard travel. The course of this disease is so acute that often there is not even time to start any kind of treatment. For treatment, seek professional help.

FOOT AND LEG PROBLEMS

Sound feet and legs, correctly set, almost always result in correct movement and freedom from all but accidental or infectious unsoundness. Since a horse, to be of value, must be in motion, it is recommended that you avoid the poorly set legs illustrated in Figures 20-1 and 20-2 as the best preventive of foot and leg disorders.

In spite of all precautions, even the structurally sound and nutritionally perfect horse occasionally has foot and leg disorders that require attention.

Figure 20-3 illustrates horse anatomy terms and points out sites of some problems common to horse owners around the world. Figure 20-4 gives illustrative terminology helpful in understanding specific foot care and treatment.

The following disorders are not restricted to poorly conformed or undernourished horses, but their occurrence is to be expected more often where faulty structure, handling, feeding, or sanitation predisposes the horse to the condition.

Bowed Tendons (Tendinitis)

Signs. Tendinitis usually occurs during forced exercise or hard work and is particularly characteristic of race horses. There is an inflammation of the tendon below the knee. In thoroughbreds, the inside front leg, right or left depending on whether they race in a clockwise or counterclockwise direction, is invariably the one that produces a strained tendon and subsequent swelling. The horse stands with the heel elevated, and the swelling is hot and painful. The swelling is obvious when comparisons are made with the other leg. This condition normally occurs in only one front leg, and it happens frequently in some horses at a less severe level. Some veterinarians have treated these chronic cases by "firing," that is, using a hot iron to burn into the area of the infected swollen tendon. The theory is that this will make a chronic condition convert to an acute condition, thus allowing a more rapid recovery. This is a questionable practice but may be employed on some occasions with chronic sufferers. Results with this treatment to date have been disappointing. Surgical treatments are being utilized in some instances, but they too are not completely satisfactory and are somewhat questionable as to the end results.

Cause. Tendinitis is normally a case of genetic weakness and/or improper "warming up" of the horse, creating a forced strain on a tendon. The problem is strictly mechanical in nature.

Prevention. There is no real prevention; tendinitis is one of those disorders that every horseman has to take a chance on in the business of racing or working horses hard. The best hope for preventing the disorder is to warm up the horses prior to an event and to maintain proper supportive therapy through the use of bandages for those horses that are known to have a weakness for the condition.

Treatment. The only treatment is absolute rest by confinement. The swelling and inflammation can be reduced in some cases by the application of cold packs, and a veterinarian may recommend the application of a plaster cast for 6 to 8 weeks.

Injections can be given by veterinarians in the inflamed area and should be repeated at weekly intervals to reduce the swelling. The material used in this case is most often Prednisolone (a cortisone). Normally a horse affected

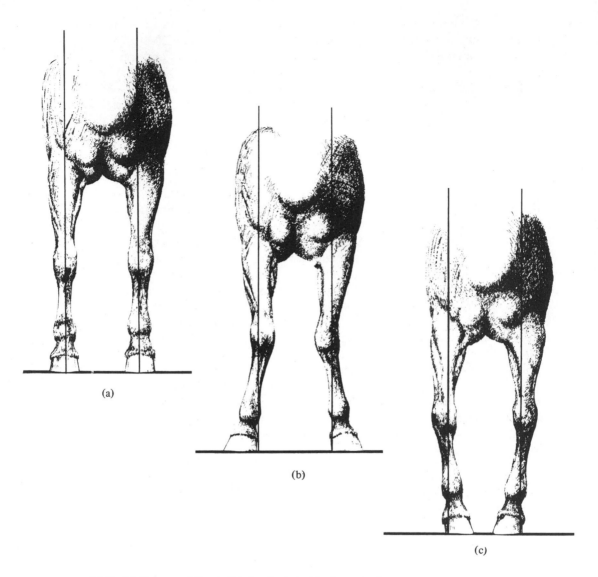

(a) Straight legs, good front; (b) slay-footed; (c) pigeon-toed.

Figure 20-1. Comparative front leg sets. *(Drawings by Tom Stallman)*

with tendinitis will be out of commission for at least a year before it can be counted on for soundness of the leg.

Bog Spavin

Signs.   A swelling on the front inner side of the hock will appear as a protrusion, having no apparent effect on the horse other than appearance.

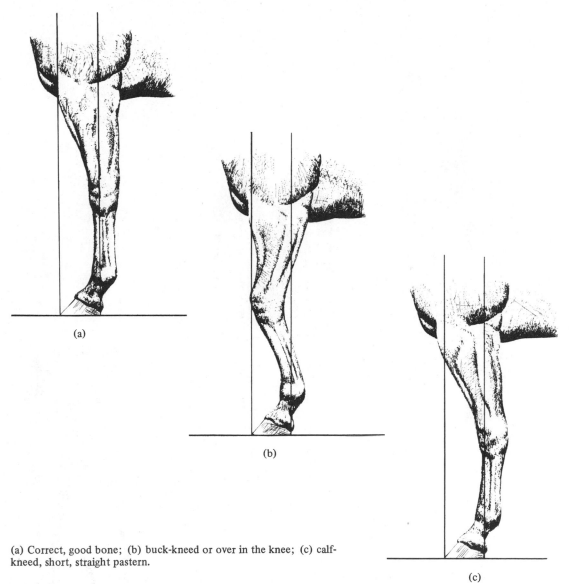

(a) Correct, good bone; (b) buck-kneed or over in the knee; (c) calf-kneed, short, straight pastern.

Figure 20-1. (*Continued*)

The bulge can be seen easily in most cases. Heat is rarely felt and lameness seldom experienced except in cases where the bulge interferes with action.

Cause. An accumulation of fluid at the hock joint capsule causes the condition. The exact reason for this is not known but it does occur fairly often in horses that are straight-hocked. It is thought to be caused from a stance inherited from parents.

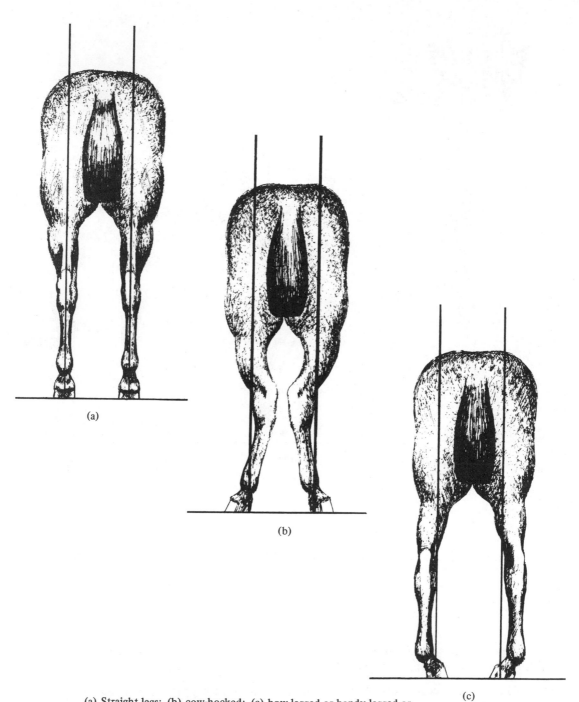

(a) Straight legs; (b) cow-hocked; (c) bow-legged or bandy-legged or "too wide," pigeon-toed.

Figure 20-2. Comparative rear leg sets. *(Drawings by Tom Stallman)*

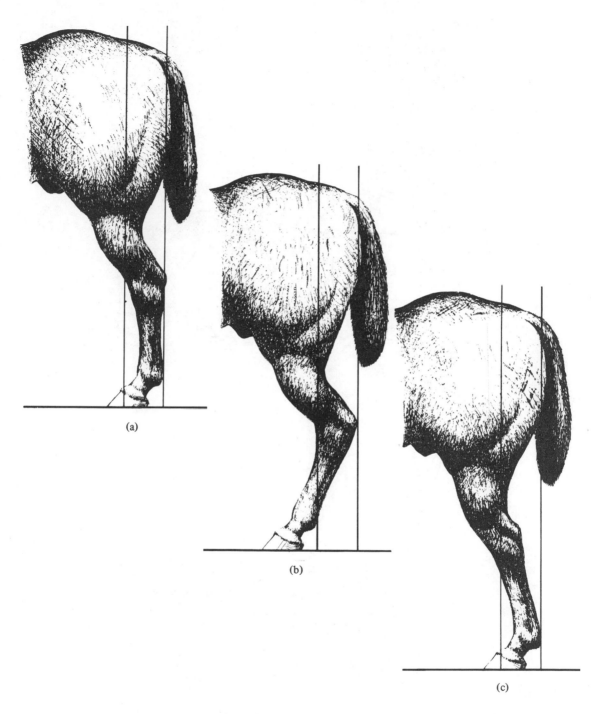

(a) Correct leg set; (b) sickle-hocked or too much set; (c) post-legged or too straight, "coon-footed."

Figure 20-2. (*Continued*).

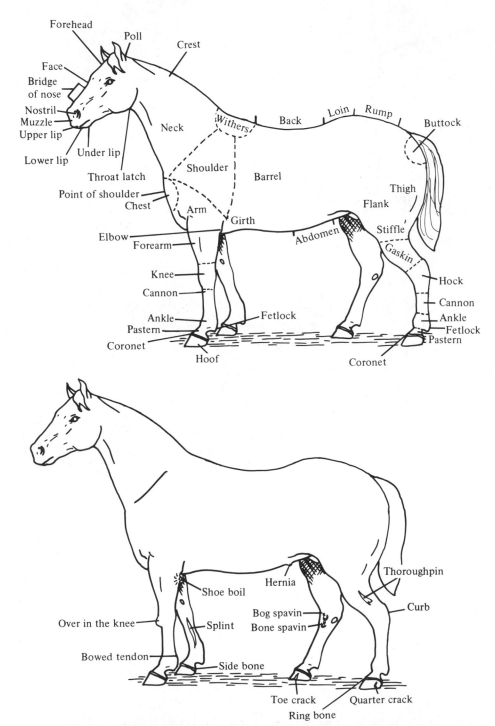

Figure 20-3. Anatomy and location of selected unsoundness in the horse. (*Courtesy of University of Missouri*)

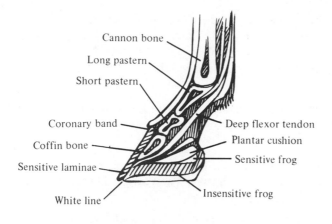

Cannon bone
Long pastern
Short pastern
Coronary band
Coffin bone
Sensitive laminae
White line
Deep flexor tendon
Plantar cushion
Sensitive frog
Insensitive frog

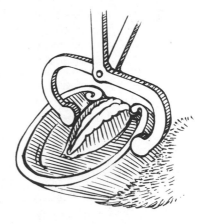

A hoof tester is used to detect pain-sensitive areas.

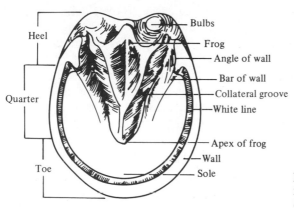

Heel
Quarter
Toe
Bulbs
Frog
Angle of wall
Bar of wall
Collateral groove
White line
Apex of frog
Wall
Sole

Figure 20-4. Anatomy of the foot of a horse. (*Courtesy of University of Missouri*)

Prevention. Young animals that are straight-hocked should not be excessively worked or exerted during their early training period. After maturity, there is less likelihood of a bog spavin developing. If signs do develop, special shoes may help to relieve the strain and prevent the condition.

Treatment. No treatment is necessary or recommended in the case of horses that are not showing lameness from the disorder. If treatment is desirable, cold applications and massage may be helpful. "Firing" may be advised in bad cases, or injections into the area by a qualified veterinarian may be advisable. The condition is normally not one to be concerned about other than from the standpoint of appearance.

Bone Spavin

Signs. Bone spavin is the worst form of spavin. It involves the inflammation of bones in the hock joint. There is an enlargement of the bone on the lower inner side of the hock. The horse tends to drag the toe as an indication of lameness in the hind leg. The lameness usually wears off after a warm-up period, but the hock still appears stiff in many cases. The spavin test may be a useful procedure in the early stages. The leg is picked up and held for a few minutes before the horse is jogged. The lameness will show up in the first few steps. This test is very dependable in older horses, but may have variable response in younger horses. Both legs should be tested if there is any sign of potential lameness.

Cause. Several theories are advanced as to the cause, including faulty hock conformation, concussion caused by excessive exercise, and mineral deficiencies.

Prevention. Bone spavin is generally thought to be related to excessive work or exertion, especially with young horses. Therefore, mild exercise with young horses is highly recommended.

Treatment. Complete rest in some cases may be necessary. Veterinarians sometimes perform "point firing" to accelerate the condition so that an acute condition develops that is often easier to treat than the chronic type. However, results have been variable and often disappointing with firing. Corrective shoeing to raise the heel and roll the toe is considered a more effective treatment.

Your veterinarian may also suggest corrective surgery called *cunean tenectomy*, which is the removal of the cunean tendon that runs across the bone where the spavin develops. This tendon is the seat of pain which, when removed, does away with the pain. This is the most common treatment.

Curb

Signs. Clinical signs are an enlargement directly below the hock of the back leg and another enlargement about 3 to 4 in. below the point of the hock. There is inflammation and heat at these spots and obvious swelling, and the horse may show lameness, although many instances occur in which there is only a disfigurement.

Cause. The cause is an inflammation on the back of the hock due to a stress brought about by very strenuous exercise and/or poor conformation. The condition is primarily a problem of faulty leg structure, creating a thickening of the plantar ligament brought on by heavy exercise. Occasionally, a horse with good conformation will get curb from a blow to the hock or from kicking something solid. Horses with good leg conformation often recover completely. Horses with poor conformation seldom recover.

Prevention. Select horses with good, strong, correct leg conformation, and the condition will probably never occur except through accidental blows. Horses with faulty leg conformation must be warmed up carefully and excessive strain on the legs prevented.

Treatment. Inflammation of the bone may produce bony growth, scar tissue, or just simple inflammation with heat. Corticosteroids and cold water treatment to reduce the swelling and pain in the early stages are recommended. A complete rest until the situation has cleared up is the best treatment. Horses with good conformation will recover fully but may have a permanent blemish. The horse with poor conformation usually has a relapse and most likely will never be cured completely because of the frequent recurrence of the condition.

Capped Hock

Signs. The chief clinical sign is an enlargement of the hock with swelling at the point of the hock, sometimes accompanied by curb.

Cause. Usually a direct injury such as a horse kicking the stall or trailer tailgate is the cause.

Prevention. Padding in stalls and trailers is the best preventive measure, along with quiet handling.

Treatment. The capped hock is usually not a cause for lameness, but it could cause a permanent blemish brought about by scar tissue forming within the bursa (the lubricating sac of the hock). The lubricating fluid protects bony friction where tendons run over the bones. An injury to a bursa causes it to fill with excessive fluid, creating the swelling. Corticosteroids and cold water treatment to reduce the swelling, followed by rest until recovery, are recommended.

Corns

Signs. A chronic lameness and obvious tenderness to the front feet are the usual signs. The condition may occur in the hind feet but is most common in the forefeet. If you will look closely at the underside of the hoof, by paring away any exposed material from the sole of the foot you may notice a corn on the inner backside of the hoof. There is usually a discoloration, either red or a reddish-yellow, at the site of the corn. There may be a corn on either side of the frog of the foot about the size of a quarter. Tapping with a light hammer over this area or applying pressure with a hoof tester will verify if there is any discomfort. The visual signs combined with obvious pain are positive indications of corns.

Cause. The disease is associated with excessive trimming of the hoof, neglect of the feet, irregular shoeing, or hooves that have not been shod for such a long time that the hoof has grown over the shoe, allowing long and irregular growth. This throws pressure on the feet, much like a tight pair of shoes would do to a human.

Prevention. Pressure on the feet should be avoided by careful shoeing, frequent shoeing, or moderate trimming of the feet if shoes are not used.

Treatment. If shoes are used, as is usually the case, they should be removed, and a professional horseshoer should be allowed to trim the feet and reshoe the horse. A bar shoe is sometimes needed to relieve pressure on the sole of the foot and to allow healing. Later, a normal shoe replaces the bar type. In severe cases where the corn has advanced, drainage may be necessary, and foot baths and antiseptic therapy may be prescribed by the veterinarian. In any case, you will need to seek the professional help of a blacksmith and/or veterinarian.

Gravel

Signs. A crack in the white line of the foot occurs first, allowing infection of the sensitive structure of the hoof. Inflammation is the result, and the infection follows the path of least resistance, breaking out in the only place where the foot has any give to it—the heel. Excessively dry feet are most commonly affected with this disorder.

Cause. A crack in the white line of the hoof allows an invasion of organisms. Founder and injury may both cause this disorder. Lameness generally appears before the drainage is visible, although the condition may go undetected until after drainage. The name *gravel* originally came from the belief that a small stone or piece of gravel worked its way into the foot, creating the problem.

Prevention. Adequate shoeing and attention to hooves, especially during dry seasons of the year, are essential in providing foot protection. Proper feeding will prevent any predisposition to gravel through a case of founder.

Treatment. The foot often does not break out in a noticeable drainage spot. Lameness may appear to be only slight, and the problem could go undetected until drainage starts. Horses may modify their gait to obtain relief, and unless you are familiar with the normal gaits of the horse, the condition may not be noticed until an obvious problem exists.

Treatment involves cleaning of the area and proper draining of the infection. Soaking the foot in Epsom salts is recommended even if drainage has begun. Tincture of iodine and antiphlogistic pastes may be applied daily, directly to the wound, under a bandage for a week, and once every 3 to 4 days afterward provided the foot stays dry. Treatment should continue until completely healed. A tetanus shot should be given.

Grease Heel (Scratches)

Signs. The pasterns and fetlocks become inflamed with a mangelike skin condition.

Cause. The cause is generally thought to be a poor sanitation measure, although horses vary in their susceptibility to the problem.

Prevention. Adequate sanitation practices, clean barns, and dry stalls, along with regular foot care, such as trimming and cleaning, are preventive measures.

Treatment. Once the condition develops, treatment consists of cleaning the fetlocks with mild soap and water and clipping the hair closely from around the affected areas. Astringents and antiseptic substances are then applied at regular intervals. The condition is relatively easy to correct if attention is given to it immediately.

Hoof Cracks

Signs. An obvious split or a crack in the hoof can be very painful to the horse. The most painful crack is usually vertical, splitting from the coronet downward. The more common cracks occur from the weight-bearing surface of the foot upward. Hoof cracks may be mild, resulting in little or no pain, or they can cause a severe lameness disorder.

Cause. The causes are excessively dry conditions, brittle hooves, or foot injuries. Faulty conformation is also a common problem resulting in hoof cracks.

Prevention. Proper trimming and/or shoeing is necessary to prevent the condition. In the case of very dry climates it may be necessary to occasionally treat the hoof with a hoof dressing to provide the necessary pliability.

Treatment. Trimming the hooves and special shoeing to allow the crack time to heal are the only recommended treatment.

Navicular Disease

Signs. A painful flexing of the front feet is usually the most noticeable sign. It is a condition not easily diagnosed. However, the horse will most often "point" the affected foot while at rest in the stable. This attempt to remove pressure from the foot is an indication that there is pain there. The involvement usually is with the deep flexor tendon of the foot, brought on by severe concussion or fracture of the navicular bone.

Cause. It is thought to be an inherited condition, but it is known that excessive pounding especially on hard surfaces develops the disorder. The name is derived from the fact that a tendon passes over the navicular bone, and in some cases this bone changes in shape and texture making it painful for the tendon to run over the surface.

Prevention. There is no satisfactory prevention other than normal care and proper trimming and shoeing.

Treatment. No satisfactory treatment has yet been discovered, but with early diagnosis, steps can be taken to relieve the pressure of the tendon when it passes over the navicular bone. This is normally accomplished by special shoes with thinly rolled toes and thick heels. Once the condition develops, it may be relieved by denerving by a veterinarian. Horses have a tendency to stumble when denerved, so you should think twice before having this done to a child's horse or a horse used for barrel racing or other fast action use. There could be a calculated risk to the rider. Otherwise, pain is relieved and years of useful service may be added to the horse's life.

Quittor

Signs. The chief clinical sign is a chronic inflammation of the hoof. There is swelling, heat, and pain over the coronary band. This condition is manifested as a deep-seated running sore, usually confined to the front feet, although it is occasionally seen in the hind feet.

Cause. The disorder is invariably caused from an injury such as a traumatic bruise or puncture wound. Circulation is reduced in the foot, bringing about the condition.

Prevention. There is no successful prevention.

Treatment. Drainage and antiseptics have been successfully used, and surgery has been tried on occasion to remove the necrotic material. This surgery has been questionable in the past and has sometimes led to hoof mutilation. Irrigation of the drainage opening with a mild antiseptic solution several times a day may be beneficial. Incisions are sometimes preferred to surgery, allowing drainage. A poultice such as Denver Mud (Demco Co., Denver, Col.) can be applied to speed healing. The foot is usually bandaged to allow the poultice to draw the infection from the foot.

Ring Bone

Signs. A bony enlargement appears on the pastern bone. There are two types of ring bone: a "low" ring bone in the coronet region and a "high" ring bone above the coronet. The high ring bone can be felt, but the low variety will require an X-ray to determine it. Lameness is constant, and a horse will flinch when finger pressure is applied to the affected area. Ring bone is seldom seen in thoroughbred horses.

Cause. Trauma is the usual cause of ring bone. Pulling, bruising, or a direct blow to the toe of the hoof leads to heat, swelling, and pain, and to new bone growth.

Prevention. Don't allow hooves to grow too long, thus saving the frog from doing the work of absorbing shocks to the feet. Horses with upright or very long pasterns are susceptible to the condition and should not be worked on hard ground unless they are properly shod. A clumsy horse should undergo corrective shoeing to prevent sharp blows and pulled ligaments that may lead to ring bone.

Treatment. Rest is the first step. Cold treatment can be used to reduce inflammation, and more permanent relief is often found in "blistering" (an irritant applied to the affected area). Cortisone is also used to reduce swelling during treatment. In some instances "firing" (the use of a hot iron or needle) may be recommended, or in more severe cases the severing of the nerve leading to the area is suggested if other methods have failed.

Side Bones

Signs. The side bone usually develops on either side of the front foot. It is seldom found in the hind feet, and almost never is seen in thoroughbred horses. Interestingly enough, mules commonly develop side bones, although the condition seldom results in lameness. An ossification (building up of bone) on either side of the back part of the hoof just above the coronet develops and can be felt if not readily seen in most cases. Lameness is unusual.

Cause. Side bones are thought to be hereditary, but often result from improper shoeing, which causes a contraction of the hoof at the heel.

Prevention. Proper shoeing is the only preventive measure. Concussions or a blow to the foot could create the condition.

Treatment. Grooving of the hoof is recommended to permit expansion of the foot and relief of pressure from within the hoof. Proper shoeing combined with grooving are the most often recommended treatments. If lameness does occur, blistering of the coronary region is often used as a therapeutic treatment for faster relief.

Splints

Signs. A bony enlargement of the splint bones, cannon bone, or enlargement between any of these bones in the foreleg is the visual sign of this condition. It usually can be seen as well as felt, and although the condition occurs occasionally on rear legs, it is usually confined to the forelegs, on the inside of the bone. When found on rear legs, it is usually on the outside of the cannon.

Cause. The condition is usually associated with hard training, malnutrition, or faulty conformation in young horses under two years old. Trauma caused by slipping, running, falling, or jumping can induce the initial injury leading to ossification (a buildup of the bony growth). Horses under two years of age are almost exclusively the victims. It occurs occasionally in horses three to four years old and very rarely in horses over six.

Prevention. Splints can be caused by blows in excessive training; therefore, boots or bandages worn during work can reduce the risk. Excessive work on immature legs should be avoided.

Treatment. Rest is recommended for at least 6 weeks. If lameness persists, the splint may be blistered or pinfired. Cold treatment or injection of cortisone can help to speed recovery. The horse should only be walked during this healing period. Usually, 30 days of rest will cause splints to heal of their own accord, but you may want to speed recovery by treating with hot and cold applications or use an antiphlogistic pack to reduce the swelling as a home remedy. This condition responds better to treatment than do most leg disorders.

Stringhalt

Signs. The clinical sign is an involuntary flexion of the hind legs, most evident when backing a horse. The foot is markedly jerked toward the abdomen and may actually hit the abdominal wall. In extreme cases, the hind foot involuntarily jerks against the belly and then violently strikes the ground. Although stringhalt is marked as a gross unsoundness, it does not materially affect the horse's ability to work.

Thoroughpin

Signs. The chief clinical sign is a puffy swelling in the web of the hock that can be confused with bog spavin. Thoroughpin "bulge" can be distinguished from bog spavin by its movement under finger pressure to the opposite side of the leg.

Cause. This disorder is usually associated with excessive strain, particularly on the hocks.

Prevention. Prevention includes avoidance of exercise that would place unnecessary strain on the hocks, especially of young horses. In the case of conformation faults, weak-hocked horses should not be used for strenuous forms of work.

Treatment. The condition is not serious, and treatment with liniments or massage may reduce the swelling. The horse should be rested, and in some cases an injection of cortisone is recommended to aid in healing. Severe cases may require drainage.

Thrush

Signs. A degeneration of the frog of the foot is the clinical sign of this disorder. It is most commonly found in the hind feet, and the first sign of trouble is a strong offensive foot odor.

Cause. The condition is generally the result of poor sanitation and lack of attention to proper cleaning of feet.

Prevention. Sanitary measures, proper trimming, and hoof care will prevent the condition. Most importantly, keep a clean, dry stall so that mud, manure, etc., will not get packed in the foot.

Treatment. Trimming away of the infected part of the frog, application of an antiseptic, and proper sanitation and rest will usually do the job. Many thrush remedies are used by owners. Among them are iodine, formalin, creolin, and carbolic acid. Copper sulfate is probably the most common treatment used.

Wind Puffs (Wind Gall)

Signs. The clinical sign is usually a small swelling just above the fetlock. It arises from a strain within the joint itself, which causes secretion of excess fluid to accumulate in a visible pocket. The condition is contributed to working on a hard surface, racing, and so forth. It is quite common in any hard-working horse, especially in one that must ride over rough terrain.

Cause. The main cause is strain and/or overwork, creating the secretion of excessive synovial fluid from the joints.

Prevention. Avoid strain and overwork, hooves that grow too long, or heels that are allowed to be too low.

Treatment. The swelling can be reduced with cold treatment or with bandages in cases where lameness results. Shoes with wedge heels are sometimes helpful, but generally are only recommended if the horse is lame. In most instances the horse is not lame, and treatment is merely an aesthetic form of management. Blistering agents, liniments, and massage may also be effective.

General Muscle Pain

Pain, soreness, and muscle spasms in the feet and legs caused from working horses hard when they are not used to it can be a problem in any age horse. The signs are about the same as in humans. When horses appear "stove up," relief can be given with the use of corticosteroids or antiinflammatory products that are not steriods (Arquel, Butazoladone, Equiproxine). Plain horse liniments, rub downs, and slow warm-up periods may be all that's needed in mild cases.

Bone Chips

Especially in young horses that are raced early, small "slab fractures" off the edges of the carpal bone in the front leg have a tendency to occur. Inflammation and arthritis usually result. Some bone chips may be reabsorbed naturally, but often a specialist and extensive surgery are needed. The recovery rate is very good, and horses have returned to the winners' circle in a matter of a few months.

Fractures of the Long Bones

You should be aware of what signs characterize a fracture of a long bone of the leg. The horse will hold the leg up, and close observation will show a deviation to one side in the leg (the leg is not straight compared to the others).

Keep the horse quiet and still until your veterinarian can arrive and apply external assistance in the form of plates, screws, splints, casts, or whatever the condition calls for. Contrary to the popular concept of having to shoot a horse with a broken leg, many fractures can be healed if the horse is kept still and quiet, to prevent further damage, until help arrives.

SKIN DISORDERS

Ringworm

Circular patches appear on the skin caused by a fungus. The disorder is not the result of a worm at all but is given the name because of the circular appearance of the fungus attack, usually resulting in most of the hair falling out inside the circle or ring.

The treatment for this condition is to paint iodine on every affected patch daily. Clipping the horse for easier application is helpful. Do not miss a single day of treatment until the condition is completely cured. Ringworm is contagious; so the horse should be completely isolated and any grooming materials kept separate from other horses. Attendants should be careful not to contaminate other horses through their clothes.

This fungus is best prevented by sterilizing or sanitizing new tack and by periodic disinfection of the stables.

Sweet Itch

Sweet itch is an irritation of the skin, mostly confined to the withers and crop. The hair will usually be rubbed off in affected areas exposing a wrinkled, inflamed skin. The condition usually occurs only in the late spring and summer.

Sweet itch is irritated by exposure to sunlight; so it is recommended that the horse be kept in a shady area by day. Zinc and sulfur ointments, sulfur and tar lotions, or calamine lotions applied to affected areas generally relieve the irritation. A veterinarian may also prescribe cortisone or antihistamines.

Nettle Rash (Hives, Urticaria)

Nettle rash is characterized by small "bumps" or swellings on the surface of the skin of the horse that do not cause irritation. The bumps will be small, soft, and numerous in most instances, occurring mostly in the early springtime when lush grass is available.

Attention to diet can often decrease the incidence of nettle rash. High-energy foods accompanied by too little exercise can bring on the disorder in other times of the year. A laxative diet and administration of antihistamines have proven to be effective in clearing up the condition. It is not painful and does not affect the horse except in appearance. It is generally accepted to be an allergic reaction to the preponderance of spring grasses and pollens. The name is derived from the fact that outbreaks are often seen from exposure to the nettle weed, which produces a toxin creating the condition.

Mud Fever

Signs. Mud fever is an inflammation of the skin on the underside of the belly and the inside of the limbs. The chief sign is a puffiness in the legs, accompanied by heat. The skin will get rough, scabby, and irritable. Occasionally, if the condition is bad enough in the legs, the horse will go lame.

Cause. It is not known specifically what causes the disorder, but it is thought to be an allergic reaction due to muddy conditions in certain parts of the country. Other dry areas of the country produce weeds during the spring of the year that precipate a similar condition. In these areas the condition is known as *weed fever*. In both cases, a horse with white-stocking feet is more susceptible than other horses to the development of the condition.

Prevention. Avoid riding in muds that are known to cause this condition, or if this is not possible, wash down the horse's legs and keep as clean as possible. The dry "weed" variety is difficult to control.

Treatment. Keep the legs clean and dry, brush often, and if irritation begins, treat with a soothing lotion or cream, such as zinc ointment, lanolin, or other material prescribed by the veterinarian.

Cracked Heel

Signs. In this disorder the back of the pastern becomes dry, cracked, and often scabby. There will be soreness and a reddish discoloration to the area.

Cause. The cause is dry stables or extremely dry pasture conditions.

Prevention. The horse's feet may be coated with lanolin, petroleum jelly, or neat's-foot oil periodically to maintain pliability of skin and hoof tissue.

Treatment. The same treatment used for mud fever will apply in this case, a soothing lotion or cream.

POISONOUS PLANTS

Poisonous plants are covered in more detail in Chapter 6, Disease. Those plants that are specifically harmful to horses are touched on briefly here for the sake of organization.

Lantana

Lantana is both an ornamental and a wild plant, growing mostly in the coastal plains of the South. It is most dangerous in the spring and summer.

A sloughing off of the skin, gastrointestinal disturbances, and a bloody, watery feces are signs of poison.

Remove the plants from the pasture or control with herbicide spray. There is no treatment other than keeping the animals out of direct sunlight after they have eaten the plant. There is an interaction with the chemical produced by lantana and sunlight that aggravates the condition.

Bracken Fern

Bracken fern is a cumulative-type poison that takes 1 to 3 months to develop. It is often difficult to convince farmers and ranchers that bracken fern is poisonous because signs are often not seen until 2 to 3 weeks after herd removal from a fern-infested area. Fern bracken is also poisonous as a contaminant in hay.

Bracken fern poisoning in horses is similar to thiamine deficiency under nutritional stress. There is muscular incoordination and a crouching stance. The neck is arched and the feet are planted wide apart. In most cases the temperature remains normal, but in some instances it has gone up to 104° F.

Bracken fern poisoning is not difficult to control. Most horses will not eat the plant unless they are forced to, due to drought or lack of grazing. An alternate grazing plan will prevent the cumulative effects from developing. Three weeks on a bracken fern pasture followed by 3 weeks on noncontaminated pastures works well to reduce the possibility of poisoning and to retard the growth of the plant by close grazing and trampling. This alternate grazing system may be repeated as needed to control the fern. Weed killers and burning a pasture have not been effective in controlling the plant.

Thiamine is usually given subcutaneously as a treatment at a dosage of 100 mg in the morning and afternoon of the first day. Thereafter 100 mg is generally prescribed daily for 7 days. In extreme cases 200 mg of thiamine have been administered for 2 weeks before recovery was assured.

Nightshade

The nightshade plant if consumed in enough quantity causes weakness, trembling, nausea, either constipation or diarrhea, and death. It is most prevalent in summer.

Treatment consists of 2 to 3 mg of Carbachol or an injection of 15 mg of strychnine.

Johnson Grass

Horses are as susceptible as cattle to Johnson grass prussic acid poisoning. Signs include slobbering, increased respiration rate, rapid weak pulse, convulsions, and death. The condition is most often seen on dark green second growth or when grass is stunted by drought or by freezing for a few hours just after a hard freeze. The plant is not toxic after it is made into hay, if it has been well cured and dried. Treatment consists of sodium nitrite or sodium thiosulfate given intravenously by a veterinarian.

Oleander

The winter and spring are the most dangerous periods of time for oleander poisoning, but it can occur throughout the year in the coastal plains of the South, where the plant is most predominant.

Signs of poisoning are nausea, depression, and bloody diarrhea. A weak and irregular heartbeat develops in the later stages before death.

There is no treatment. The condition may be caused through absorption in wounds and inhalation from smoke.

Castor Bean

The castor bean is potentially dangerous any time of the year. Horses forced to consume the plant will develop blood poisoning, nausea, vomiting, diarrhea, and a severe thirst. Death is quite common.

Gastric preparations to clean out the digestive system are helpful. Provide warmth and sedatives if necessary.

Death Camas

This poisonous plant is most dangerous during the spring. It resembles an onion, except it has flat leaves and no odor.

Signs of death cama poisoning are salivation, vomiting, incoordination, coma, and death.

Even the hays with dried camas in them are poisonous.

Atropine sulfate and picropoxin are injected by veterinarians as an antidote.

Thistle

The yellow star thistle is most dangerous in the summer and fall and is particularly perilous to horses.

Signs are involuntary chewing movements, twitching of the lips, and a peculiar flicking of the tongue. The mouth commonly will be held open, although affected horses are unable to eat or drink. Eventual death occurs from starvation or thirst. There is no treatment.

Loco Weed

Loco weed is especially poisonous in the early spring, but may occur during all seasons throughout the desert Southwest where it grows profusely. Mild winter temperatures make it a threat at all seasons.

The signs are a staggering gait, wild-eyed appearance, and easy excitability.

There is no treatment.

Groundsel

Signs of excessive consumption of groundsel are aimless walking, slight staggering, a blank expression, and running into objects.

Control may be had by spraying pastures with herbicides. Supplemental feeding is helpful as a preventative. Horses usually will not eat groundsel unless they are forced by starvation or drought.

PARASITE CONTROL

There are various chemical wormers available for the horse owner of today that have a greater variety of effects than at any other time in our history. Yet parasite problems continue to be as bad or worse than they have ever been.

Although chemical wormers help to control parasites, they are only part of the answer in reducing infestation. Parasites are always going to be with us; so we must learn to prevent undue damage. A good sanitation and health program is indispensable to the parasitic control program.

Some of the disadvantages of relying strictly on chemical dewormers are that they are often dangerous when administered indiscriminantly, treatment is time-consuming and expensive, and in some cases ill horses or pregnant mares cannot be treated at all.

Ideally, stool samples should be checked every 60 to 90 days to determine if parasite eggs are present. Naturally, by the time the eggs show up, the damage has already been done, but it is a good technique to monitor droppings in order to check the chemical treatment.

It has been recognized for many years that worming only two times per year is insufficient to control most parasites. It is necessary to repeat chemical wormers 3 to 4 weeks after the initial dosage in order to cause expulsion of immature parasites that may have developed since the first worming. Horses should be wormed at least four times per year. Many places find that six to twelve treatments per year are required. The normal recommendation is to worm early in the spring and repeat the treatment 3 weeks later. Then, worm again 6 months from that date and repeat 3 weeks following. In this manner the adults as well as the immature stages should be fairly controlled. Use two or three worming agents alternately to get a more effective kill and to help prevent the development of drug-resistant parasites. Don't rely on worming agents added to the feed. It is usually best to tube a horse so you will be assured of sufficient dosage. With very valuable animals or in cases of severe parasite problems, deworm every 3 months instead of 6.

Of the several factors that reduce an animal's ability to stave off attacks by parasites, nutrition is the number one factor in maintaining a healthy horse that will be able to withstand an attack by parasites and subsequent chemical expulsion.

There are some climates, especially those that are humid and hot, that predispose the horse to parasites. Areas that are fortunate enough to have freezing temperatures during the winter, or better yet, alternate freezing and thawing, have much less problems from parasitic organisms because nature destroys many of the eggs.

Some horses develop an immunity to certain parasites. In most cases all older horses are somewhat less susceptible to parasitic damage than the very young; however, all horses are susceptible to most parasites. The younger horses are simply more easily affected by them. For instance, it is known that young horses develop roundworm problems much more often than older animals.

Overcrowding of horses always produces the danger of cross-inoculation of parasites and an outbreak of parasitism.

The greatest single factor in predisposing a horse to parasitic attack, however, is sanitation. Stalls should be cleaned daily; many bloodworm eggs as well as other parasites require less than a week to develop and infect a horse. Manure piles should be kept far enough away from the barn so as to cause no contamination, and should be made inaccessible to horses. Young colts as well as older animals often will nose around and eat from these manure piles, thus picking up the organism and spreading the infection anew.

Pasture management is extremely important in reducing parasite attack. Several simple rules will enable most horse managers to have a sound sanitation program.

1. All horses should be wormed at the same time. This reduces the possibility of reinfestation.

2. If possible horses should be segregated by age. Because older horses are more immune to parasitic attack, they should not be allowed to graze with very young horses nor should they go before younger animals in a pasture rotation.

3. Another preventive measure is to harrow the pasture with a spring-tooth harrow or some mechanical device to spread the manure out and allow the sunlight to sterilize worm eggs as much as possible. Most organisms do not grow and thrive in dry, hot environments.

4. Pastures should not be grazed too closely because of the horse's ability to get his teeth and lips right next to the ground thus picking up the organisms that you are trying to avoid.

5. Another suggestion for reducing the parasite population is to consider a pasture rotation with two different species, such as cattle and horses because they normally do not carry the same parasites.

6. Pastures should not be rotated at less than 60-day intervals and preferably use 90-day intervals. At least two grazing pastures will be required under this method. Cattle would graze for 60 to 90 days in one pasture, then be moved into a clean pasture, and horses would follow behind them. Because of some differences in selective grazing, this plan works out well to also control some species of plants.

TYPES OF PARASITES

Internal Parasites

Horse Bots. Horse bots is caused by a fly that in itself is not parasitic and only lives about 2 weeks. But this fly, living off the energy stored from pupal stage, lays eggs on the hairs of the horse, especially about the neck, shoulder, and legs. The horse licks the leg areas, and the moisture from the lips activates the egg to produce a larva that hatches in the mouth and is mobilized in the saliva. This takes about 2 to 3 days. The larva remains in the horse's mouth for about 30 days and eventually migrates to the stomach, where it attaches itself to the lining of the stomach or small intestine to feed off the blood of the horse. It will remain attached to the stomach lining for 8 to 10 months and will grow to about the size of a pencil eraser. The larvae become numerous, can almost completely cover the lining of the stomach, and, in an autopsy, look like bees in a honeycomb. They are extremely hard on the digestive system of the equine, bringing about digestive disturbances and in severe cases even rupture of the stomach.

The eggs laid by the flies are quite visible to the naked eye. Proper grooming to remove these eggs by scraping or sponging with warm water will be helpful in controlling initial outbreaks. Sponging with warm water causes the eggs to hatch, and the larvae can be washed away 2 to 3 days later.

The only control for bots is to use an effective wormer annually. Trichlorfon (1.8 gm/100 lb) can be used as a drench about 1 month after a killing frost has destroyed the flies.

Ascarids (Roundworms). Roundworms infect young foals especially, and the source of contamination is almost exclusively solid contamination from eggs that come from foals of the previous year. The adult roundworm develops in the upper intestine, producing eggs. These worms interfere with digestion and produce hyperactivity of the intestinal tract, which can produce both diarrhea and a "telescoping" of the gut. If the roundworms occur in heavy concentrations, the upper intestine can be completely blocked, the gut ruptured, and death can occur. Foals show unthriftiness, loss of energy, and digestive disturbances. Diagnosis is based on worm eggs in the feces.

The source of infestation is from eggs being passed onto the ground in the stool. Horses grazing on the pasture ingest the eggs and larvae, which then hatch in the intestine. The larvae penetrate the intestinal wall, migrating to the liver, then to the lungs. This migration to the lungs creates a tickling sensation, which causes a hacking, dry cough. The larvae are then coughed up by the horse and are swallowed, to develop in the intestine to the adult stage.

Treatment should be started when foals are 8 weeks old and should be repeated at 8-week intervals until they are yearlings. Numerous products are available for ridding the worms from foals. One of the more common products is piperazine given at the rate of 4 gm/100 lb. Table 20-1 lists numerous other products that are equally as effective.

Stomach Worms. The signs of the large stomach worm in horses are gastric irritability, poor digestion, and sometimes colic, which may be brought about by the presence of as few as 200 to 300 adult worms.

The stomach worm is spread by the house or stable fly, which serves as an intermediate host. Horses are infected by the larvae, which travel from the housefly to the lips of the horse. For this reason, control of stable flies is especially important in controlling stomach-worm infestation in horses. In a fly-free environment there is little chance of stomach-worm infestation.

Diagnosis of stomach worms is difficult because the thin-shelled eggs passed out in the stool are readily destroyed with common diagnostic techniques.

Treatment should be in the form of a regular program of worming, using such products as piperazine (4 gm/100 lb).

Strongyles (Bloodworms, Palisade Worms). Infection of strongyles is by ingestion only; so it is very important to break the cycle. Larvae develop to the infective stage 7 days after eggs are passed in the feces and are quite resistant to drying and low temperatures, making infection a real threat.

Eggs from the infected pasture develop in less than 1 week. The female worm may lay as many as 5000 eggs per day, any of which can be picked up by a grazing horse. The larvae enter the intestinal tract, penetrate the wall of

Table 20-1. Common Deworming Agents and Their Effectiveness in Removing Horse Parasites

Wormer	Dose Level	Bots	Roundworms	Strongyles (Bloodworms, palisade worms)	Pinworms
		AVERAGE REMOVAL EXPECTANCY (%)			
Dichlorvos[1]	1.6 gm/100 lb	80–100	95–100	70–100	90–100
Pyrantel[2]	.33 gm/100 lb	0	90–100	75–100	60–70
Thiabendazole[3]	2 gm/100 lb	0	10–30	90–100	90–100
Thiabendazole plus piperazine	2+2.5 gm/100 lb	0	95–100	95–100	30–40
Piperazine	4 gm/100 lb	0	95–100	10–60	50–70
Phenothiazine plus piperazine plus carbon disulfide	1.25+4 gm/100 lb	78–85	95–100	95–100	50–70
Phenothiazone plus piperazine	1.25+4 gm/100 lb	0	95–100	90–100	50–70
Piperazine plus carbon disulfide	4 gm/100 lb	78–85	95–100	40–60	40–60
Trichlorfon	1.8 gm/100 lb	90–100	95–100	0–10	90–100

Adapted from Gabby Hoeppner, D.V.M., *Horse and Horseman*, April 1977. Reprinted with permission.

Note: Trade names 1. Atgard, Shell Chemical Co.; 2. Banminth, Pfizer and Co.; 3. Thibenzole, Merck and Co.

the intestine, and migrate through the blood vessels creating damage to arteries. The name *bloodworm* comes from this fact. The larvae may migrate to internal organs such as the heart, liver, and lining of the abdominal cavity. The larvae are not susceptible to deworming agents until reentry into the intestine as adults. The adults attach themselves to the intestinal wall, suck blood, and produce eggs. These eggs are then passed out in the stool to be picked up again, completing the cycle.

Strongyles are active bloodsuckers, and anemia is the most characteristic sign. Other signs of strongyle attack include weakness, emaciation, and diarrhea.

Thiabendazole at the rate of 2 gm/100 lb of body weight is a recommended dewormer. It is one of the best drugs because it is highly effective against immature worms and is on the lower scale of toxicity to the horse. Treatment, generally, should be repeated at least four times per year for effective control. This corresponds to treatment for ascarids, previously discussed, so that these two internal parasites may both be treated at the same time. Consult Table 20-1 for recommendations for deworming agents that will control other internal parasites as well.

Pinworms (Oxyuris). The characteristic sign of pinworms is the rubbing of the tail and buttocks by the horse on fences, posts, trees, etc. In severe cases, all of the hair may be rubbed off surrounding this "itching" spot.

The adult worm lives in the intestinal tract near the rectum and anus. The females migrate to the anus and deposit their eggs around the opening. The eggs drop out with the stool to contaminate bedding, feed, or water, and are then ingested by the horse. The eggs then develop to larvae in the large gut. They do not migrate. The main problem is irritation causing the horse to rub its tail.

External Parasites

The control of parasites such as flies, mosquitoes, lice, and mange mites is best accomplished by destroying the breeding sites. Even a small amount of water, no more than a handful, can be a fertile breeding ground for mosquitoes, horseflies, and deerflies. Other pests need rotting organic matter or manure in which to breed; so it is important to drain areas where horses are kept and to maintain stalls and stables clean and free of rotting debris.

Usually, the first sign of external parasite problems is a poor haircoat. This is especially true in the case of lice and mites, which are generally seen on the neck, head, and flank first. However, these pests can become severe enough to infect the entire horse.

Remember that flies transmit intestinal parasites to the lips of the horse, and mosquitoes are transmitters of diseases such as sleeping sickness.

Mites and lice cause injury to the horse because of itching and subsequent scratching to ease the irritation. Control must start with cleanup and adequate sanitation, then the use of chemical preparations such as repellents.

Numerous repellents are on the market and can be purchased at any local feedstore; all do an adequate job.

MISCELLANEOUS INJURIES

Tooth Wear

Horses normally wear their teeth or molars down, producing sharp points that make it painful for them to eat, and they also lose lots of grain from their mouth while eating. These sharp points are removed by a veterinarian filing off the points in a routine procedure known as *floating*. This corrects the condition. If your horse appears to have difficulty eating or goes off feed for no reason, yet is obviously hungry, this could be the problem. The procedure is easily done by a veterinarian and is relatively painless to the horse.

Wounds

The horse is especially subject to wounds from loose nails, projecting boards, sharp objects, barbed wire, and the heels and teeth of other horses. Horses are known to panic under stressful situations such as being in a tight spot, which increases the danger of an open wound or injury. Proper cleaning of wounds, suturing when needed, and tetanus shots should be given at the first sign of a wound. If wounds are not cleansed and closed immediately, the horse is especially prone to slow healing.

21

Reproduction in Horses

MALE REPRODUCTIVE TRACT

The male reproductive tract of the horse is illustrated in Figure 21-1. The sperm is produced by the testes, and secondary sex glands produce the bulk of the seminal fluid. The minor differences that occur between the horse and other species are not worthy of expanding for our purposes.

FEMALE REPRODUCTIVE SYSTEM

The female reproductive system of the horse is similar to that of the cow, but is T-shaped rather than curled (see Figure 21-2). The placenta (sac) is not zonary in its attachments, which means that the afterbirth (placenta, sac) is attached by small cotelydons over the entire surface of the uterus like the sow. The ovaries normally shed one ovum (egg) at a time, but multiple ovulation is seen in about 18% of the cycles. Occasionally, twins are born to horses as in cattle, but 90% of the twins in horses are aborted.

ESTROUS CYCLE

The mare has an estrous (heat) cycle that is normally 21 days, just like that of the cow, although there is more variation in the mare than in any other species. The peculiar breeding habits of the horse make it one of the more difficult species to breed with any regularity and efficiency. The estrous cycle may range from 10 to 37 days. The mare will remain in estrus (heat), on the average, 4 to 6 days, but that too may range from as little as 1 day to as much as a continuous heat, in the case of some fillies. Some clues of impending estrus in horses are nervousness, nickering, walking up and down

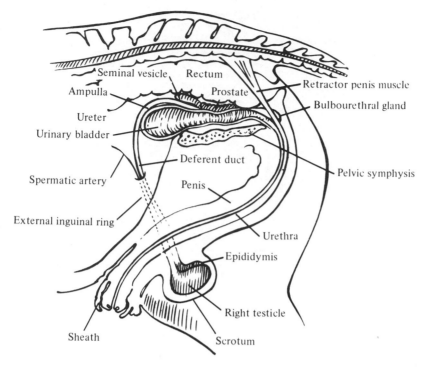

Figure 21-1. Reproductive organs of the stallion. (*Drawing by P. G. Garret, DVM*)

the fence line, a desire for company, frequent urination, and a swelling of the external genitals.

Some mares in heat do not exhibit any of these clues. Therefore, a necessary technique in breeding mares as opposed to other species is the use of a teasing system to definitely determine heat and to insure maximum conception at the time of breeding. Bringing the mare into close proximity of a stallion separated by a teasing board (strong wall) may cause her to exhibit more natural outward signs. The stallion may be on one side of a teasing board restrained by a halter in the field, or he may be just led through the barn when mares are in separate stalls. Those mares who are approaching or experiencing estrus will "show" (nicker, nervous, urinate), so that they can be spotted by the handler. Some establishments use very small stallions or Shetland ponies to reduce the chance of an accidental mating. Although the national average is only a 50% foal crop, under natural pasture conditions and well-managed farms, it is possible to get more than a 90% foal crop annually. By teasing mares to detect estrus, a good handler may get 85 to 95% of the mares in foal. Through the use of hormones, ovary palpation, and examination of the cervix via a speculum, even higher conception rates can be obtained.

Under wild conditions, the horse's reproduction rate approached 90% efficiency or more; but under the domestic conditions imposed by man, the

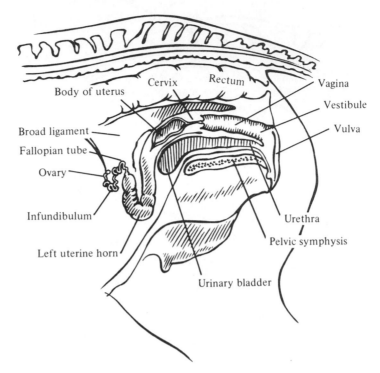

Figure 21-2. Reproductive organs of the mare. (*Drawn by P. G. Garrett, DVM*)

rate usually has fallen far short of this mark. The chief reasons for this failure appear to be poor management, disturbing the normal reproductive environment. For instance, under a higher concentration system of pasture breeding, some mares are sensitive to organisms that they are exposed to during mating, and these may reduce conception capabilities. For this purpose it is very important that strict sanitation measures be observed. The stallion's and the mare's genitals should be washed with warm water and soap. A tail bandage made of flannel or gauze should be applied to the tail of the mare to prevent any of the tail hairs from interfering with the natural mating or introducing an organism that would prohibit conception. Because of the spirited nature of the horse, in the wild, there is a great deal of kicking and rough play during the act of mating. Under man's unnatural handling of the situation, it is advisable to restrain the mare by twitch and hobbles to prevent injury to the stallion. These precautionary measures are needed only about 10% of the time but are recommended as a safety precaution.

Ovulation occurs during the later stages of the estrous period. The egg in the mare is viable for about 6 hours, and sperm from the stallion will remain viable for 24 to 96 hours. Therefore, it is normally recommended that mares be bred every other day beginning with the third day of estrus. It is generally believed that the sperm must be present prior to ovulation for conception to occur.

The average gestation (pregnancy) period is 336 days for the mare, with normal variations ranging from 315 to 350 days. Mares tend to follow a pattern over a period of years, with some consistently foaling at 315 days, others foaling at the later stages, etc. Once the pattern is determined, an experienced handler can make more accurate predictions.

The time of approaching birth is one of particular importance in horses. With other species, we have not been greatly concerned other than being available in the event assistance is needed. In the case of the horse, although assistance is not often needed, when it is necessary, it must be given promptly and correctly. The experienced handler will take every precaution to be available and to be prepared to assist in foaling. It is universally true that mares foal almost exclusively during the dark hours. The proper care and sanitation should be available through a careful calculation of the mare's foaling date and observation just prior to parturition. One of the first signs that the mare is about to give birth is the "making of a bag," the gradual enlargement of the mammary glands. Also, if you will look closely on the end of the teats, there will appear a waxy substance usually within 12 to 24 hours of birth. This "waxing" will soften and fall away just prior to foaling. Milk may even drip or stream from the teats in the case of good producers. It should be mentioned that these signs may occur 2 to 3 days prior to the actual foaling date.

Also, about this same time, there will begin a noticeable relaxation of the ligaments in the hindquarters and in the muscles around the vulva. The muscles and ligaments associated with the pelvis begin to relax at this point, so that they may stretch far enough to allow natural passage of the foal when the time comes. This makes the mare appear very loose about the hips, and to the trained observer this is an obvious sign of approaching parturition. Another sign of a less physical nature is the mare seeking solitude, leaving the herd if in a pasture to find a quiet place to be alone. The mare may also appear to show flares of temper, pinning her ears back and kicking when approached by other horses. The mare may also carry her tail slightly away from her body, urinate frequently, bite at her sides showing that she is exhibiting some pain, and alternate in lying down and then standing up. Unlike other animals, the horse is capable of sweating, and may begin to sweat profusely, which is normal at foaling time. The placenta (water bag or sac) usually breaks, allowing 2 to 5 gallons of fluid to escape, lubricating the birth canal for the foal. If the foal is in the right position (head and feet first), involuntary muscle contractions of the uterus (womb) will cause expulsion of the foal in a surprisingly short period of time. If the foal is in a breech condition, the handler is necessary in most instances to save the mare. Because of the complicated conditions of a difficult birth and the likelihood of tetanus and other problems developing, a trained veterinarian is highly recommended in the event a difficult birth (dystocia) is obviously developing. In most cases, delivery should not take longer than 30 minutes. If no foal is delivered in 20 minutes after placental rupture (breaking of water bag), the mare probably needs help.

FOALING PROBLEMS

A clean, well-bedded box stall, a source of light, clean hot water, soap (Ivory is suggested as excellent and easily available), tail bandages, approved disinfectants, and suitable navel dressings such as iodine or Merthiolate should be available for foaling. Because of the peculiar digestive disorders that occur in horses, it is also recommended that an enema bag and a locally obtained laxative such as milk of magnesia be kept available.

When there is no doubt that the mare is about to foal, the attendant wraps her tail in flannel or gauze and stands back to let nature take its course. Occasionally assistance will be necessary, but none should be given unless it is obvious that help is needed. If the foal is presented in the natural position (head tucked between the front feet), help is not usually required; but in a small percentage of cases it may be necessary to tie a soft, thick rope around the foal's forelegs and pull gently to assist the mare. Birth may take from 10 minutes to 30 minutes.

If within 15 minutes after placental rupture, the muzzle or one or more legs of the foal cannot be seen, soap and water should be used to wash the hands and arms of the attendant and the vulva of the mare, and an antiseptic solution should be poured over these areas to reduce contamination. Then the examiner, preferably a veterinarian, should enter the vulva to determine the position of the foal. In a small percentage of the cases the foal can be merely rotated through hand manipulation to a normal position. If the foal is in a breech presentation, the time for birth must be extremely short once passage through the birth canal starts because oxygen can be cut off through a crushing of the umbilical cord, resulting in separation of the placenta, terminating gaseous exchange with the foal. This time period should be limited to about 3 minutes for birth to occur without the danger of suffocation to the foal.

If the newborn foal is born without assistance, it should be checked for any membranes covering the nose and mouth, and these should be cleared away for normal breathing.

A time lapse of 2 to 3 hours for the foal to gain strength before it nurses is considered normal, but most foals will stand and nurse in 20 minutes. If the foal does not nurse by 3 hours, the handler should assist it in nursing. Colostrum milk supplies the foal with the necessary antibodies, plus an added boost in energy to start and maintain its life functions. This colostrum is extremely important in horses because of the many diseases and organisms they are exposed to under the confinement system imposed by man. The antibodies are absorbed during the first 15 to 24 hours of life and offer protection against diseases for 6 to 12 weeks. The horse, unlike other animals that receive a substantial amount of immunity through the blood circulation of its dam, must rely almost entirely on colostrum for the development of its immunities. It is also a common practice to administer a tetanus antitoxin and a penicillin-streptomycin shot to the foal.

Meconium, a waste product in the bowels of the foal, is normally expelled shortly after birth and is usually no problem, but rumors among oldtimers have referred to it as "poison." Meconium is not particularly toxic; it is formed throughout gestation as the foal swallows amnionic fluid. It is a normal fetal waste product, but it can result in constipation, causing the foal to colic, which could be fatal. For this reason the precautionary measure of giving $4\frac{1}{2}$ oz of Fleet Enema (commercial name) or an enema with warm, soapy water should be a part of the birth procedures, along with a dose of milk of magnesia if signs of constipation are observed.

The navel cord normally breaks by itself. In the event it does not after 30 minutes postpartum (after birth), it can be cut 2 in. from the abdomen, and the stump should be treated with 2% iodine to prevent a case of navel infection. The cord should not be tied off because this sometimes brings on the infection. The treated navel stub should receive additional treatments daily until it has dried up and obviously no longer constitutes a threat of invasion by external organisms.

The placenta (sac, afterbirth) should ideally be shed without assistance during the first 3 hours. This is important in horses because of the potential threat of a retained placenta to cause founder or infection in the mare. The placenta is usually expelled intact. Its integrity is easily determined by filling it with water through the tear in the placenta through which the foal emerges. If the sac is watertight, nothing was retained. If any part of the placenta is retained, examination by a veterinarian and subsequent treatment are recommended.

REBREEDING

Another unusual difference in handling horses as compared to other species covered in this book is that rebreeding should occur as soon as possible because of the inefficiency of reproduction under stable management. Mares will exhibit a foal heat (heat occurring a few days after foaling), more often called *nine-day heat*, and will often rebreed at this time if there are no complications. This nine-day heat can actually occur from 5 to 15 days after birth. Also, some mares will experience foal heat but won't "show" because they are too worried about the teaser hurting the foal.

Foal heat is one time when early rebreeding is recommended in order to gain the primary objective, that of improving breeding efficiency. This time should be used to advantage, however, only if there are no visible signs of lacerations or bruises in the reproductive system of the mare, internally or externally. Conception rate at this time averages about 50%, especially if AI is used. Any slight advantage is appreciated by breeders. Most mares who do not conceive at foal heat will return to estrus within 21 days, and the regular cycle of 21 days will continue as previously described.

ABORTIONS

Abortions are quite common in horses compared to other species, and the cause should be determined by a veterinarian if possible. There are some abortions caused by virus and bacteria that are preventable through the use of vaccines.

Two types of abortions occur more frequently in horses than in other species. The first is an abortion caused by a twisting of the navel cord of the developing fetus (foal). The second cause of abortion is the unusual incidence of twinning, which causes the mare to abort in 90% of the cases. Therefore, although there is an 18% incidence of multiple ovulation, twins born alive to a mare are an extreme rarity.

There are two reasons why the mare usually aborts:

1. The surface of the uterus is inadequate for perfusing two placentas and keeping both fetuses alive.

2. Local autoimmune responses occur at the interface of the two placentas due to the different genetic makeup of the fetuses.

PREGNANCY TESTING

Mares may be examined rectally and diagnosed in foal by a skillful examination as early as 18 days after conception. There are biological tests as well as palpation to determine pregnancy in horses. Biological tests can be used from 40 to 120 days, and include the use of rabbits or frogs. The tests can determine a very accurate positive diagnosis of pregnancy, but false positive readings can be formed in mares that have aborted after 40 days.

ARTIFICIAL INSEMINATION (AI)

Artificial insemination has been practiced since the early beginnings of the horse. Legend has it that Arab chieftains used to steal into an enemy camp and get semen from an admired stallion, bringing it back to their own camps to artificially inseminate their mares without running the larger risk of stealing the stallion. Although this story may be mythical, artificial insemination has been a common practice in breeding horses since 1938 in this country. When a young stallion is properly fed and managed, he may be ready for service as early as 24 months of age. An artificial vagina is the preferred method of semen collection from stallions. The semen then may be diluted, but must be used fresh on the farm of origin. (You can freeze it, but the resulting pregnancy rate will be less than 10%.)

Horse Herd Management

VACCINATION AND DEWORMING SCHEDULE FOR HORSES

January–March

Pregnant Mares.   Deworming with thiabendazole is safe up to 9 to 10 months of gestation. Deworm mare during foal heat about 8 days after foaling, then every 9 to 12 weeks. Tetanus toxoid should be given 2 to 4 weeks prior to parturition.

Six weeks after parturition take the following steps:

1. Deworm.

2. Repeat tetanus toxoid.

3. Vaccinate for encephalomyelitis (eastern, western, and VEE).

4. Vaccinate for distemper (problems like flu and strangles), according to the advice of your local veterinarian.

Breed at foal heat if possible.

Stallions.   Begin preparation for breeding season:

1. Examine for fertility.

2. Inject with a tetanus toxoid and vaccinate for encephalomyelitis (eastern, western, and VEE).

3. Vaccinate for distemper in areas where this is a problem.

4. Check teeth and float if necessary.

Newborns.   Give a tetanus antitoxin at birth. Deworm at 6 weeks of age and every 8 weeks until 2 years old, and inject a tetanus toxoid. Treat the navel with 2% iodine at birth. Give a mild enema if no bowel movement is forthcoming within 12 hours after birth.

Yearlings. Inject with a tetanus toxoid. Deworm every 8 weeks. Vaccinate for encephalomyelitis (eastern, western, and VEE). Vaccinate for distemper in areas where this is a problem.

April–June

Pregnant Mares. Deworm with a mild, broad-spectrum anthelmentic. Examine for pregnancy at 18 to 20 days, 30 days, and 45 days, and check in fall for abortions.

Stallions. Deworm and check teeth and float if necessary.

Newborn. Deworm at 2 months of age and every 8 weeks until 2 years. Inject with a tetanus toxoid. Vaccinate for encephalomyelitis (eastern, western, and VEE).

Yearlings. Deworm. Alternate with different broad-spectrum deworming agents in order to kill out those parasites that may have developed a resistance to the previous deworming material.

July–September

Mares. Deworm and check teeth.

Stallions. Deworm and check teeth.

Yearlings. Deworm. Alternate with different broad-spectrum deworming agents in order to kill out those parasites that may have developed a resistance to the previous deworming material.

Under One Year of Age. Deworm (start deworming at 8 weeks of age and deworm every 8 weeks thereafter until one year old). Vaccinate any animal missed in the April–June schedule due to age.

October–December

Mares. Deworm. You may alternate paste and tube worming, and should use a boticide every second or third worming until the last trimester of pregnancy.

Stallions. Deworm.

Yearlings. Deworm.

Index

OTHER AGRICULTURAL BOOKS
AVAILABLE FROM DOANE

Estate Planning for Farmers–A 248 page Doane guide to help you make sure your estate–the money and property you've worked a lifetime to build–isn't hit by thousands of dollars of unnecessary estate taxes, probate and settlement costs. Estate Planning for Farmers shows how to transfer your farm to sons or daughters in an equitable way; how to cut federal estate taxes; how to guarantee your wife a lifetime of security; how to organize your farm business to assure worry-free retirement years; how to use wills, trusts, insurance as estate planning tools; and much more. Contains 16 chapters.

Facts & Figures for Farmers–Here's a complete reference that brings together all the facts, calculations, mathematics, tables and charts you need in the everyday operation of your farm. It's full of facts to help you calculate inputs, measure land, figure silo capacities, balance rations, calibrate sprayers, analyze budgets, estimate space requirements, machinery costs and capacities . . . to name just a few. Contains 348 pages of concise, easy-to-use information on livestock, crops, buildings and equipment, accounting, tax management, weed and pest control and much, much more.

Farm Management Guide–The soft-cover, bound version of Doane's famous Reference Volume. Contains 336 pages, packed with valuable production, management and marketing information. Thirteen detailed chapters cover: types of farming; acquiring the farm; records, planning and financing; taxes and insurance; soils and crop production; forage production; livestock production; dairy production; livestock feeds and feeding; agricultural chemicals; buildings, equipment and machinery; water and irrigation; marketing. Makes an excellent "carry around" farm reference guide, or a wonderful gift for farm friends, neighbors, ag students.

Do It Right the First Time–This 250 page book is a practical guide for making legal and business arrangements for a farm operation. It discusses questions like incorporating a family farm, sources of operating and real estate loans, the mechanics of borrowing at the lowest rate, leasing of farmland, farm appraisals, insurance, legal liabilities when a salesman or somebody else is visiting your farm, and much more. It is a book filled with grassroots advice regarding what you should look out for to prevent legal problems as you conduct the business end of farming.

For information on any of the above books, simply contact Doane.

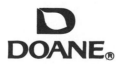

Doane Agricultural Service, Inc.
8900 Manchester Road
St. Louis, Missouri 63144

DATE DUE

SEP 3 0 1990			

#47-0108 Peel Off Pressure Sensitive